MANAGEMENT
GUIDELINES
FOR NURSE
PRACTITIONERS
WORKING WITH
WOMEN

New Editions of F. A. Davis's
Management Guidelines for Nurse Practitioners Series

Unique clinical references created to help nurse practitioners manage problems they encounter with clients throughout the life span

❖ *Management Guidelines for Nurse Practitioners*
Working with Adults, 2nd Edition
By Lynne M. Dunphy
ISBN 0-8036-1117-X

    ❖ *Management Guidelines for Nurse Practitioners*
    Working with Children and Adolescents, 2nd Edition
    By Nancy L. Herban Hill and Linda M. Sullivan
    ISBN 0-8036-1102-1

❖ *Management Guidelines for Nurse Practitioners*
Working with Women, 2nd Edition
By Kathleen M. Pelletier Brown
ISBN 0-8036-1116-1

PDA versions of these books, including a free trial available at www.fadavis.com

    ❖ *Management Guidelines for Nurse Practitioners*
    Working with Older Adults, 2nd Edition
    By Laurie Kennedy-Malone, Kathleen Ryan Fletcher,
    and Lori Martin Plank
    ISBN 0-8036-1120-X

Each book:
• Is pocket-sized for on-the-spot consultation
• Focuses on health promotions, anticipatory guidance, and disorder guidelines
• Focuses on recommendations and guidelines, not theory
• Includes ICD-9 codes for all the disorders
• Includes diagnostic test information tables with test name, results indicating disorder, and CPT codes
• Lists one or two "Signal Symptoms" for each disorder that helps nurse practitioners quickly target potential differential diagnoses.

Recently Published:

    ❖ *Management Guidelines for Nurse Practitioners*
    Working in Family Practice
    By Alice F. Running and Amy E. Berndt
    ISBN 0-8036-0810-1
    • Organized by anatomical areas, it covers 310 disorders
    and conditions, with rationales and causes provided for
    abnormal test values.

Purchase copies of one or all of the books in F. A. Davis's
Management Guidelines Series
as well as **related PDA software**
from your local health science bookstore or directly from F. A. Davis
by shopping online at www.fadavis.com
or calling 800-323-3555 (US), 800-665-1148 (CAN).

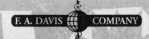

F. A. DAVIS ⊕ COMPANY

MANAGEMENT GUIDELINES FOR NURSE PRACTITIONERS WORKING WITH WOMEN

Second Edition

Kathleen M. Pelletier Brown R.N., MSN, NP, PhD
Professor of Nursing
University of Pennsylvania
School of Nursing
Philadelphia, Pennsylvania

 F. A. DAVIS COMPANY | Philadelphia

F. A. Davis Company
1915 Arch Street
Philadelphia, PA 19103

Printed in Canada

Last digit indicates print number: 10 9 8 7 6 5 4 3 2 1

Acquisitions Editor: Joanne Patzek DaCunha, RN, MSN
Developmental Editor: Diane Blodgett
Cover Designer: Louis J. Forgione

As new scientific information becomes available through basic and clinical research,
recommended treatments and drug therapies undergo changes. The authors and
publisher have done everything possible to make this book accurate, up to date, and
in accord with accepted standards at the time of publication. The authors, editors, and
publisher are not responsible for errors or omissions or for consequences from
application of the book, and make no warranty, expressed or implied, with regard to
the contents of the book. Any practice described in this book should be applied by the
reader in accordance with professional standards of care used with regard to the
unique circumstances that may apply in each situation. The reader is advised always
to check product information (package inserts) for changes and new information
regarding dose and contraindications before administering any drug. Caution is
especially urged when using new or infrequently ordered drugs.

Library of Congress Cataloging-in-Publication Data

Pelletier-Brown, Kathleen, 1950-
    Management guidelines for nurse practitioners working with women/Kathleen M.
Pelletier-Brown.–2nd ed.
    p.; cm.
Prev. ed. of: Management guidelines for women's health nurse practitioners, c2000.
Includes bibliographical references and index.
ISBN 0-8036-1116-1
    1. Gynecologic nursing. 2. Nurse practitioners. I. Pelletier-Brown, Kathleen, 1950-
Management guidelines for women's health nurse practitioners. II. Title.
    [DNLM: 1. Genital Diseases, Female. 2. Nurse Practitioners. 3. Women's Health. WP 140
P388m 2003]
RG105.P44 2003
618.1'0231–dc22

2003049377

To the readers, who provide the best care possible for women, in an increasingly complex health-care environment.

To all the women with whom I have interacted in my professional life. You taught me everything that I know, and I am now passing that knowledge on to others.

KPB

PREFACE

Management Guidelines for Nurse Practitioners Working with Women was written as a reference guide for Women's Health NPs in clinical practice. It is my hope that it will be useful for NPs who interact with women.

Chapter One deals with health promotion including up-to-date recommendations for health-related screening for women of all ages. This chapter also includes recommendations for the promotion of health in women.

In Unit II, Managing Illness, common clinically presenting symptoms and problems of women are discussed followed by a system by system discussion of women's health-related issues.

Unit III discusses reproductive concerns, contraception, antenatal, and postpartum care as well as menopause and reproductive concerns of women in detail.

The book, which is written in a monograph easy-to-follow format, includes many useful tables, figures, and boxes. The monograph format and the use of tables and figures make the book an easy-to-use reference source for the NP working with women.

The book contains handouts that can be copied and given to female patients. These handouts may be modified as desired by the NP and given to women who may find them useful.

This book was written by a Women's Health NP with 20 years of clinical experience. The author is sharing with the reader her experience in providing individualized care for women. Twenty years of active listening and "practicing," in the true sense of the word, is passed on to the reader. The book provides the practicing NP with helpful guidelines for everyday clinical situations. It assists the NP in forming plans of care, provides guidelines for referral to other health-care professionals, gives suggestions for counseling and teaching, and provides useful NP appendixes and patient handouts.

KPB

ACKNOWLEDGMENTS

A special acknowledgment to Bruce Kaufmann, MD, without whom my clinical life would not have been possible.

Thanks to Diane Blodgett for her patience and her encouragement in writing this book. Not only is she my editor, but she is now a friend.

CONSULTANTS

Ellen M. Chiocca, RNC, MSN, CPNP
Assistant Professor
Loyola University Chicago
Marcella Niehoff School of Nursing
Chicago, Illinois

Gretchen Hope Miller Heery, APRN, BC
Occupational Health Nurse Practitioner
WorkForce Wellness Program
Family Nurse Practitioner
Gnaden Huetten Memorial Hospital
Lehighton, Pennsylvania

Anita Hunter, RN, PhD, PNP
Assistant Professor
Clemson University School of Nursing
Clemson, South Carolina

Marjorie Thomas-Lawson, PhD, RN-CS, FNP
Associate Professor
University of Southern Maine
Portland, Maine

Donna G. Nativio, PhD, CRNP, FAAN
Associate Professor
Director of the Family Nurse Practitioner Program
University of Pittsburgh School of Nursing
Pittsburgh, Pennsylvania

Kristy Kiel Martyn, PhD, RN
Assistant Professor
University of Michigan School of Nursing
Ann Arbor, Michigan

CONTENTS

Unit *I*
THE HEALTHY WOMAN

Chapter *1*
PROMOTING
HEALTH

INTRODUCTION

Today women are the majority of consumers and providers of health care. As women become increasingly more knowledgeable, independent, and assertive, they view health care providers as consultants, teachers, and resources for current information about health concerns. Women expect to be active participants in their health care, from identifying signs and symptoms to deciding on a treatment plan. They believe, and rightly so, that they know more about their bodies and lifestyles than anyone else, and therefore can best decide which treatment option is most suitable for them. The nurse practitioner (NP) adequately informs about all relevant health issues and supports a woman's decisions. The NP determines the type and amount of information a woman requires and the degree of participation and responsibility the woman is willing to assume in health-care decisions. The NP is familiar with current diagnostic and treatment techniques. The NP keeps current on research in the field of women's health and must be able to explain clearly to a woman the screening options, diagnoses, treatments, potential consequences, side effects, risks, and benefits. Alternative treatments that may fit the woman's lifestyle should also be considered. Supporting the woman's right to choose and the choices that she makes is an important function of the NP.

LEVELS OF PREVENTION

Primary prevention involves activities directed toward decreasing the probability of becoming ill. Health promotion activities, such as regular exercise, are labeled as *primary prevention*. These activities are directed toward sustaining or increasing a level of well-being. *Secondary prevention* focuses on direct screening to promote early diagnosis and treatment of disease. *Tertiary prevention* minimizes disability.

Up-to-date guidelines on the schedule for adult immunizations recommended by the Department of Health and Human Services Centers for

Table 1–1   Levels of Prevention

Primary	Secondary	Tertiary
Decreasing probability of illness	Screening to promote diagnosis and treatment	Minimizing disability

Disease Control may be accessed at *http://www.cdc.gov/nip/recs/adult-schedule.pdf*. *See also Box 1–1* for important information regarding the administration of immunizations.

Box 1-1
Specific Immunization Considerations

Do Not Immunize When ...

Adult immunization is an important but frequently overlooked part of patient care. High-risk adults should be immunized against vaccine-preventable diseases; travelers may require special vaccines. Adverse reactions to vaccination are rare and are usually local. A history of previous serious allergic reaction is the only absolute contraindication to vaccination in general. However, pregnancy and immunocompromised status may prohibit vaccination.

Likely candidates for adult immunization are:
- Persons with chronic disease
- Immunocompromised patients
- Alcoholics or drug abusers
- Heath-care workers
- Nursing home residents
- Homeless people
- International travelers
- Migrant workers
- Child-care employees
- Institutionalized persons

Factors that are *not* contraindications to vaccination:
- Mild to moderate reaction to a previous vaccination
- Current antibiotic therapy
- Contact with pregnant women
- Recent exposure to illness
- Personal history of allergies
- Family history of allergies

Contraindications to vaccination:
- Influenza—allergy to eggs
- Tetanus-diphtheria—none
- Polio—pregnancy, compromised immune status, malignancy, HIV infection, household contact with HIV-infected persons
- Pneumococcal—pregnancy
- Hepatitis A—none
- Hepatitis B—allergic reaction to baker's yeast
- Measles, mumps and rubella—pregnancy, allergy to eggs or neomycin, compromised immune status (should not be given to women who plan to be pregnant within three months of vaccination)
- Varicella—pregnancy, compromised status, receipt of blood products in the last 5 months, allergy to neomycin

Adapted from National Coalition for Adult Immunization, 4733 Bethesda Avenue, Suite 750, Bethesda, MD 20814-5228.

Screening Tests

Screening tests are tests administered to large populations of asymptomatic people with the hope of identifying disease or potential disease. The disease being screened for should be associated with significant morbidity or mortality in the population; there must be effective treatment for the disease; and the screening test must be accurate, simple, acceptable, and safe for the screened population. Table 1–2 lists screening tests for women who are generally at low risk for disease.

Accuracy of the test is measured by sensitivity, which is the proportion of positive tests among those known to have the disease. Specificity reflects the portion of negative tests among those who have the disease. The positive predictive value refers to the likelihood that people with positive results actually have the disease in question. This latter category is how the practitioner interprets test results: What is the probability that this positive result is a true one?

When screening is applied to large numbers of people, follow-up for positive results is an important consideration. There must be a commitment of resources to a follow-up screening program. There must be ability to notify patients of positive test results and the ability to further evaluate and test those with positive results. Figure 1–1 indicates the decision process needed for patient evaluation and subsequent promotion of a healthy lifestyle.

Age Considerations

The National Center for Health Statistics provides up-to-date information on the role of a woman's age as an important consideration in providing health care (see Box 1–2). Age is related to risk factors, morbidity, and mortality. Young women are at greatest risk for death from accidents and violence. For middle-aged women, accidents and violence continue to be important causes of death, but heart disease, cancer, and suicide also become important causes of female mortality. As women age, heart disease, cancer, stroke, diabetes, pulmonary disease, and liver disease increase in frequency as causes of death. In elderly women the principal

Table 1–2   Screening Tests for Low-Risk Women

Age 18–40	Age 40–50	Age 50–65	65 and Older
BSE monthly	BSE monthly	BSE monthly	BSE monthly
BE by practitioner annually ————————applies to all age groups ————————>			
Annual Pap	Annual Pap	Annual Pap	Pap as indicated
Physical examination q3yr	Physical examination q3yr	Physical examination q3yr	Annual physical
BPq2yr	BPq2yr	BPq2yr	BP as indicated
Serum cholesterol q^{5}yr ——————————applies to all age groups—————————>			
Periodic fasting glucose ——————————applies to all age groups—————————>			

Abbreviations: BSE=Breast self-examination; BE=Breast examination; BP=blood pressure.

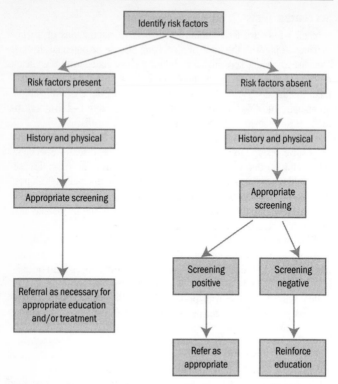

Figure 1–1. Decision tree for screening of, and promoting healthy lifestyles in, women patients.

causes of death are cancer, cardiovascular disease, pneumonia, diabetes, and respiratory disease (see Figure 1–2).

Screening Recommendations

Breast Cancer

Breast cancer is the second leading cancer killer in American women. In 2000, 40,800 women died of breast cancer (American Cancer Society). Screening tests for breast cancer include breast self-examination (BSE), clinical examination by a practitioner, and mammogram. All women over the age of 20 years should do breast self-examination every month. According to the American Cancer Society, all women between the ages of 20 and 39 should have a clinical breast examination by a health professional every three years. After age 40, women should have a clinical breast examination every year. The clinical examination should take place before mammography so that any abnormality detected can be evaluated more carefully.

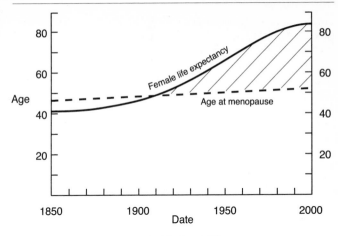

Figure 1–2. The female lifespan.

Mammography plays a central role in the early detection of breast cancers. Mammography can show changes in the breast up to two years before a patient or an NP can palpate a carcinoma. Screening mammography also increases the detection of small abnormal growths confined to

---

Box 1–2
Age-specific Health Goals for Women

Adolescence
- Maintain physical, mental, emotional, and social growth at optimum levels.
- Develop positive health behavior patterns in physical fitness, nutrition, exercise, work, recreation, sex, and relationships.

Young Adulthood
- Move from dependent adolescence to independent adulthood.
- Achieve employment.
- Develop healthy social relationships.

Middle Adulthood
- Develop good health habits; detect disease early and treat disease.
- Reevaluate values, family situations, and career choices.
- Evaluate goal achievement.

Older Adulthood
- Adjust to menopause.
- Detect and treat any chronic illness.
- Continue achievement of life goals.

Elderly Years
- Prepare for retirement.
- Prepare for biologic, psychologic, and social changes.

Advanced Years
- Maintain independence.
- Continue to be physically and mentally active.

the milk ducts (ductal carcinoma). The Food and Drug Administration says that mammography can detect 85% to 90% of breast cancers in women over 50. Current guidelines from the American Medical Association, the American College of Radiology, and the American Cancer Society recommend annual mammograms beginning at the age of 40 years. The amount of radiation exposure during mammography is regulated by federal guidelines. Screening mammograms are believed to be safe.

Colon and Rectal Cancer

Screening tests include a rectal examination, fecal occult blood testing, sigmoidoscopy, colonoscopy, and double contrast barium enemas. Fecal occult blood testing determines the presence of blood in stools, presumably from an early cancer. Positive tests can be produced by recent consumption of rare red meat and by some medications, such as aspirin and iron, as well as by hemorrhoids. Follow-up for positive tests is colonoscopy or a combination of sigmoidoscopy and barium enema. The American Cancer Society does *not* recommend repeat fecal occult blood testing for positive results.

The American Cancer Society recommends annual rectal examination of all adults beginning at age 40, fecal occult blood testing annually beginning at age 50, flexible sigmoidoscopy every 5 years beginning at age 50, and colonoscopy every 10 years beginning at age 50. Special attention should be paid to people at high risk for colon cancer, that is, those with one or more of the following risk factors: significant family history; personal history of breast, endometrial, or ovarian cancer; polyps; or ulcerative colitis.

Cervical Cancer

The screening test for cervical cancer is the Papanicolaou (Pap) smear. The risk factor for cervical cancer is sexual activity, particularly that with multiple partners. A consensus was developed by a number of professional organizations, including the American Cancer Society, the National Cancer Institute, the American College of Obstetricians and Gynecologists, and the American Medical Association, recommending annual Pap smears for all women who are sexually active or have reached the age of 18. When three Pap smears have been "normal," Pap testing may be done less frequently, with the usual recommendation being every 3 years. Women over the age of 65 do not seem to benefit as much from screening if previous smears have been consistently normal.

Ovarian Cancer

Ovarian cancer has a high mortality rate. Unfortunately, no effective screening modality has been identified. Pelvic examination is inadequate for detecting the disease in an early phase.

Endometrial Cancer

The American Cancer Society recommends endometrial sampling for high-risk women at menopause. Risk categories include infertility, obesity, history of ovarian failure, abnormal uterine bleeding, unopposed estrogen therapy, and tamoxifen treatment.

Women should be encouraged to report any postmenopausal vaginal bleeding or spotting to a health care provider.

Skin Cancer

The major concern in skin cancer is malignant melanoma. The screening modality is complete physical examination of the skin. High-risk groups are people with a history of skin cancer, those who work outdoors, and those exposed to chemical skin carcinogens.

The American Cancer Society recommends a thorough skin examination every three years for people over 20 and a thorough skin examination every year for people over 40.

Diabetes

Diabetes is relatively common in women and is often asymptomatic. Routine screening for nonpregnant women can lead to early detection. Urine testing for glucose is a poor screening tool. Periodic fasting serum glucose measurement in high-risk individuals, that is, women who are obese, have a significant family history of diabetes, or have gestational diabetes, should be performed as recommended by the American Diabetes Association.

Osteoporosis

Osteoporosis is a disease of low bone mass and structural deterioration of the bone. Ten million people are diagnosed with this disease (Osteoporosis Resource Center, 2001), with 80% of those people being women. Osteoporosis is a silent disease that requires screening. Risk factors for osteoporosis are: a diet low in calcium and vitamin D, lack of weight-bearing exercise, and consumption of cigarettes and alcohol. The risk for osteoporosis increases with age. The screening tool for osteoporosis is bone densitometry testing.

HEALTH PROMOTION RECOMMMENDATIONS

Exercise

Regular exercise is part of a healthy lifestyle. Fitness describes the positive changes in cardiovascular endurance, muscle strength, coordination, and flexibility produced by exercise.

The goal of most exercise programs is to obtain cardiovascular fitness that permits sustained activity over a period of time. Optimally, aerobic activity should be performed for at least 30 minutes three to four times per week. The goal of such exercise is to reach and maintain a specific heart rate over a period of time. By utilizing this method, each exercise session can be monitored to reach the goal (see Box 1–3).

Box 1-3
Target Heart Rate

Target heart rate = (220 − age × (60% to 80%). The resulting number is the target range.
Sample: 220 − 48 (age in years) × 70% = 172 × 0.70 = 120 beats per minute .

Each exercise program should have at least a 5-minute warm-up to prevent muscle injury and a 5- to 15-minute cool-down period after exercise to allow for recovery to normal resting heart rate.

Coordination, balance, and flexibility also improve as a result of an exercise program. As muscles work together, they become efficient as a group. However, any level of conditioning is reversible, making a long-term commitment to exercise necessary.

Exercise can reduce and maintain weight. Weight programs that are combined with exercise are more effective than diet alone.

For any muscle to strengthen, it must work repetitively against fixed resistance, which causes the fibers to hypertrophy. For muscle strength to occur, one must develop a program for a specific muscle group. Depending on the type of program, some cardiovascular fitness effect may also occur. For example, circuit training, a very popular exercise program, develops muscular strength and cardiovascular fitness simultaneously.

Bone density can increase in women involved in an active exercise program. Pressure on the bones results in increased calcium deposition as a result of increased osteoblastic activity. Exercise designed to prevent osteoporosis involves the use of large muscles attached to the long bones. *Any weight-bearing exercise, including walking, helps prevent osteoporosis.*

Exercise should be a regular part of every woman's daily activity. Any athletic program will have long-term benefits for women and will contribute to a healthy lifestyle.

Stress Management

The physical reaction to stress is the same regardless of the stressor. Dr. Selye, the father of discussion about stress, taught us that stress creates a physiologic response that he describes in phases or stages. The first stage is alarm—your body recognizes the stressor and prepares for "fight or flight." The body increases heart rate, respiration, and blood sugar levels. The person perspires, the pupils dilate, and digestion slows. A person then chooses whether to use these physiologic responses to run or stay and fight. After fight or flight, the body repairs any damage from the stress. If the stressor is not removed, repairs cannot be made and the body enters an exhaustion stage, in which it becomes susceptible to diseases of stress such as headache and irritable bowel.

Teaching women to deal with stress involves two components. The first is the recognition of stressors. If the woman does not perceive the stress as a stressor, she will not enter into fight or flight. Self-talk becomes important here. She must convince herself that the potential stressor is not a stressor at all; rather, it is a challenge or an opportunity. The second component involves stress management techniques. A simple but effective technique for stress management is deep breathing. Relaxation techniques reduce chronic stress response. These include such techniques as progressive relaxation and meditation (see Figure 1–3).

In progressive relaxation, you concentrate on relaxing body parts in sequence—relax your right arm, your left arm, your shoulders, your jaw,

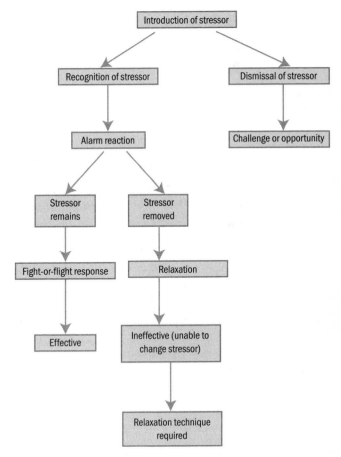

Figure 1–3. Stress management.

etc. The hope is that as the muscles of the body relax, the mind will follow and relax as well. With the use of meditation, you concentrate on eliminating all thoughts except thoughts about relaxing. In this case, the mind becomes relaxed and the body follows. Commonly used relaxation techniques involve thinking about relaxing with images such as feeling warm and heavy, going down in an elevator, or lying on a warm beach.

Women identify stress as a major factor in their lives. Women who are working while fulfilling the roles of wife and mother find their organizational skills taxed and their ability to deal with stress challenged.

Nutrition

Women have special nutritional considerations. Women require increased amounts of calcium, and iron is an important consideration for menstruating women. Nutritional considerations that are important for all adults such as sufficient amounts of Vitamin C warrant review with all women. The typical daily diet of each woman seeking care from an NP should be reviewed and recommendations given as appropriate. (See also Figure 1–4.)

Discussion topics for consideration include:
- Eating breakfast
- Making fruits and vegetables readily available for consumption
- Decreasing fat intake
- Healthy snacks
- Ordering wisely in a restaurant
- Achieving and maintaining a healthy weight

Smoking Cessation

Cigarette smoking plays a major role in the mortality of American women. Since 1980, when the Surgeon General's Report of women and smoking was released, about three million women have died prematurely of smoke-related diseases. Women smokers who die of smoking-related diseases lose an average of 14 years of potential life. Women who stop smoking greatly reduce their risk of dying prematurely. Smoking cessation is beneficial to women of all ages. Women ceasing to smoke reduce their risk for lung cancer, cancer of the oropharynx and bladder, cancer of the liver and colorectal area, and cervical cancer. Stopping smoking decreases the risk for cardiovascular diseases including stroke, peripheral vascular disease, and coronary artery disease (Figure 1–5). Stopping smoking reduces the risk for COPD.

Women who smoke expose their children to reduced and impaired lung function. Some studies suggest that smoking may alter menstrual function by increasing the risk for painful menstruation and secondary amenorrhea. Women who smoke have an increased risk for conception

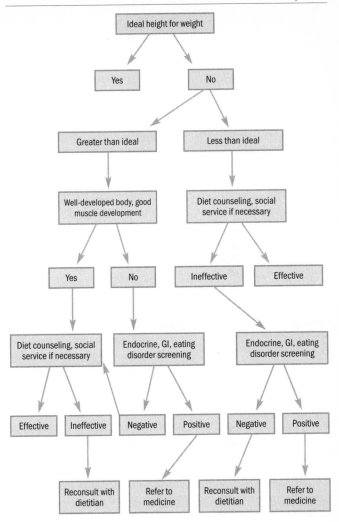

Figure 1–4. Malnutrition.

delay. Pregnant women who smoke risk pregnancy complications. Postmenopausal women who smoke have lower bone density than women who do not smoke.

For all of these reasons, each therapeutic interaction with every woman should include screening questions related to smoking. If the woman smokes, help resources for stopping should be provided.

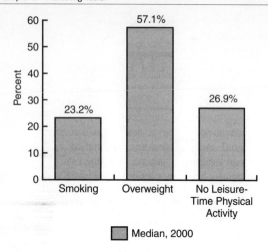

Figure 1–5. Preventing Heart Disease and Stroke at a Glance 2002 (Source: *www.cdc.gov/nccdphp/cvd.cvdaag.htm;* accessed in 2002).

SUMMARY

Health prevention and promotion are important aspects of NP care. The complex lives of modern women in American culture require that NPs work to assist women in maintaining their health and in preventing future illness. Women look to NPs to provide accurate information regarding the health aspects of their lives. Every NP should be prepared to discuss methods that prevent disease and activities that promote wellness with every client. The first goal is to help women stay healthy by educating and counseling them about general health strategies such as healthy eating, exercise, and stress management as well as cessation of smoking and decreased consumption of alcohol. The next goal is to involve them in screening programs so that identification of disease at an early stage will allow effective intervention and treatment.

For 18 years, the Center for Disease Control has conducted surveys about wide ranges of behavior that affect health. The following behaviors are linked to heart disease, stroke cancer, and diabetes, the nation's leading killers:

Not enough physical activity
Eating a high-fat and low-fiber diet
Using tobacco and alcohol
Not getting lifesaving medical care (mammograms, Pap smears, colorectal cancer screenings, and flu shots).

NPs should address each of these areas with every woman she encounters in her practice arena.

Table 1–3   Promoting Health in Women

Health-Related Issue	Assessment Tool
Body weight	Calculate BMI or metabolic syndrome
Nutrition	Evaluate daily dietary habit
Physical activity	Assess activity level
Stress prevention	Determine stressors
Smoking/alcohol/drugs	Evaluate history of activities
Injury prevention	Determine work and leisure activities
Prevention of sexually transmitted infection	Assess sexual activity history

The following Leading Health Indicators reflect the major public health concerns in the United States according to *Healthy People 2010,* published by the Office of Disease Prevention and Health Promotion, U.S. Department of Health and Human Services.

- Physical activity
- Overweight and obesity
- Tobacco use
- Substance abuse
- Responsible sexual behavior
- Mental health
- Injury and violence
- Environmental quality
- Immunizations
- Access to health care

NPs in women's health can make a very real difference in the lives of women via health promotion and prevention discussions at every clinical encounter (see Table 1–3).

REFERENCES

Association of Women's Health Obstetric and Neonatal Nursing: *www.npwh.org*

American Cancer Society: *www.cancer.org*

American Heart Association: *www.americanheart.org*

American Medical Association: *www.ama-assn.org*

Centers for Disease Control and Prevention: *www.cdc.gov*

Healthy People 2010 Fact Sheet: *www.health.gov*

National Center for Health Statistics: *www.cdc.gov/nchs*

National Diabetes Association: *www.diabetes.org*

National Institutes of Health, Department of Health and Human Services: *www.nih.gov*

National Women's Health Information Center: *www.4woman.gov*

Osteoporosis and Related Bone Diseases National Resource Center: *www.osteo.org*

Unit *II*
MANAGING
ILLNESS

Chapter 2

SYMPTOM-BASED PROBLEMS

ABDOMINAL PAIN

SIGNAL SYMPTOM ▶ "belly pain"

Abdominal pain   ICD-9-CM: 789.00 (the 5th digit is changed depending on site)

Definition: NPs in women's health are frequently challenged when a woman presents with abdominal pain. A woman's definition of abdominal pain, particularly lower abdominal pain, includes both the abdomen and the pelvis. Women do not consider the abdomen and pelvis as separate areas, so they frequently visit the women's health NP with a complaint of "belly" pain. The pain that may be diffuse or localized is frequently associated with nausea and vomiting. The woman's previous experience with pain, her culture, and her educational background influence her interpretation of pain. All of these factors make diagnosis a challenge.

The three categories of abdominal pain include:

Visceral pain. This pain tends to be localized and is perceived as dull, burning, diffuse, and sometimes crampy. It can produce nausea, vomiting, and diaphoresis.

Somatic pain. This pain is described as sharp, knifelike, and well localized.

Referred pain. This is pain located in an area other than the source; for example, pain under the diaphragm can be related to a ruptured ovarian cyst.

Etiology: Cholecystitis, diverticulitis, pancreatitis, colitis, perforated ulcer, obstruction, appendicitis, irritable bowel, constipation, cancer of the colon, and inflammatory bowel disease are all possible etiologies (see Table 2–1).

Occurrence: Depends on etiology.

Age: See Table 2–1.

Table 2–1 Etiology of Abdominal Pain

Disease	Age	Symptoms	Diagnostic Aides
Cholecystitis	30–60	Pain commonly starts a few hours after a meal that includes fatty foods. Nausea and vomiting are common. Pain is located in right upper quadrant (RUQ) and may radiate to the scapulae or shoulder. Deep inspiration increases the pain.	Ultrasound
Diverticulitis	50–60	Pain in the left lower quadrant (LLQ). Nausea is common. Elevated WBC count.	CT scan
Pancreatitis	30–50	Commonly associated with chronic alcoholism or biliary tract disease. Pain is epigastric and radiates to the back. Nausea and vomiting are common. Severe tenderness on palpation. Elevated amylase and WBCs.	Abdominal ultrasound and CT scan
Perforated ulcer	Any age	Pain is sharp, epigastric, and radiates out over the entire abdomen. Shoulder pain may be present. Nausea and vomiting are common. Fever. Serum amylase and WBCs are elevated. The abdomen is rigid with rebound tenderness in all four quadrants.	Abdominal x-ray and CT scan
Large bowel obstruction	More than 40 years	Pain has a gradual onset accompanied by constipation, absence of flatulence, and abdominal distention. Abdomen is tympanic.	Abdominal x-ray or CT scan
Appendicitis	Teens to early twenties	Pain begins in the periumbilical area and migrates toward the right lower quadrant (RLQ). Atypical location can and does occur during pregnancy and retrocecal appendix. In these cases, pain is in the RUQ. Mild fever may be present. WBCs may be elevated.	Abdominal ultrasound

Ethnicity: Gallstone formation is more common in Native American women over 30 years of age than in other American women.

Contributing factors: High-fat diet; gallstones occur more frequently in women who have been pregnant than in nonparous women. Women who use oral contraceptives for at least 4 years have a two-fold increased incidence of cholecystitis.

Signs and symptoms: Fever suggests sepsis, pelvic abscess, pelvic inflammatory disease (PID), appendicitis, or pyelonephritis. Diarrhea is associated with colitis. The patient will be able to identify where the pain is most intense. Auscultation of the abdomen may reveal increased or decreased bowel sounds. Palpation of the abdomen may reveal direct, rebound, or referred tenderness. Masses may be present. Note any guarding and rigidity. Direct and/or rebound tenderness points to an inflammatory process (see Figure 2–1).

Right Upper Quadrant

Cholecystitis
Pancreatitis
Perforated ulcer
Appendicitis
Pneumonia
Ischemic bowel
Intraperitoneal bleeding

Left Upper Quadrant

Gastritis
Pancreatitis
Perforated ulcer
Pneumonia
Ischemic bowel
Gastric ulcer disease
Intraperitoneal bleeding

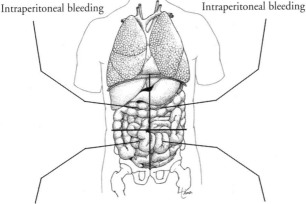

Right Lower Quadrant

Large bowel obstruction
Appendicitis
Irritable bowel
Ectopic pregnancy
PID/Tubo-ovarian abscess
Ruptured ovarian cyst
Mittelschmerz
Ureteral calculi
Ischemic bowel
Intraperitoneal bleeding

Left Lower Quadrant

Large bowel obstruction
Diverticulitis
Irritable bowel
Ectopic pregnancy
PID/Tubo-ovarian abscess
Ruptured ovarian cyst
Mittelschmerz
Ureteral calculi
Ischemic bowel
Intraperitoneal bleeding

Figure 2–1. Possible sources of abdominal pain.

Tests:

Test	Results Indicating Disorder	CPT Code
CBC	Elevated white blood cells, decreased hemoglobin	85025
Urinalysis	Negative for infection	81001
Pregnancy test (urine)	Negative	81025
Pelvic ultrasound	Negative	76856
Abdominal ultrasound/CT	Mass, inflammation, obstruction	76700 Ultrasound 74160 CT with contrast 74150 CT without contrast 74170 CT with and without contrast

History is the most important diagnostic test for abdominal pain. Carefully elicit the nature, onset, location, severity, duration, quality, radiation pattern, and effect on activity. The woman should describe her activities prior to onset of the pain, including whether the onset of pain was gradual or sudden. Ask the patient how eating, urination, and defecation affect the pain. Obtain a detailed description of the pain. In addition, obtain the menstrual history.

Differential diagnosis:

- PID (lower bilateral/pelvic pain, vaginal discharge, spotting, dyspareunia, dysuria)
- Ectopic pregnancy (one-sided lower abdominal pain with possible radiating pain to shoulder)
- Acute gastroenteritis (crampy, diffuse abdominal pain relieved by vomiting or defecation)
- Ruptured ovarian cyst (midcycle, sharp, abdominal pain, may be associated with bleeding or spotting)
- Mittelschmerz (pain in mid menstrual cycle, may be right- or left-sided)

Treatment: Depends on diagnosis. Hospitalization may be required. Surgical or medical therapy may be indicated.

Follow-up: Surgical therapy requires frequent, but short-term,

Table 2-2 Pelvic Pain

Acute	Chronic
PID	Primary dysmenorrhea
Torsion of tube or ovary	Secondary dysmenorrhea
Ovarian cysts	Irritable bowel syndrome
Appendicitis	Pelvic adhesions
Kidney stones	Pelvic relaxation
UTI	Interstitial cystitis
Diverticulitis	Levator spasm
Intestinal abscess	
Mittelschmerz	

follow-up visits. Medical therapy requires long-term follow-up for adjustment of diet and medication.

Sequelae: Depends on the severity of the illness.

Prevention/prophylaxis: Low-fat diet, weight control, stress management.

Referral: Abdominal pain requires referral to either a surgeon or a medical doctor. Any evidence of peritoneal irritation or obstruction is an indication for immediate hospitalization and surgical consultation.

Education: Stress the importance of follow-up after diagnosis and treatment, counseling for low-fat diet if prescribed, methods of weight reduction or maintenance, and strategies for stress reduction.

DYSMENORRHEA

SIGNAL SYMPTOMS ▶ lower abdominal pain; lower back pain; pain in upper thighs during menses

Dysmenorrhea	ICD-9-CM: 625.3

Definition: Dysmenorrhea is painful menstruation. Dysmenorrhea is divided into two types: primary and secondary. Primary dysmenorrhea occurs with menses from menarche. Secondary dysmenorrhea occurs with menses after menarche. Primary dysmenorrhea does not imply underlying pathology. Secondary dysmenorrhea, especially if it occurs after years of minimal or no discomfort, can indicate an underlying pathology (see Table 2–3).

Etiology: Dysmenorrhea is caused by an increase in prostaglandin levels. Increased uterine tone and dysrhythmic contractions create a "cramping" sensation with menses.

Occurrence: Dysmenorrhea affects one half of menstruating women. Of menstruating women, 10% report being incapacitated by dysmenorrhea. In the United States, work absenteeism due to dysmenorrheal is estimated to be 600 million work hours per year with economic consequences of two billion dollars per year (Howard, 2000).

Age: Dysmenorrhea can occur in any menstruating female.

Table 2–3 Chronic Pelvic Pain

Source	History	Examination
Endometriosis	Increasing dysmenorrhea	Pelvic tenderness
Primary dysmenorrhea	Pain with menses from menarche	Negative
Secondary dysmenorrhea	Pain with menses	Uterine and/or adnexal tenderness
Pelvic adhesions	Starts months after surgery, localized	Thickening on exam, pain with motion

Ethnicity: Not significant.

Contributing factors: Endometriosis, PID, adenomyosis, ovarian cysts.

Signs and symptoms: Painful menses, "crampy" in nature, occurring with the onset of menses and lasting 48–72 hours. The cramping is felt in the suprapubic area, lower back, and inner thighs.

Diagnostic tests:

Test	Results Indicating Disorder	CPT code
Pelvic examination	Uterine tenderness; no enlargement or masses	Included in exam code
CBC	Low hemoglobin indicates anemia	85025
Urinalysis	Negative for infection	81001
Serum HCG	Negative	84702
Pelvic ultrasound	Adenomyosis, leiomyomata, masses, polyps	76856
GC/ *Chlamydia* culture	Negative	87850/87110

Differential diagnosis:

- PID: lower bilateral/pelvic pain, vaginal discharge, spotting, dyspareunia, dysuria
- Ectopic pregnancy: one-sided lower abdominal pain with possible radiating pain to shoulder
- Torsion of the ovary
- Ruptured ovarian cyst: midcycle, sharp, abdominal pain, may be associated with bleeding or spotting
- Acute abdomen
- Pelvic mass: confirmed by ultrasound

Treatment: Nonsteroidal anti-inflammatory agents are effective for relief of dysmenorrhea. Oral contraceptives reduce dysmenorrhea (Figure 2–2).

Follow-up: Follow-up visits for efficacy of therapy are advised for dysmenorrhea.

Sequelae: None.

Prevention/prophylaxis: Aerobic exercise has been demonstrated to reduce dysmenorrhea.

Referral: Secondary dysmenorrhea requires consultation for further diagnosis and treatment.

Education: Dysmenorrhea is a common complaint among menstruating women. Cramping with menses that interferes with usual activity is an indication for evaluation and treatment. Cramping with menses in women who have no prior episodes of dysmenorrhea is an indication for evaluation.

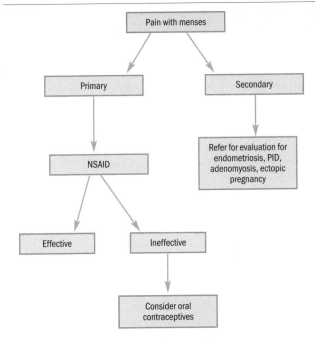

Figure 2–2. Dysmenorrhea.

DYSPAREUNIA

SIGNAL SYMPTOM ▶ pain during or immediately after sexual intercourse

| Dyspareunia | ICD-9-CM: 625.0 |
| Psychogenic dyspareunia | ICD-9-CM: 302.76 |

Definition: Dyspareunia is pain with intercourse; it is a pain syndrome, not a sexual dysfunction. Many conditions can create dyspareunia, including infection and allergy.

Etiology: There are two types of dyspareunia. The first type—in which pain is present on insertion—is caused by lack of lubrication, lack of stimulation, or vulvar irritation and inflammation. The second type—in which pain occurs on deep penetration—is caused by endometriosis, ovarian cysts, adhesions, or PID (see Figure 2–3).

Occurrence: Of women surveyed, 60% report experiencing dyspareunia at least once in their lives; 30% of women surveyed labeled dyspareunia as a chronic problem.

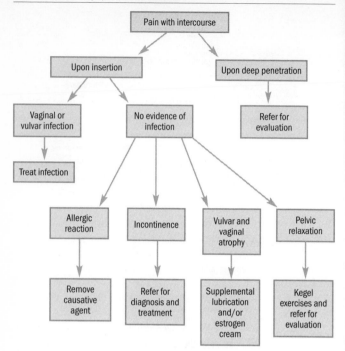

Figure 2–3. Dyspareunia.

Age: Dyspareunia can occur in any sexually active female.

Ethnicity: Not significant.

Contributing factors: Vaginal infections; allergens, such as deodorants, soaps, douching agents, bubble bath, and contraceptive foams and creams; obesity; incontinence; shaving in the pelvic area; history of sexual abuse.

Signs and symptoms: Infection or allergy (erythematous and edematous vulva; rashes such as macules, papules, scaling, ulcers, other lesions; lice; palpable inguinal lymph nodes); evidence of incontinence; vulvar atrophy; pelvic relaxation (see Chapter 15); vulvodynia (chronic vulvar discomfort with burning and stinging producing irritation and "rawness"); Bartholin's cyst and abscess (which presents as a tender, cystic mass in the area of Bartholin's gland).

Dyspareunia can be situational, in which the woman describes pain that is limited to a specific partner or situation.

Diagnostic tests:

Test	Results Indicating Disorder	CPT Code
Cervical and vaginal culture	Positive for infection	87070
Urine culture	Negative	87088
Vaginal wet prep	Positive for *Monilia* or bacterial infection	87210

Differential diagnosis:
- Infected episiotomy—redness, swelling, purulent drainage from episiotomy
- Retained suture material—material present on inspection
- Urethritis or cystitis (dysuria, frequency, urinary urgency; urethritis: involvement of urethra only)—diagnosed by urine culture
- Vulvar cancer—diagnosed via biopsy

Treatment:
- Treat bacterial infection with topical or systemic antibiotics.
- Treat fungal infection with antifungal medication.
- Treat atrophy with supplemental lubrication, Kegel exercises, position changes for intercourse, and/or estrogen cream.
- Treat Bartholin's cyst or abscess with warm soaks to encourage drainage. (see Figure 2–4).

Follow-up: All women with pelvic pain should have a follow-up visit (or visits). The multiple causes of this condition require follow-up for assurance of correct diagnosis, treatment, and resolution.

Sequelae: Resolution occurs in most cases with appropriate therapy. Vulvodynia occurs in 9% of women with vulvar symptoms. This syndrome has no known etiology and is, therefore, difficult to treat. Vulvodynia is a chronic condition.

Prevention/prophylaxis: Supplemental lubrication in the menopausal period. Prevention of vaginal infection.

Referral: Women with deep dyspareunia require referral for diagnosis of any of the etiologic agents, such as PID, ovarian cysts, adhesions, or endometriosis.

Women with vulvodynia, a diagnosis made by exclusion, should be referred to a provider specializing in this disease.

Pelvic relaxation should be referred to a gynecologist for treatment.

Sexual dysfunction, particularly if the partner also has a dysfunction, should be referred to a specialist.

Women with a history of sexual abuse should be referred to a provider skilled in dealing with this issue.

Bartholin's cysts that do not respond to local therapy or require incision and drainage (I&D) should be referred for therapy. Therapy includes I&D or marsupialization or insertion of a Word catheter.

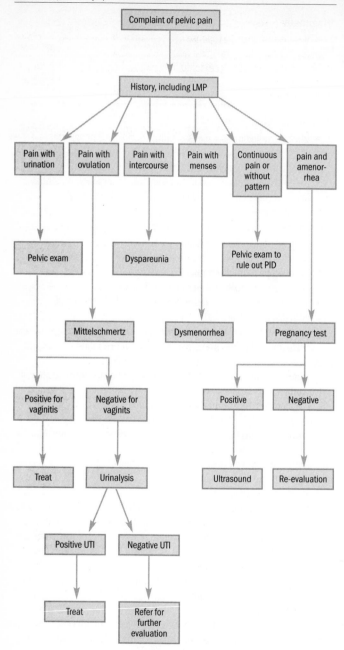

Figure 2–4. Pelvic pain.

Education: As a part of their education process, all women should learn about the human sexual response cycle. Pain with intercourse is not a "normal" occurrence, and may indicate an underlying disorder. Pain during intercourse can lead to anticipation of pain in future sexual encounters. Resolution of the cause of pain with intercourse must be achieved in order to prevent sexual avoidance.

CYCLIC MASTALGIA

SIGNAL SYMPTOM▶   breast discomfort prior to menses

Cyclic Mastalgia   ICD-9-CM: 611.71

Definition: Cyclic mastalgia is the most common breast-related complaint seen in women's health practice. The breast is a complex organ that is sensitive to hormones. Estradiol and progesterone stimulate breast tissue. Breast pain that positively correlates with menses is called cyclic mastalgia. Cyclic mastalgia and fibrocystic changes are not the same (see Chapter 4). One can exist without the other. Cysts and pain are different entities that may or may not occur together.

Etiology: Premenstrual breast tenderness and swelling in the luteal phase most commonly occurs 1–4 days premenstrually. It may occur anywhere from 5–14 days premenstrually. The severity and intensity can vary.

Occurrence: In a study of more than 1000 women reporting to an ob/gyn clinic, 69% described premenstrual breast discomfort; 36% reported seeking help for this condition; and 20% reported seeking out more than one healthcare provider for advice related to this symptom. Cyclic mastalgia, when defined as a part of premenstrual syndrome, is better established than mood disorders.

Age: Cyclic mastalgia can occur in any menstruating female.

Ethnicity: Not significant.

Contributing factors: Caffeine consumption, hormone replacement therapy, oral contraceptives.

Signs and symptoms: Breast pain prior to menses. The pain may interfere with normal activities. Women report wearing loose clothing and avoiding touching of the breasts during sexual activity premenstrually. The pain does not usually interfere with work or school or with social activities.

   Physical examination does not reveal mass or discharge. The breast is tender upon palpation.

Diagnostic tests: None are indicated; however, women less than 36 years old with cyclic mastalgia are five times more likely to have a positive mammogram than asymptomatic women.

Differential diagnosis:

- Breast infection—red, swollen, painful breast
- Duct obstruction—reddened area on the breast following the duct
- Breast cancer with inflammatory mass—peau d'orange present on breast
- Periareolar infection—redness and swelling around the nipple
- Trauma—history of trauma, bruising

Treatment: Support bra, avoidance of caffeine, vitamin E supplementation up to 400 IU daily. Reassurance is part of the treatment plan for cyclic mastalgia. Medications such as danazol, tamoxifen, and bromocriptine have been utilized for breast tenderness. These medications have many adverse reactions, such as hot flashes, hirsutism, and dysfunctional uterine bleeding. They should be utilized only in the most severe cases of cyclic mastalgia.

Follow-up: Follow-up is at the discretion of the patient.

Sequelae: The extent to which cyclic mastalgia influences breast screening, self-medication, and use of alternative medicine is unknown.

Prevention/prophylaxis: Decrease caffeine consumption. Careful selection of oral contraceptive agents for each woman desiring this medication.

Referral: Severe cases of cyclic mastalgia require referral to a physician.

Education: Types of food and drinks containing caffeine should be reviewed. Hazards of overconsumption of vitamin E, a fat-soluble vitamin, should be reviewed.

HEADACHE

SIGNAL SYMPTOM ▶ headache

Headache, unspecified	ICD-9-CM: 345
Variants of migraine (includes cluster/histamine)	ICD-9-CM: 346.2
Classical migraine	ICD-9-CM: 345
Variants of migraine	ICD-9-CM: 345.90
Migraine, unspecified	ICD-9-CM: 346.9
Tension headache	ICD-9-CM: 345.90

Definition: Less than 1% of headaches in women indicate serious intracranial disease. Most headaches generally fall into one of three classes:

Migraine: common in women, moderate to severe in intensity, unilateral, often accompanied by nausea and increased sensitivity to light and sound, increasing with activity

Cluster headache: multiple recurrent attacks of severe unilateral pain occurring most frequently in men

Tension type: mild to moderate dull, steady bilateral pain brought on by stress and/or depression

Etiology: Headache can be caused by intracranial or extracranial factors. Intracranial factors are derived from cranial nerves, dura, and cranial arteries. Extracranial factors are derived from skin; muscles; eyes; blood vessels; extracranial arteries; mucous membranes of nose, ears, sinuses; or the temporomandibular joint. Hormones greatly influence the frequency and severity of headache in women.

Occurrence: 18 million American women report severe incapacitating headache (Winner, 1998). Throughout adulthood, women experience a greater prevalence of both migraine and tension headaches compared with men. Twice as many women report migraine headache than men. The majority of women experience chronic headaches, with the prevalence of migraine at 25% and tension headaches at 88% (Marcus, 1999).

 Clinical Pearl: Headache worsens around the menstrual period for 60% of women.

 Clinical Pearl: 16% of women report their first migraine in the perimenopausal years.

 Clinical Pearl: Onset of migraine occurs 10 times more often in women using oral contraceptives.

Age: The peak onset of migraine with aura in girls is 12 to 13 years. Migraine without aura in girls has a peak onset of 14 to 17 years. Onset of migraines in girls is closely related to menarche (see Table 2–4).

Ethnicity: Not significant.

Contributing factors: Menstrually related migraines occur as the levels of estrogen and progesterone decline. Headaches worsen during estrogen decline (ovulation, menstruation) and improve with estrogen increase (pregnancy).

Stress, food allergies, sinus infection, temporomandibular joint dysfunction, systemic infection, hypertension, and eye muscle strain can influence the frequency and severity of headache.

Signs and symptoms: Headache can be mild, moderate, or severe; unilateral or bilateral; generalized or localized; and with sudden or gradual onset.

Table 2–4 Characteristics of Migraine Headaches

Prodrome	Aura	Headache	Termination	Postdrome
Irritability	Visual symptoms	Unilateral	24–48 hours	Fatigue
Nausea	Vertigo	Throbbing		Irritability
Difficulty concentrating	Aphasia			

Source: Sturm, J, and Donnan, G: Diagnosis and investigation of headache. Aust Fam Physician 27(7): 587, 1998.

A new pattern of headache that is occipitonuchal in location and/or begins after age 55 may indicate intracranial pathology.

In women with very frequent or daily headache, analgesic overuse is a likely diagnosis. Detailed history of both prescription and non-prescription drugs is needed.

Headaches of long duration (several days) are usually tension headaches. Those of moderate duration (less than 24 hours) are usually migraine, and brief headaches (1–2 hours) usually are cluster headaches.

Diagnostic tests: Use the following evaluations to rule out other disorders.

Tests	Results Indicating Disorder	CPT Code
Blood Pressure	Hypertension	93770
Temperature	Afebrile or febrile	Included in exam code
Neurologic exam	Negative	Included in exam code
CT scan (head)	Negative	70470 with and without contrast 70460 with contrast 70450 without contrast
Diary	Pattern of headache related to menses	Included in history code

History, including a description of the intensity of the headache, presence of aura, character of the pain, precipitants, aggravating and alleviating factors, and a medication history determine the diagnosis of migraine.

Differential diagnosis:

- Sinus infection: Sinus infection creates headache that is throbbing, acute at onset, worse upon awakening, better after rising, and worse as the day progresses. Sinus headache is accompanied by purulent nasal discharge.
- Temporomandibular joint dysfunction: This condition creates headache from tension induced by jaw clenching and nocturnal teeth grinding. Masticator muscles fatigue and spasm, creating a chronic, dull, aching headache and difficulty opening the mouth in the morning.
- Ocular headache: Ocular headache occurs from eye muscle strain or acute glaucoma.
- Masses: Masses in the head can create headache. When masses create headache, the headache is in one location, progressive, and increases in duration and severity. Eventually changes in mental status occur.
- Meningitis: This inflammation creates a severe, generalized, and constant headache.
- Systemic fever and infection: Systemic fever and infection create cranial vasodilatation and a diffuse throbbing headache.

- Hypertension: High blood pressure creates an occipital headache that is worse in the morning.

Treatment: Acute care treatments are used for infrequent headache. Preventative medications are used for frequent headaches. The most effective acute treatments are combination analgesics (e.g., analgesic plus caffeine). Acute care treatments are limited to a maximum of two to three days per week. The woman should have at least four to five days per week requiring no treatment at all. Analgesic overuse creates a mild, bilateral, daily headache. Preventative therapies include antidepressants, beta-blockers, calcium channel blockers, and antiepilepsy medication.

Menstrual migraines can be treated with anti-inflammatory medication. Preventative medications can also be utilized for three or four days prior to menses. A low-dose estrogen patch may be worn during the week prior to menses.

Discontinue oral contraceptives in women with migraines related to this medication. Discontinuing relieves the headache although it may take months for complete resolution.

Use of oral contraceptives in women who have a history of migraines is associated with increase in headache from 18% to 50%. (Marcus, 1999). Some women notice no change at all.

Approximately one half of the women with a history of migraine note an improvement in their condition during pregnancy; however, migraine worsens in the week following delivery. Only a limited number of medications used to treat migraine headache may be used during pregnancy. Migraine improves spontaneously in many women after menopause.

Relaxation, biofeedback, and exercise programs result in lessening of headache frequency and severity in 50% to 75% of women.

Tension headache is treated with nonsteroidal anti-inflammatory medication or acetaminophen. The causative factor of the headache can, at times, be removed, thus eliminating the headache in ocular headache, hypertension headache, and headache related to infection and fever.

Follow-up: Migraine headache requires frequent follow-up for management of medication.

Sequelae: Appropriate follow-up and careful management of medications for women with chronic headache should eliminate any negative sequelae.

Prevention/prophylaxis: Women with a history of migraine headache should carefully consider the use of oral contraceptives and supplemental estrogen.

Referral: Headache must be quickly referred if it is sudden, severe, or persistent. A new headache of acute onset or a headache that progresses over days or weeks, or any headache with an abnormal neurological examination requires immediate referral. Neck stiffness, altered mental state, ataxia, and severe nausea and vomiting all require immediate referral.

Education: Frequency of analgesic use, whether prescription or over-the-counter, should be assessed in all women who complain of headache.

REFERENCES

Abdominal Pain

Barrenetexa, G, et al: Abdominal mass in a young woman. Pitfalls and delayed diagnosis. Eur J Gynaecol Oncol 17(6):507, 1996.

Goroll, A, et al: Primary Care Medicine. JB Lippincott, Philadelphia, 1995.

Howard, F: Pelvic Pain. Lippincott Williams & Wilkins, Philadelphia, 2000.

McFadyen, B, et al: Laparoscopic management of the acute abdomen. Surg Clin North Am 72(5): 1169, 1992.

Seltzer, V, and Pearse, W: Women's Primary Health Care. McGraw-Hill, New York, 1995.

Silen, W: Early Diagnosis of the Acute Abdomen. Oxford University Press, London, 1991.

Taylor, K, and Kelner, M: The emerging role of the physician in genetic counseling and testing for heritable breast, ovarian, and colon cancer. CMAJ 154(8):115, 1996.

Cyclic Mastalgia

Adler, D, and Browne, M: Prevalence and impact of cyclic mastalgia in a United States clinic based sample. Am J Obstet Gynecol 177(1):126, 1997.

Tavaf-Motamen, H: Clinical evaluation of mastalgia. Arch Surg 133(2):211, 1998.

Dysmenorrhea

Apgar, B: Dysmenorrhea and dysfunctional uterine bleeding. Primary Care Clin Office Pract 24(1):161, 1997.

Howard, F: Pelvic Pain. Lippincott Williams & Wilkins, Philadelphia, 2000.

Jamieson, D, and Steege, J: The prevalence of dysmenorrhea, dyspareunia, pelvic pain, and irritable bowel syndrome in primary care practices. Obstet Gynecol 87(1):55, 1996.

Steege, J: Office assessment of chronic pelvic pain. Clin Obstet Gynecol 40(3):554, 1997.

Dyspareunia

Baggish, M, and Miklos, J: Vulvar pain syndrome: A review. Obstet Gynecol Surv 50(8):618, 1995.

Fisher, G: The commonest causes of symptomatic vulvar disease: A dermatologist's perspective. Aust J Dermatol 37(1):12, 1996.

Hill, D, and Lense, J: Office management of Bartholin gland cyst and abscesses. Am Fam Physician 57(7):1619, 1998.

Howard, F: Pelvic Pain. Lippincott Williams & Wilkins, Philadelphia, 2000.

Jamieson, D, and Steege, J: The association of sexual abuse with pelvic pain complaints in primary care populations. Am J Obstet Gynecol 177(6): 1408, 1997.

Lecks, K: Vulvodynia: Diagnosis and management. J A Acad Nurse Pract
10(3):129, 1998.

Headache

Marcus, D: Focus on primary care: Diagnosis and management of headache in
women. Obstet Gynecol Sur 54(6):395, 1999.

Marks, D, and Rappoport, A: Practical evaluation and diagnosis of headache.
Semin Neurol 17(4):307, 1997.

Ryan, R: Headache diagnosis. Clin Cornerstone 1(6): 11, 1999.

Warshaw, L and Lipton, R: Migraine: a woman's disease Women and Health
28(2): 79, 1998.

Winner, P: Migraine: diagnosis and rational treatment Internat J Fertil Women's
Med 43(2):104, 1998.

Chapter *3*
INTEGUMENT DISORDERS

SKIN CONDITIONS INFLUENCED BY THE ENVIRONMENT

SIGNAL SYMPTOMS ▶ painful skin, soreness, itching: change in a mole; lesions, masses, tumors on the skin

Contact dermatitis	ICD-9-CM: 693
Urticaria	ICD-9-CM: 708.9
Impetigo	ICD-9-CM: 684
Folliculitis	ICD-9-CM: 704.8
Fungal infection	ICD-9-CM: 117.9
Monilia NOS, Candidiasis NOS	ICD-9-CM: 112.9
Dermatitis, drug-related	ICD-9-CM: 693
Herpes simplex	ICD-9-CM: 054.2
Melanoma	ICD-9-CM: 172.9
Basal cell carcinoma	ICD-9-CM: 173.9
Neoplasm, skin, malignant	ICD-9-CM: 173.9
Burns	ICD-9-CM: 949

Description: Skin conditions affected by the environment include dry skin, contact dermatitis, superficial infection of the skin, and sun-related skin damage (see Figure 3–1).

Diagnosing skin disorders

Etiology: Photodamage is skin damage caused by chronic exposure to ultraviolet (UV) light. It is the leading cause of extrinsic aging or alterations in the skin due to environmental exposure. Photodamage causes changes in the skin (such as drying) and also increases the risk for skin cancer.

- Various bacteria, including *Staphylococcus* and *Streptococcus*, can invade the skin.
- Fungus or yeast may infect the skin.
- Contact dermatitis is caused by exposure of the skin to an irritant.
- Many chemicals and drugs may cause side effects that include reactions in the skin.

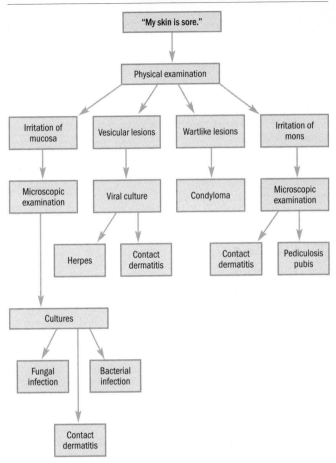

Figure 3–1. Diagnosing skin disorders.

- Folliculitis can be caused by bacteria, but can also be caused by oil-based cosmetics and by shaving.

Occurrence: Incidence of infection or rashes related to contact dermatitis or drug reaction is unknown.

Skin cancer accounts for one third of all cancers in the United States. One out of six Americans develops skin cancer.

Age: The incidence of cancer of the skin increases with age. The incidence of skin cancer increases fourfold in elderly females.

Ethnicity: Women with fair skin, light hair, and blue, green, or gray eyes are most susceptible to skin cancer.

Contributing factors: Exposure to an allergen. Women who work as hairdressers, restaurant workers, hospital employees, in metal industries, and in gardening positions commonly develop contact dermatitis.

Exposure to the sun. Approximately one half of a women's UV exposure occurs before the age of 18 years.

Candidiasis commonly flares with antibiotic usage.

Immunosuppression commonly results in infection of the skin.

Infection of the skin is more likely to occur in skin that is broken or open.

Diabetes mellitus predisposes women to fungal infections.

Heredity is an important factor in contact dermatitis. There is genetic predisposition to this condition.

Signs and symptoms:

 Clinical Pearl: The location of the skin abnormality often suggests the cause; e.g., facial involvement may indicate irritation due to soap or cosmetics.

- Thin-walled vesicles or pustules
- Erosions or ulceration of the skin
- Erythema of the skin
- Tenderness of the skin
- Inflammation surrounding a hair follicle
- Scaling or crusting of the skin
- Fissures in the skin
- Itching of the skin
- Urticaria
- Hyperkeratosis of the skin

Diagnostic Tests:

Tests	Results Indicating Disorder	CPT Code
Viral culture	Positive	87253
Bacterial culture	Positive	87070
Scraping of the lesion	Positive for bacteria and WBCs under microscope	88348 (electron microscopy)
Scraping of the irritated area	Positive for hyphae with budding spores; 10% KOH solution will enhance visualization	87210
Biopsy	Positive for malignancy	11100 + 11101 for each site
Patch testing	Patch testing can be done after the contact dermatitis is resolved. To determine allergy sensitivity.	95044

Differential Diagnosis:

- Cellulitis (redness, warmth, streaking, edema)
- Hematologic malignancy
- Eczema (intense itching, red vesicles or blisters in the acute stage)

- Abcess (fever, chills; painful)
- Molluscum contagiosum (small round, umbilicated, elevated masses)
- Lichen planus (small pruritic red papules that change to rough, scaly patches)
- Psoriasis (silvery, scaly plaques, can be generalized)
- Scabies (pruritic papules and burrows on hands, waist, genitalia)
- Insect bite (history of exposure to pets/animals, insects)

Treatment:

Bacterial infection of the skin can be treated with topical antibiotic ointment or cream. Systemic antibiotics are rarely required to treat superficial infection.

Contact dermatitis: Most episodes of contact dermatitis are self-limiting and resolve in two or three weeks unless bacterial infection complicates the recovery. Women with contact dermatitis must identify the allergen and avoid further contact. Contact dermatitis can be treated with topical agents such as Burow's solution, topical corticosteroids, and oral antihistamines to reduce itching and irritation.

Folliculitis caused by shaving or other forms of irritation can be treated by avoiding the source of irritant. Bacterial folliculitis can be treated with antibacterial topical ointment.

Yeast infection: Treatment for yeast infection in the genital area includes antifungal creams or ointments or oral antifungal therapies.

Follow-up:

Two-day follow-up for re-examination for severe infections
One-week follow-up examination for mild infections

Sequelae:

- Unresolved infection
- Unresolved or recurrent contact dermatitis
- Untreated bacterial infection can develop into cellulitis

Prevention/prophylaxis: Common irritants and allergens responsible for contact dermatitis include: soap, detergents, organic solvents, topical medications, perfumes, certain metals, poison ivy.

Minimizing moisture by avoiding tight clothing and wearing cotton underwear will help reduce the incidence of yeast infection in genitalia. Women with diabetes mellitus will experience fungal infection with less frequency if blood sugar levels are in good control.

Avoid all but minimal exposure to sunlight, particularly during midday. Intact skin is less likely to develop infection.

Referral:

Basal cell carcinonoma grows slowly and seldom metastasizes. It is most common in fair-skinned women over the age of 40 years and usually appears on the face. Initially there is a translucent nodule

leaving a depressed center and a firm elevated border. Referral for biopsy and treatment is necessary.

Squamous cell carcinoma usually appears on sun-exposed fair-skinned women over 60 years of age. It may develop within keratosis. It grows quickly and is firm and reddish. The face and the back of the hands are often affected. Referral for biopsy and treatment is necessary.

Malignant melanoma manifests itself as a noticeable growth or color change in a benign mole. This is a highly malignant tumor most commonly seen in fair-skinned women. Suggestive signs are variation in color, irregular perimeter, raised and irregular surface, ulceration, and crusting. Referral for biopsy and treatment is necessary.

Bacterial or viral infection: refer unresolved cases of contact dermatitis for medical evaluation.

Education:

If oral antihistamines are part of the treatment plan, drowsiness may be associated. Activities requiring concentration should be avoided.

Avoid tight fitting clothing, add chlorine to hot tubs, and shave underarms and legs with clean razors.

Instruct women to do monthly examination of the skin.

Decrease exposure to the sun, particularly in midday. Stress the importance of sunscreen. Encourage wearing skin-protective clothing and hats with a wide brim.

HAIR LOSS

SIGNAL SYMPTOM diffuse hair loss

Hair Loss	ICD-9-CM: 704.00

Definition: Some degree of alopecia (hair loss) with aging is inevitable in both men and women. The exact underlying mechanism is not well understood. Women may experience diffuse hair loss after menopause.

Etiology: The etiology of hair loss is not clear. Some cases are managed best with reassurance and education. Other cases require referral for treatment. Hair loss can be divided into three categories: hair shaft abnormalities, permanent alopecia, and nonpermanent alopecia.

Occurrence: Hair loss is a common problem in both men and women.

Age: Hair loss can occur at any age. Hair loss in women is most common after menopause

Ethnicity: Unknown in women.

Contributing factors:

Permanent alopecia can be caused by trauma, or fungal or bacterial infection.

Hormonal balance can influence hair loss.

Nutritional disorders can influence hair loss.

Androgenic alopecia is an inherited disorder.

Sign and symptoms:

In hair shaft abnormalities, the woman presents with diffuse or patchy areas of short hair and a history of hair that will not grow beyond a certain length.

Permanent alopecia is irreversible hair loss associated with destruction of the bulge area in the midportion of the follicle. Androgenic alopecia or common baldness is prominent central pattern scalp alopecia induced by androgens and may affect genetically predisposed people at any time after puberty. Androgenic alopecia is an autosomal dominant disorder that affects men and women equally.

Nonpermanent alopecia is hair loss with chances of regrowth. Causes are hair pulling or plucking. The primary sign presented by the woman is shedding of hair. Decreased hair volume is noted by the woman after approximately 20% loss. Daily shed counts are high—usually around 150 to 200.

Diagnostic Tests:

Tests	Results Indicating Disorder	CPT Code
Gentle hair pulling	20 to 50 shafts dislodge	None available
Bacterial culture	Positive	87070
Culture for fungus	Positive	87101
Hormonal screening	Perimenopausal changes; androgen excess	80418 and 80415
Thyroid function	Abnormal	84443, 84479, 84481, and 84439

Differential Diagnoses:

- Hepatic and renal disorders (history, appropriate lab tests)
- Syphilis (positive VDRL)

Treatment: Cause or causes must be isolated in order to effectively treat. Having the woman keep a calendar may be helpful. Record in the calendar amount of shedding; stress; illnesses; and drug intake.

Treatment for alopecia can include steroids (topical or systemic), minoxidil, immunotherapies. Choices are based on the extent of the disease and the woman's age.

Hair transplantation can be effective for women with androgenic alopecia.

Sequelae: None.

Prevention/prophylaxis: Adequate nutrition, balance of hormones, decreased stress levels, lack of trauma to the hair.

Referral: Reassurance may be all that is required when a woman complains of hair loss. Reassurance that hair changes occur with aging and that complete baldness will not occur may be all that is required.

If signficant loss is noted after tracking of hair loss symptoms via a calendar, referral should be given.

All cases of permanent alopecia and androgenic alopecia in women should be referred.

Education: Traction can physically damage hair and alter the growth cycle. Practices such as tight braiding, wearing ponytails, wearing elastic bands, or using rollers can damage hair.

HERPES INFECTION

SIGNAL SYMPTOMS▶ painful genitalia; lesions on external genitalia

Herpes zoster	ICD-9CM: 053.9
Herpes simplex, oral	ICD-9CM: 054.4
Herpes simplex, genital	ICD-9CM: 054.1

Definition: Herpes is a viral infection that affects men, women, and children. Genital herpes infection is a lifelong disease that may result in painful recurrent lesions that may have psychosocial effects. Genital herpes can produce serious negative outcomes in neonates born to women infected at the time of delivery.

Etiology: The cutaneous lesions of herpes simplex virus (HSV) infections are produced by HSV 1 (most commonly oral) and HSV 2 (commonly associated with genital infection). Each of these viral types can infect any skin area. Recurrence in the genital area from type 1 is less common than from type 2. Many women seek clinical assistance to confirm the herpes infection they suspect or to reduce frequently recurring symptoms.

Occurrence: Unknown.

Age: Genital herpes occurs in sexually active women.

Ethnicity: Not significant.

Contributing factors: Sexual activity. Reactivation of the latent herpes virus can be stimulated by sunlight, trauma, or immunosuppression.

Signs and symptoms: Primary HSV 1 usually presents as severe pharyngitis or gingivostomatitis with fever and lymphadenopathy. Primary HSV 2 presents as painful vulvovaginitis with ulcerations and lymph node enlargement. Fever and malaise also occur in the majority of women. Small, maculopapular-vesicular blisters occur 12–24 hours after contact with a herpes virus. Eventually there is re-epithelialization of the skin, usually without scarring.

During the initial 3–4 days of primary infection, some woman autoinoculate themselves to other areas (commonly mouth to genitalia), but secondary infections are usually mild, brief, self-limiting, and incapable of establishing disease in other areas.

After acute infection, the virus lies dormant in the dorsal root ganglion and circulates to the skin when there is a breakdown in host defenses.

The result is a localized, self-limiting form of the illness. It may begin with tingling or discomfort. Most women experience the maculopapular-vesicular rash. Recurrent infections can occur in different distributions, but along the same ganglia.

Diagnostic Tests:

Tests	Results Indicating Disorder	CPT Code
Viral culture with DNA probe	Positive	83896 + infectious agent code (87000 level code)

In most cases, the diagnosis is a clinical one.

Differential Diagnosis:

- Contact dermatitis (erythematous papules with scaling, itching)
- Condyloma acuminatum (fleshy growth on extremities)
- Chancroid, excoriation (highly contagious STD; papule that increases in size, ulcerates and forms vesicles or bullae)
- Bacterial infection (positive culture)

Treatment: The goals of therapy are to speed healing and reduce symptoms, reduce the frequency and severity of recurrences, and decrease the risk for complications. Acyclovir, the mainstay of treatment, is effective against both types. It shortens viral shedding time and reduces the time to heal. The earlier the treatment begins, the better. Treat symptomatic lesions with oral acyclovir, 200 mg five times daily or 400 mg every eight hours. Treatment should continue for five to ten days. Titrate the dosage depending on the patient response. Acyclovir can be given in 800-mg doses two to four times daily.

Chronic acyclovir prophylaxis can be given to women who experience more than six outbreaks per year. Use the smallest dose of acyclovir that will prevent infection. Good local skin care and the use of a drying agent help speed the transition from acute vesicle to crusting.

Follow-up: Follow all herpes genital infections closely during pregnancy. All primary infection should be followed closely for resolution.

Sequelae: Secondary bacterial infection can occur. Chronic pain associated with this disease has been identified. Women can have post-herpetic neuralgia without evidence of skin lesions. Both hemorrhagic cystitis and dyspareunia can occur as a result of this disease. HSV has been associated with retina necrosis. Secondary infection can occur.

Prevention/prophylaxis: Herpes infection is a risk associated with sexual activity. Using condoms can reduce the risk but does not always prevent transmission of the disease.

Referral: Refer all infected women who are also pregnant to an obstetrician. Women with suspected eye involvement should be referred to an ophthalmologist.

Education: Herpes has acquired an unjustifiable reputation. The only substantial risk associated with HSV is during childbirth. Risk of infection to the fetus can be reduced by culturing any possibly herpetic lesions and performing caesarean birth if necessary. The stigma associated with the disease must be reduced. Reassuring a frightened patient is important therapy.

Women must be educated about transmission. The risk of transmission is greatest during the first 96 hours after the appearance of the lesions. Silent shedding must be explained, as should the fact that condoms reduce the probability of infecting others with the disease.

HUMAN PAPILLOMAVIRUSES

SIGNAL SYMPTOMS▶   "bumps" on genitalia

Viral warts NOS and verruca vulgaris	ICD-9-CM: 078.10
Condyloma acuminatum	ICD-9-CM: 078.11

Description: Warts result from skin infection with the human papillomavirus (HPV).

Etiology: HPV, a DNA virus with more than 60 types identified, causes tumors of the epidermis. At least five types are potentially oncogenic, with two implicated in cervical carcinoma and three in squamous cell carcinoma. Warts can be transmitted by direct contact or autoinoculation.

Occurrence: Unknown.

Age: During the sexually active years.

Ethnicity: Not significant.

Contributing factor: Sexual activity.

Signs and symptoms: Anogenital warts and condylomata acuminata, which result from sexual transmission of HPV, grow on mucous membrane. They range in size and are often asymptomatic.

Diagnostic Tests:

Test	Results Indicating Disorder	CPT Code
Pap smear	HPV on description in Pap smear result	88142

Appearance is generally sufficient for diagnosis. Acetic acid in a 5% solution can be used to enhance visualization of small condylomata. The colposcope can provide magnification.

Differential Diagnosis:
- Condyloma acuminatum of syphilis (fleshy growth on extremities)
- Squamous cell carcinoma (confirmed by cytology)

- Molluscum contagiosum (small round, umbilicated, elevated masses)
- Lipomas (fatty tumor in subcutaneous layer, smooth, soft)

Treatment: Trichloracetic acid (TCA) in solution can be applied to external condylomata. TCA does not require removal. TCA should be applied carefully in order to protect unaffected areas. Petroleum or KY jelly can be applied to the unaffected area surrounding the condylomata during TCA application.

Podofilox 0.5% (Condylox) can be applied to external lesions by the woman infected with the disease. The manufacturer's directions and restrictions must be followed carefully.

A carbon dioxide laser can be used for extensive external disease and for HPV of the cervix.

Liquid nitrogen can be applied to resistant external lesions.

Follow-up: Lesions can become numerous and large, requiring more extensive treatment. The woman with this disease should be examined at least every 4 weeks for evaluation until resolution of the disease. A Pap smear should be performed in women treated for external condylomata every 6 months for at least 2 years.

Sequelae: Recurrences occur in approximately one third of women.

Prevention/prophylaxis: Prevention entails avoiding others with warts. Removing condylomata prevents further infection.

Referral: A Pap smear showing cervical dysplasia and the evidence of HPV requires referral. Women with extensive condylomata may require referral for possible laser treatment or use of liquid nitrogen.

Education: Condylomata may disappear spontaneously. For some women, the treatment is lengthy, time-consuming, and expensive. Bolstering the immune system with adequate sleep and rest, excellent nutrition, and vitamin therapy may reduce the viral reserve. When a diagnosis is made, sexual partners should be examined for the disease.

PEDICULOSIS PUBIS

SIGNAL SYMPTOMS▶   pubic itching; visualization of nits

Pediculosis Pubis	ICD-9-CM: 132.2

Description: Human lice are wingless, blood-sucking insects of two types: *Pediculus humanus,* which infests the head and body, and *Phthirus pubis,* which infests the pubic area. These insects are elongated or rounded and 3–4 mm in length or diameter.

Etiology: Transmission is by contact with infested clothing or bedding, and/or by sexual transmission. The adult louse lives and lays eggs in clothing, often in the seams, and travels onto the skin for feeding. The second and third pairs of legs serve as claws that clasp hair tightly. The nits hatch and evolve into adults in 2–3 weeks. Lice live approximately 1 month. *Phthirus* affects primarily the pubic hairs; however, the eyelashes and axillary, chest, and thigh hair can be involved.

Occurrence: Unknown.

Age: Lice can be transmitted to a woman of any age.

Ethnicity: Not significant.

Contributing factors: Close contact with lice through clothing, bedding, or sexual activity.

Signs and symptoms: Itching, which is the cardinal symptom, is caused by the lice injecting saliva, digestive juices, and feces into the skin.

Diagnostic tests: Diagnosis is made by direct examination of egg cases in the involved area. They are usually visible to the naked eye, but a hand lens and light may help. Microscopic examination of nits or adult lice is also diagnostic.

Differential diagnosis:

- Contact dermatitis (erythematous papules with scaling, itching, inflammation, irritation of skin from contact with irritating substance)
- Bacterial infection (positive culture)
- Viral infection (positive viral culture)

Treatment: Lindane 1% shampoo used for 4 minutes and washed off, followed by permethrin 1% cream used for 10 minutes and then rinsed off. Lindane should not be used during pregnancy or lactation.

To prevent reinfestation, treat asymptomatic close contacts simultaneously. Wash bed sheets and clothing worn in the last few days in hot soapy water and dry-clean any nonwashable items.

Treat eyelashes by applying occlusive ophthalmic ointment to the eyelids twice daily for 10 days.

Follow-up: Evaluate patients in 1 week. Treatment can be repeated if the parasites are still present.

Sequelae: Secondary infection can occur. Reactions to medicated shampoo can occur.

Prevention/Prophylaxis: Avoidance of the parasites.

Referral: Treatment failure should be referred. Coexisting dermatologic conditions should be referred.

Education: Tell sexual partners that they must be treated simultaneously to prevent reinfestation. Family and household members who are infected should also be treated simultaneously.

REFERENCES

Skin Conditions Influenced by the Environment

Bergfeld, W: A lifetime of healthy skin: implications for women. International J Fertil Women's Med 44(2):83, March-April 1999.

Goroll, A, et al: A. Primary Care Medicine. JB Lippincott, Philadelphia, 1995.

Hansen, J: Common cancers in the elderly. Drugs and Aging 13(6):467-478, 1998.

Hair Loss

Avram, M: Hair transplantation in women. Semin Cutan Med Surg. 18(2):172, June 1999.

Mulinari-Brenner, et al: Hair loss: An overview. Derm Nurs 13(4):269, August 2001.

Rubin, M: Androgenic alopecia. Postgrad Med 102(2):129, August 1997.

Herpes Infection

Barton, SE, et al: Asymptomatic shedding of herpes simplex virus from the genital tract. Int J STD & AIDS 7(4):229, 1996.

Brugha, R, et al: Genital herpes infection: A review. Int J Epidemiol 26(4):698, 1997.

Roberts, SW, et al: Genital herpes during pregnancy: No lesions, no caesarean. Obstet Gynecol 85(2):261, 1995.

Shelley, WB, and Slehhey, ED: Stat single dose of acyclovir for prevention of herpes simplex. Cutis 57(6):453, 1996.

Human Papillomaviruses

Casper, K, and Mehta, B: Healthy skin for women: a review of conditions and therapies. J Am Pharm Assoc 42(2):206, Mar–Apr 2002.

Swygart, C: Human papillomavirus: disease and laboratory diagnosis. Br J Biomed Sci 54(4):299, Dec. 1997.

Pediculosis Pubis

Brown, S, Becher, J, and Brady W: Treatment of ectoparasitic infection: Review of English language literature. Clin Infect Dis 20(Suppl 1):104, 1995.

Chapter 4
CHEST DISORDERS

Evaluation of the chest plays an important role in women's health examinations. Breast cancer is associated with high rates of morbidity and mortality for women. A combination of breast self-examination, practitioner examination, and screening tests enhances early detection and therefore reduces mortality. Physical examination detects early disease and provides an excellent opportunity for teaching breast self-examination and discussing the importance of mammography.

Depending on the definition used, 15%–25% of adult Americans have hypertension. Every woman should have a blood pressure check at every clinical visit.

Cardiovascular disease is by far the leading cause of death among women in the United States. It is also a chronic condition that affects millions of American adults. More women die of cardiovascular disease than from all other causes combined. The responsibility for screening and intervention lies with all practitioners. In any practice setting, efforts should focus on the prevention of cardiovascular disease through risk reduction and on early identification of cardiovascular disease in patients with symptoms.

This chapter discusses prevention, diagnosis, and treatment for benign and malignant breast disease and screening and prevention of cardiovascular disease.

CARDIAC DISEASE

SIGNAL SYMPTOM▶   **chest pain**

Coronary Artery Disease	ICD-9-CM: 414.1 (CAD)
Cardiovascular Disease	ICD-9-CM: 429.2

Description: Cardiovascular disease, specifically coronary heart disease (CHD), is the leading cause of death in women in the United States. In women, deaths from cardiac disease total more than twice the number of deaths from cancer. Nearly twice as many women in the United States die of heart disease and stroke as from all forms of cancer (American Heart Association, 2002). Gender differences exist in both the diagnosis and the treatment of CHD. Morbidity from cardiac disease is higher in women than it is in men. There is a growing body of knowledge related to preventive strategies, diagnostic testing, responses to medical and surgical therapies, and other aspects of cardiovascular disease in women, but current information is still insufficient. Because of the under-representation of women in previous clinical trials, few comparisons of long-term outcomes between men and women with CHD have been made.

Etiology: The major cause of heart disease in women is coronary artery disease (CAD). Although other forms of heart disease exist in women, including valvular disease and heart disease during pregnancy, the incidence is significantly less and therefore these diseases will not be discussed in this chapter. Please refer to a general text for discussion of valvular disease, peripheral vascular disease, and stroke.

Occurrence: Cardiovascular disease hospitalizes 2.5 million women per year and claims the lives of 500,000 annually. These numbers exceed those of men. Cardiovascular disease accounts for 37% of the deaths in all women and 50% of the deaths in postmenopausal women. CAD remains the leading cause of mortality in women, accounting for 28% of deaths. Morbidity from cardiovascular disease is higher in women than in men. The higher morbidity and mortality rates in women can be partially explained by the tendency for women to be older, sicker, and to have more advanced disease at time of diagnosis.

Age: Increased incidence of CHD in women occurs after age 54. In women 55 years of age and older, there is a tenfold increase in CHD. The increased risk for men in the same age group is 4.6. This change in risk in women is thought to be largely related to the onset of menopause.

Ethnicity: Black women have a greater risk of heart disease and stroke than do white women.

Contributing factors (see Box 4–1):

Box 4-1
Risk Factors for Cardiac Disease

Cigarette smoking
Diabetes
High blood pressure
Elevated cholesterol
Obesity
Sedentary lifestyle
Postmenopause
Family history

Family history may predispose women to heart disease. Of significance is any first-order relative, male or female, with a history of heart disease.

Blood pressure is a more common risk factor in women than it is in men. Hypertension affects an estimated 70% of women over 65 years of age.

Smoking has well-established deleterious health effects. Women who smoke more than one pack of cigarettes per day increase their coronary artery risk to two to four times that of non-smoking women. Concerns for smoking women include the anti-estrogenic effect of smoking, earlier onset of menopause in smokers, and interaction with oral contraceptives. Women smokers taking oral contraceptives have a 20-fold increase of myocardial infarction because of the enhanced risk of thrombosis.

Hyperlipidemia is an important risk factor in women. Levels of high-density lipoprotein (HDL), which are inversely associated with CHD, are higher throughout a woman's life than a man's. After menopause, however, HDL levels drop slightly, and the risk for CHD rises. The risk for CHD in women increases when the HDL level falls to less than 45 mg/dL. In men the risk is higher at levels under 35 mg/dL. Levels of low-density lipoproteins (LDL) rise after menopause, surpassing those of men, whose LDL levels tend to plateau at age 50.

Diabetes presents a very unfavorable risk factor for women, who in general experience a two-fold greater risk for CHD than diabetic men. In addition, mortality from myocardial infarction and congestive heart failure is two times higher for diabetic women than for diabetic men. Diabetes creates a 3- to 7-times greater risk for heart disease in women.

Obesity, with incumbent higher waist size–to–hip size ratios, has been shown to increase the risk for CHD in women.

History of previous heart attack or *stroke* is a risk factor.

Lack of physical activity is a risk factor for heart disease.

Signs and Symptoms:

Gender plays an important role in manifestation of CHD. In men, the three major presentations include angina, sudden death, and myocardial infarction. In women, angina appears to be the most common manifestation. Women are twice as likely as men to present with angina and less likely to present with sudden death or infarction. In the acute care setting, women are more likely than men to have heart failure and cardiogenic shock associated with infarction, perhaps in part because women present with an infarction on an average of 5 hours later than men. Women have a higher mortality rate than men during hospitalization, and at 6 weeks and 1 year after infarction. Four years after infarction, mortality rates were 36% for women and 21% for men.

Heart disease typically develops in women seven to ten years later than in men. Chest pain is the most common initial manifestation of CHD. However, women can present as older men do, with shortness of breath, dizziness, and atypical pain involving the neck, shoulders, back, arm, upper abdomen, and jaw rather than classic chest pain. The greater prevalence of diabetes in women may also interfere with perception of pain.

Chest pain compatible with angina warrants evaluation for coronary artery disease in both men and women. The higher prevalence of angina as the presenting symptom places a greater burden on diagnostic strategies than the more easily recognized myocardial infarction. History is important for diagnosis. In one study, women who had typical anginal pain had a 70% incidence of angiographically documented CAD as compared to 2%–7% of those with atypical chest pain (Oettgen and Douglas, 1994).

Diagnostic Tests:

Tests	Results Indicating Disorder	CPT Code
Exercise electrocardiogram (ECG)	Change in electrical activity (poor at detecting or excluding CAD in asymptomatic women)	93000
Stress ECG with pharmacologic stimulation	Change in electrical activity (75% sensitivity in women)	93015
Exercise ECG with thallium scintigraphy	Area of diminished isotopic activity (85% sensitivity in women)	93024
ECG-gated single photon emission computed tomography	The slices of myocardium evaluating isotopic activity in conjunction with diastole and systole. Increased specificity	93543
Angiography	Direct visualization of degree of narrowing in the vessels. Gold standard for assessment of CHD in women.	93571 + 93572 with each added vessel

Differential Diagnoses:
- Muscular disorders, including muscle spasm or strain
- Skeletal disorders, including costochondritis, rib fracture, and metastatic disease
- Neurologic disorders, including herpes zoster and nerve root compression
- Pleuropulmonary disorders, including pneumothorax, pulmonary embolism, and bronchospasm
- Esophageal disorders, including spasm and reflux, cholecystitis, and peptic ulcer disease
- Psychogenic disorders, including anxiety and depression

Treatment: Women with suspected CAD are referred less frequently for coronary angiography and coronary bypass surgery. Male patients are 6.5 times more likely to be referred for catheterization than female patients. This seems paradoxical in light of the fact that the noninvasive tests are less accurate in women and the need for a gold standard such as angiography would be more desirable in women to define the presence or absence of disease.

Invasive diagnostic and therapeutic procedures are underutilized in women. Women are treated less frequently with thrombolytics, even though thrombolytic therapy for acute MI has equal benefit for both men and women. In a 1996 study, Villablanca concluded that women with acute MI were half as likely as men to be treated with angioplasty, thrombolysis, or coronary artery bypass graft surgery (CABG). In a 1999 study, women with unstable angina were less likely than men to receive cardiac catheterization, coronary angioplasty, and CABG (Emory Center, 2000). In a study of gender differences in response to coronary artery bypass graft surgery, perioperative complications and recurrent angina were more frequent in women (Nurse Practitioner Study, 2001).

It is unclear whether women's poorer outcomes after coronary events are related to differential treatment or to differences in presentation. Following MI, women have higher rates of hospital mortality, reinfarction within the first year, and mortality within the first year. The mortality rate for women younger than 50 is twice that of men of the same age. The difference decreases with age and is no longer significant after age 74.

Use of pharmacologic agents in women with CHD is being investigated. Women are as likely as men to receive beta blockers; however, women are more likely than men to receive ACE inhibitors.

Follow-up: Exercise rehabilitation benefits both men and women. Physicians refer fewer women with CAD than men for exercise rehabilitation.

Sequelae: Women have higher operative mortality rates and they are twice as likely as men to have continued symptoms after coronary angioplasty.

Prevention/prophylaxis:

- Smoking cessation
- Weight reduction
- Physical exercise
- Excellent control of hypertension
- Good control of diabetes
- Reduced dietary intake of fat
- Early diagnosis of rheumatic heart disease

The American Heart Association (2002) recommends that risk factor screening for heart disease begin at age 20 years. Every two years, blood pressure, body mass index, waist circumference, and pulse should be noted by a practitioner. Every five years, a cholesterol profile and glucose testing should be recommended by a practitioner.

The Women's Health Initiative Trial as published in the Journal of the American Medical Association, July, 2002, states that as a result of the trials "hormone therapy should not be initiated for the purpose of preventing a second heart attack or death among women with heart disease." Ongoing trials may indicate that overall health risk may be present in women taking combined estrogen and progesterone.

The U.S. Prevention Services Task Force, June 2002, recommends that practitioners routinely screen women over the age of 45 for lipid disorders. Lipid measurement can identify asymptomatic women who are at risk for coronary artery disease. The recommendation for screening includes measurement of total cholesterol and high density lipoprotein. The National Heart, Lung and Blood Institute in 2001 recommended measuring levels of total cholesterol, low density lipoprotein and high density lipoprotein, and triglycerides.

Referral: Any indicator for heart disease warrants a referral for evaluation.

Education: Inform the patient that:

- The risk of CHD can be reduced in women by 14% within 2 years of stopping smoking. Three to five years after cessation of smoking, the risk for coronary artery disease between a former smoker and a woman who has never smoked is the same.
- Weight gained after the age of 18 years is associated with increased risk.
- A correlation exists between the intake of vitamin E and protection against CHD.
- Small doses of aspirin per day reduce the risk of CHD.
- Four randomized clinical trials have demonstrated no effect of hormone replacement therapy on coronary health.

 Clinical Pearl: Dietary fat intake less than 30% of total calories, aerobic exercise (three to five thirty-minute sessions per week), and cessation of smoking are the cardinal prevention mechanisms for heart disease.

CARCINOMA OF THE BREAST

SIGNAL SYMPTOM ▶ lump in breast; breast cancer is often asymptomatic

Malignant neoplasm of the female breast	ICD-9-CM: 174
Nipple and areola	ICD-9-CM: 174.0
Central portion	ICD-9-CM: 174.1
Upper-inner quadrant	ICD-9-CM: 174.2
Lower-inner quadrant	ICD-9-CM: 174.3
Upper-outer quadrant	ICD-9-CM: 174.4

Lower-outer quadrant	ICD-9-CM: 174.5
Axillary tail	ICD-9-CM: 174.6
Unspecified	ICD-9-CM: 174.9
Carcinoma in situ of breast	ICD-9-CM: 233.0
Mastodynia	ICD-9-CM: 611.71
Breast lump/mass	ICD-9-CM: 611.72

Description: Breast cancer is the leading cause of death in women aged 35 through 54. More than 178,000 women develop breast cancer each year in the United States. Of these, 40,800 will die of the disease (American Cancer Society, 2000). The lifetime probability that an American woman will develop breast cancer is 10%. Four out of five women have a relative or acquaintance who has developed breast cancer.
Etiology: Unknown.
Occurrence: Breast cancer incidence and death rate vary by race (see Figure 4-1). The incidence for white women in the United States from 1992 until 1998 was 115 per 100,000.
Age: Between 1973 and 1998, incidence rates of invasive breast cancer increased for women over age 40. Incidence rates did not increase for women under age 40. The risk of developing breast cancer increases with age. Women under 40 years of age account for 20% of breast cancer cases. The median age at the time of diagnosis is 54 years, whereas 45% of the cases occur after age 65 years. Half of breast cancer deaths are in women over age 65.

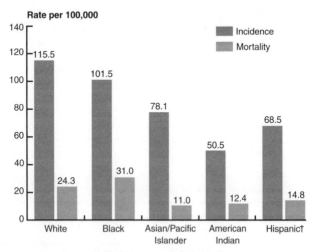

*Rates are age-adjusted to the 1970 US standard population.
† Persons of Hispanic origin may be of any race.
American Cancer Society, Surveillance Research, 2001.
Data sources: NCI Surveillance, Epidemiology, and End Results Program, 2001, and National Center for Health Statistics, 2001.

5-Year Survival Rates* by Stage at Diagnosis and Race (%)

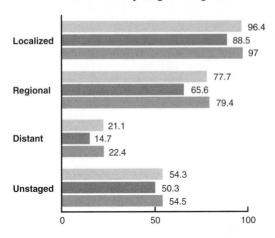

Percent Diagnosed by Stage and Race

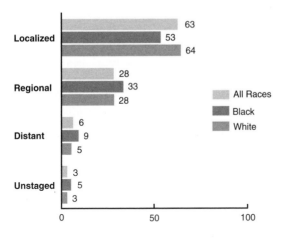

*Survival rates are based on follow-up of patients through 1997.

American Cancer Society, Surveillance Research, 2001.

Data source: NCI Surveillance, Epidemiology, and End Results Program, 2001.

Figure 4-1. Female breast cancer incidence (Sources: NCI Surveillance, Epidemiology and End Results Program, 2001, American Cancer Surveillance Research, 2001).

Ethnicity: Breast cancer is more common in white women than in black women, but the mortality rate for breast cancer is higher in black women than it is in white women. Between 1992 and 1998, incidence rates have remained relatively unchanged in women of all racial and ethnic groups.

Contributing factors: A number of factors have been associated with increased risk of breast cancer, including:

- Personal or family history of breast cancer. The risk for women who have a first-degree relative with breast cancer is two to three times higher than in the general population.
- Biopsy positive for hyperplasia
- Nulliparity and delayed childbearing
- Early menarche
- Late natural menopause

Other factors that may be associated with breast cancer, but about which the literature is still inconclusive, are diet, exogenous hormones, alcohol consumption, breast trauma, viral infection, higher socioeconomic status, and obesity.

Breast feeding may decrease the risk for breast cancer.

Signs and symptoms: Breast examination is an integral part of a woman's health care. Every woman should be taught to perform breast self-examination.[*] A diagnostic evaluation for breast cancer begins with physical examination and history. Any firm mass suggests malignancy. Fixation to the skin, skin edema, nipple retraction, or deep fixation is further evidence of carcinoma. When a mass is suspected or detected, history should be recorded, with particular emphasis on date of onset, size, and exact location.

Incidence rates of in situ breast cancer have increased considerably over the last 25 years. Most of the increase can be explained by the detection of ductal carcinoma with a mammogram. Most cases of ductal carcinoma are detectable only through mammography. Since 1998, invasive breast cancer rates have remained level, but ductal carcinoma incidence continues to increase. This shift is thought to reflect earlier detection rather than a true increase in occurrence.

Nonpalpable lesions presenting as asymptomatic clusters of microcalcifications require repeat mammography or biopsy. Although most of these lesions are benign, 15%–20% represent early cancer. Consultation with a radiologist is essential to determine the significance of this finding.

A woman with a BRCA1 or BRCA2 altered gene is more likely to develop breast or ovarian cancer than a woman without these alterations. However, not every woman who has these genes will develop a carcinoma. Therefore, an altered gene alone is not sufficient to cause cancer. Most breast cancer cases do not involve altered genes. At most, one in ten

---

[*]In 2003, The American Cancer Society described breast self-examination as optional.

breast cancers involve an altered gene. Finding an altered gene indicates an increased risk for developing cancer but it will not indicate that it will occur. Knowing that a woman is at risk suggests increased surveillance via mammograms, breast examinations, and ultrasound of the ovaries. Women considering genetic testing should speak to a professional trained in genetics before deciding whether or not to be tested. Information on genetic testing and referral centers can be found via the National Cancer Institute at 1-800-4-CANCER or *www.cancer.gov.*

Diagnostic Tests:

Test	Results Indicating Disorder	CPT Code
Breast self-examination	Palpable mass present	None
Clinical breast examination	Palpable mass present. Skin changes may be present	Included in exam code
Mammograms	Mass, developing density, calcifications, skin thickening, and architectural distortion.	76091 Bilateral 76090 Unilateral
Biopsy of mass	Cytological examination confirms the diagnosis of breast cancer *	19100 (needle) 19101 (incisional); 19102 (with imaging) 88172 (cytology of biopsy)

* Cytologic detection by biopsy is most useful in the diagnosis of breast cancer. A malignant cytologic finding permits immediate planning of treatment and discussion of treatment alternatives. Open biopsy can be performed, as can needle biopsy under radiologic guidance.

Differential diagnosis: Nonmalignant breast mass (breast pain)

Treatment: Clinical staging determines the therapy for breast cancer. The woman's wishes, the size and histology of the lesion, the size of the breast, and the skill and experience of the oncology team determine the course of surgical treatment. The use of radiation and/or chemotherapy is determined based upon the staging of the disease.

Follow-up: Follow-up depends on the course of therapy. Women may have courses of chemotherapy or radiation therapy before or after surgery. After therapy, women are seen at regular intervals. One regimen involves clinical evaluation every 3 months with annual pelvic examination, mammogram, chest x-ray, and liver function tests. This program continues for 2 years, with an increase to 4-month intervals in the third and fourth years, and every 6 months thereafter.

Sequelae: The 10-year survival rate for early-stage lesions (up to 2 cm and no node involvement) is 75%–85%. This figure drops to 40% survival if there is node involvement. Recurrent disease occurs most often in the first 2 years following treatment, but because women continue to die of breast cancer for periods exceeding 15–20 years following treatment, follow-up must continue indefinitely.

There has been an important reduction in breast cancer deaths in recent years. Between 1950 and the late 1980s overall breast cancer mortality was relatively stable. Between 1989 and 1995, the death rate decreased by 1.6%. Between 1995 and 1998 the decrease accelerated to a decline of 3.4% annually. This decline has been attributed to improvements in cancer treatments and to the benefits of mammography screening. During the 1990's, the death rate declines have been most notable in white women. Death rates for women under 50 declined an average of 3.1% annually between 1990 and 1998. The decline for older women was 2.1% annually.

Prevention/prophylaxis: The combination of breast self-examination, physical examination by a health-care provider, and a mammogram provides the most effective means of screening for breast cancer.*

The Breast Cancer Prevention Trial is currently investigating whether tamoxifen can prevent the development of breast cancer in healthy women at risk for the disease. The U.S. Preventive Services reported in 2002 in the *Annals of Internal Medicine* that tamoxifen and raloxifene reduce the incidence of estrogen receptor–positive breast cancer in women. The absolute risk reduction varies by risk factors for breast cancer and must be balanced against potential harm.

Referral: All palpable masses that do not resolve after menses should be referred for further evaluation. Women with palpable findings should be referred for evaluation regardless of mammogram results. Breast tissue is considerably denser in young women, making a negative mammogram result not always negative for malignancy.

Education: Teach breast self-examination* to all women. Menstruating women should perform breast self-examination approximately 7 days after the onset of menses. For women who do not experience menses, a day of the month should be chosen for breast self-examination.

Many women in the United States have breast implants. Examination of the augmented breast should include examination of the natural tissues as well as evaluation of the implant. During the examination, the implant is displaced with one hand and the breast tissue palpated with the other. Integrity of the implant is evaluated.

NONMALIGNANT CONDITIONS OF THE BREAST

SIGNAL SYMPTOM ▶ lump in the breast; breast pain

Cystic breast, fibrocystic breast disease	ICD-9-CM: 610.1
Solitary cyst of breast	ICD-9-CM: 610.0

---

*Breast self-examination should focus on general breast health. It is a way for women to know how their breasts normally feel and to notice changes. So far, the mammogram is the only screening method that has proven to reduce deaths from breast cancer. Breast self-examination should supplement mammography and clinical breast examination.

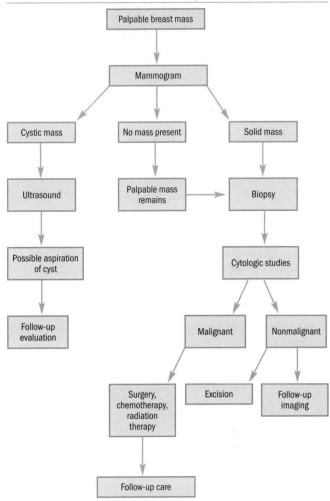

Figure 4–2. Lump in breast.

Description: The nurse practitioner is in a favorable position to educate, screen, counsel, and treat women with breast disease. Every woman should be taught breast self-examination. Any and all symptoms of breast disease must follow a protocol to rule out carcinoma (see Figure 4–2). When a benign condition is diagnosed, treatment should be within the realm of the nurse practitioner's expertise.

Etiology:

Breast pain can be caused by edema, ductal dilatation, and/or inflammatory response.

Cystic change refers to dilatation of the ducts. Most common is the development of microcysts (2 mm or less), but 20%–40% of microcysts progress to form palpable macrocysts. Macrocysts may regress with menses, may persist, or may disappear and reappear.

Fibrous change, occurring in the menstrual years, is characterized by a firm, palpable mass usually located in the upper quadrant of the breast that develops following an inflammatory response to ductal irritation.

Hyperplasia, a layering of cells, is associated with a five-fold increase in the risk of breast cancer.

Adenosis is related to changes in the acini in the distal mammary lobule. These small ducts become surrounded by a firm, hard, plaquelike material. This is most commonly seen in women in their 30s and 40s.

Papilloma is a lesion seen in later menstrual years. It is a small palpable mass adjacent to the areola and accompanied by serosanguineous nipple discharge.

Ductal ectasia is the presence of dilated, distended terminal collecting ducts.

Subareolar abscesses are seen most commonly in younger women. This condition is not related to mastitis.

Fat necrosis is associated with trauma to the breast and usually presents as a hard, tender mass.

Occurrence: Fibrocystic change, the most common benign condition of the breast, occurs in approximately 10% of women under the age of 21, but becomes much more common in the premenopausal period. There is usually a regression of some of the signs of fibrocystic change during menopause.

Age: Depends on diagnosis.

Contributing factors: Caffeine ingestion has been associated with fibrocystic changes of the breast.

Signs and Symptoms: The common symptoms of fibrocystic change are pain and tenderness, usually bilaterally, and most often in the upper outer quadrants of the breasts. Premenstrual pain is most often noted. Solid painless masses in the breast are detected with breast self-examination. Ductal ectasia presents as a mass near the areola with burning and itching. There may be a greenish to black nipple discharge. Subareolar abscess presents with pain and inflammation (see Figure 4–3).

Diagnostic Testing:

Tests	Results Indicating Disorder	CPT Code
Physical breast examination	Skin changes and/or the presence of a mass.	Included in exam code

(Continued on the following page)

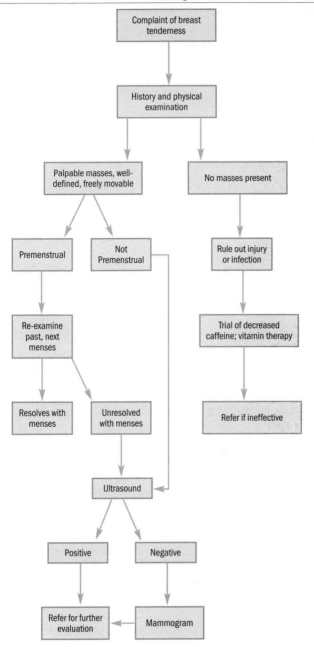

Figure 4–3. Complaint of breast tenderness.

Tests	Results Indicating Disorder	CPT Code
Mammograms (screening and diagnostic)	Alterations in the density of the breast tissue, calcifications, and thickening of the skin, fibrous streaking, and nipple changes. Mammography can also aid in the identification of fibroadenoma, lymph nodes, galactocele, or fat necrosis.	76091 (screening bilateral) 76096 (Needle)
Ultrasound of the breast	Cystic mass	76645
Excisional biopsy of lump	Cytologic evaluation*	19101
Needle aspiration	Fluid obtained in cysts	19100

*Biopsy is required if any of the following findings are present: bloody fluid on aspiration, failure of the mass to disappear after aspiration, recurrence of a cyst after two aspirations, solid mass not diagnosed as a fibroadenoma, bloody nipple discharge, nipple ulceration, and the presence of skin edema or erythema.

Differential Diagnosis: Breast cancer (positive cytology)

Treatment:

Dietary modifications may be helpful, particularly reduction in caffeine for cystic changes. Administration of vitamins A and E has been shown to reduce the discomfort of cystic formation in breasts.

Macrocysts can be drained of fluid to confirm diagnosis and decrease discomfort.

Fibroadenoma, hyperplasia, adenosis, and papilloma, which require biopsy for diagnosis, may require excision for therapy.

Ductal ectasia is treated with excisional biopsy.

Subareolar abscess is treated with antibiotics and at times incision and drainage.

Follow-up: Depends upon diagnosis and treatment.

Prevention/prophylaxis: A combination of breast self-examination, examination by a health-care provider, and mammography screening.

Referral: Any suspicion of breast cancer demands referral.

Education: Teach all women breast self-examination.

REFERENCES

Cardiac Disease

Binder, E, et al: Effects of endurance exercise and hormone replacement therapy on serum lipids in older women. J Am Geriatr Soc 44:231, 1996.

Emory Center for Outcomes Research. Cardiol Rev 8(1): 65, 2000.

Major Findings from the Nurse's Health Study, 1976–1998.

Manson, J, et al: Heart Disease in older women. Patient Care for the Nurse Practitioner, May 2001.

Oettgen, P, and Douglas, P: Coronary artery disease in women: Diagnosis and prevention. Adv Int Med 39:467, 1994.

Rockhill, B, et al: Physical activity and mortality: A prospective study among women. Am J Public Health 91(4): April 2001.

Sams, R: Chest pain. Adv Nurse Practit 9 (12): Dec. 2001.

University of Tampa: Women and coronary heart disease. Nurse Practit: 26(8): 12, 2001.

U.S. Prevention Service Task Force: Screening guidelines for lipid disorders in adults. Am J Nurse Practit 6 (6): June 2002.

Villablanca, A: Coronary heart disease in women. Postgrad Med 100(3):191, 1996.

Weis, J, Scott, L: Detecting Diabetes and Heart Disease. Lifelines Oct/Nov. 2001, pp. 71–75.

Wenger, N., et al: Cardiovascular health and disease in women. N Engl J Med 329(4):247, 1993.

Web Sites

American Heart Association *www.americanheart.org*

National Center for Health Statistics *www.cdc.gov/nchs*

Breast Disease

Carty, N, et al: Management of fibroadenoma of the breast. Ann Royal Coll Surg Engl 77(2):127, 1995.

Dahlbeck, S, et al.: Differentiating inflammatory breast cancer from acute mastitis. Am Fam Physician 52(3):929, 1995.

Healthy People 2010: National Health Promotion and Disease Prevention Objectives. United States Printing Office, Washington, D.C., DHHS PUB No. 91-50212.

McKeon, VA: The Breast Cancer Prevention Trial. Advanced evidence-based practice. Women's Health, Supplement to JOGNN, 28(6):1, 2000.

Shapiro, TJ, and Clark, P: Breast cancer: What the primary care provider needs to know. Nurse Practit 20(3):36, 1995.

Sheps, C: Chemoprevention of breast cancer. Ann Intern Med 137(1):59, 2002.

Nonmalignant Conditions of the Breast

American College of Obstetricians and Gynecologists: Nonmalignant conditions of the breast. ACOG, Washington, DC, 1997.

Deschamps, M, et al: Clinical determinants of mammographic dysplasia patterns. Cancer Detect Prev 20(6):610, 1996.

Dixon, J, et al: Assessment of the acceptability of conservative management of fibroadenoma of the breast. Br J Surg 83(2):264, 1996.

Issacs, J: Benign tumors of the breast. Obstet Gynecol Clin North Am 21(3):487, 1994.

Levi, F, and Randimbison, L: Incidence of breast cancer in women with fibroadenoma. Int J Cancer 57(5):681, 1994.

Web Sites:

American Cancer Society *www.cancer.org*

National Center for Health Statistics *www.cdc.gov/nchs*

American College of Obstetricians and Gynecologists *www.acog.org*

Chapter 5
HEPATIC AND RENAL DISORDERS

ACUTE PYELONEPHRITIS

SIGNAL SYMPTOMS▶ flank pain; fever; frequency of urination; urgency of urination; painful urination

Acute pyelonephritis	ICD-9-CM: 590.1
Acute pyelonephritis without lesion of medullary necrosis	ICD-9-CM: 590.10
Chronic pyelonephritis	ICD-9-CM: 590.0

Description: Acute pyelonephritis is an infectious disease involving the collecting system and the renal parenchyma of the kidney.

Etiology: Bacterial infection, usually with a gram-negative organism. *Escherichia coli* is the most common causative agent.

Occurrence: Surveys of office practices and hospital admissions demonstrate 250,000 episodes of acute pyelonephritis annually in the United States.

Age: Between the ages of 15 and 24, the prevalence of bacteriuria is about 2%–3%, increasing to about 10% by age 60, 20% after the age of 65, and 25%–50% after age 80.

Ethnicity: Not significant.

Gender: Infection of the urinary tract is more common in women than in men by a ratio of 8:1.

Contributing factors: Advanced age, inefficient bladder emptying, decreased functional ability (dementia, incontinence, neurologic deficits), nosocomial infections, pregnancy, diabetes, sickle cell trait, cystic renal disease.

Signs and Symptoms: Chills, fever, unilateral or bilateral costovertebral angle tenderness, dysuria, frequency of urination, urgency of urination, cloudy malodorous urine. At times, women experience nausea and vomiting.

Diagnostic Tests:

Test	Results Indicating Disorder	CPT Code
Urinalysis	WBCs present	81001
Urine culture	+ for organisms >105	87088

Differential diagnosis:
- Cystitis (pain with urination)
- Other causes of flank pain

Treatment: For mild symptoms, use oral fluoroquinolone for 10–14 days. For severe symptoms, women may require hospitalization for treatment with parenteral antibiotics.

Follow-up: No follow-up is necessary for a mild infection that resolves prior to completion of the course of antibiotics. Severe infections require a repeat urine culture at 5–7 days after initiation of therapy, and at 4–6 weeks after discontinuation of therapy. Recurrence of symptoms requires a renal ultrasound or CT scan.

Sequelae: In 30% of patients with acute pyelonephritis, bacteria invade through the mucosa into the bloodstream, causing bacteremia.

Prevention/prophylaxis: Prompt treatment of pyelonephritis is essential.

Referral: All cases of acute pyelonephritis require consultation for management.

Education: Between 10% and 30% of all patients relapse after a 14-day course of therapy. Individuals who relapse are usually cured with a second course of antibiotics.

ASYMPTOMATIC BACTERIURIA

SIGNAL SYMPTOM none

Asymptomatic bacteriuria	ICD-9-CM: 791.9
In pregnancy	ICD-9-CM: 646.5

Description: Asymptomatic bacteriuria, the persistent colonization of the urinary tract without urinary symptoms, poses a significant health risk for pregnant women. If untreated, 20%–40% of pregnant women develop acute pyelonephritis.

Etiology: In most pregnancies, dilation of the upper collecting system occurs and extends down to the level of the pelvic brim. The dilated ureters may contain over 200 mL of urine and contribute to persistence of bacteriuria in pregnancy. In elderly women, the etiology is unknown.

Occurrence: Occurs in 5%–10% of pregnant women.

Age: The incidence in young women is 1%–2%. The incidence in women more than 60 years of age is 6%–10%. The incidence in institutionalized elderly women is 25%–50%.

Ethnicity: Not significant.

Contributing factors: Diabetes, hypertension, obstruction of the urinary tract, disseminated infection, pregnancy.

Signs and Symptoms: None.

Diagnostic Tests:

Test	Results Indicating Disorder	CPT Code
Urine culture	+ for organisms > 105 *	87088

*Voided urine is easily contaminated by urethral and perineal flora. Cultures must be obtained on clean voided urine and quantified.

Differential diagnosis:

Contaminated urinary specimen for culture

Treatment:

Treatment should be initiated when clinical evidence suggests lower UTI even before results of urine culture are available. Studies show that a 3-day treatment regimen for uncomplicated lower UTI is effective. A single-dose regimen is less effective. (See Table 5–1 for recommended antibiotics for therapy.) Treatment is chosen based upon cost, safety, side effects, effect on bowel and vaginal flora, and patient allergy. Treatment should also include the recommendation to increase intake of fluids. Intravaginal estrogen may be a recommendation for perimenopausal or postmenopausal women.

Treatment of urinary infection in diabetic women may decrease long-term morbidity. Treating asymptomatic bacteriuria in pregnant women has proved beneficial; therefore, pregnant women should be routinely screened with both dipstick and culture (see Chapter 12). Treatment of asymptomatic bacteria in the urine in the institutionalized elderly woman has not demonstrated a decrease in morbidity. Dipstick tests for bacteria can be inaccurate if the organism does not produce nitrate, the specimen is not the first morning voiding, or the urine is dilute. Sensitivity for

Table 5–1 Medications for Urinary Tract Infection

Three-Day Therapy for Nonpregnant Women	
Drug	Dosage
Nitrofurantoin	100 mg bid
Ciprofloxacin	250 mg bid
Ofloxacin	200 mg bid
Norfloxacin	200–400 mg bid
Sulfamethoxazole-trimethoprim	160–800 mg bid

dipstick urinalysis is 72%–97%; specificity is 64%–82%. Dipstick screening can indicate the need for urine culture in asymptomatic women (see Figure 5–1).

Follow-up: Repeat urine culture after therapy.

Sequelae: Among women with bacteriuria identified early in pregnancy, up to 40% develop pyelonephritis if not treated. Women with bacteriuria are nearly twice as likely to deliver a low-birth-weight infant. No short-term or long-term adverse outcomes exist that are attributable to asymptomatic bacteriuria in nonpregnant women.

Prevention/prophylaxis: Screening for asymptomatic bacteriuria is recommended for pregnant women, all women who have been recently catheterized, and women with known renal calculi or other structural abnormalities of the urinary tract.

Referral: All women with asymptomatic bacteriuria require consultation for management.

Education: Pregnant women should be aware of the importance of early prenatal care.

 Clinical Pearl: Asymptomatic bacteriuria poses a significant health risk to pregnant women.

CYSTITIS

SIGNAL SYMPTOM ▶ pain upon urination

Cystitis	ICD-9-CM: 595
Acute cystitis	ICD-9-CM: 595.1
Chronic cystitis	ICD-9-CM: 595.2

Description: Acute cystitis is a superficial mucosal infection of the bladder.

Etiology: Bacteria reach the bladder by ascending through the urethra.

Contributing factors: Bacteria that commonly cause cystitis are found at the introitus in 20% of cases. Entry of bacteria into the relatively short female urethra can happen spontaneously. Infection depends on the virulence of the organism, the number of organisms, and the state of the host's defensive system. The most important host defense mechanism is the ability of the bladder's mucosal surface to phagocytize bacteria coming in contact with it. Sexual intercourse and diaphragm and spermicide use have been correlated with cystitis.

Occurrence: Surveys of office practices estimate 7 million episodes of acute cystitis occur annually in the United States.

Age: Between 20% and 30% of women have cystitis in their lifetime.

Ethnicity: Not significant.

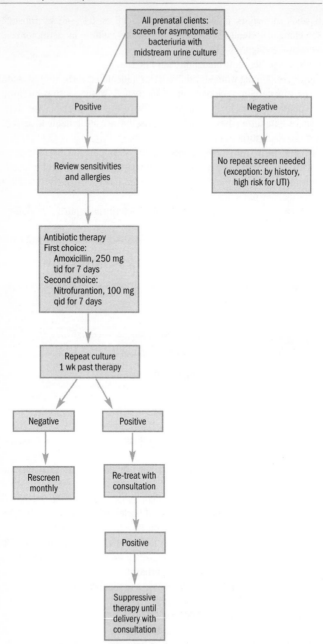

Figure 5–1. Asymptomatic bacteriuria in pregnancy.

Signs and Symptoms: Dysuria, frequency, urgency, and suprapubic discomfort. Of women with cystitis, 40% have hematuria.

Diagnostic Tests:

Test	Results Indicating Disorder	CPT Code
Urinalysis	WBCs noted	81001
Urine culture and sensitivity on a clean voided specimen	+ for organisms >105	87088 (culture) 87181 (sensitivity)
Microscopic examination of urine sediment	Leukocytes, erythrocytes, bacteria	81015

Urine screening should be done on an early morning specimen and collected via "clean catch." First, cleanse the vulvar region, followed by a cleansing of the urinary meatus with moistened cotton balls. Avoid the use of soap. Use a clean container and collect the specimen "mid-stream." Perform the urinalysis as soon as possible after collecting the specimen.

Microscopic examination of urine from women with urinary tract infection may reveal the presence of leukocytes (10 white blood cells [WBCs] per high-power field), erythrocytes, and bacteria. The specimen may or may not be gram-stained. The presence of any or all of these factors assists in the diagnosis of urinary tract infection.

Urine culture confirms urinary tract infection. The presence of an organism in amounts greater than 102 or 105 (the higher value is used in some laboratories) indicates infection with high sensitivity, specificity, and predictive value (see Figure 5–2).

Differential diagnosis:

- Urethritis diagnosed by negative urinary culture
- Vaginitis diagnosed by pelvic examination
- Local trauma or irritation

Treatment: A 3-day course of antibiotics achieves a higher rate of cure than single-dose therapy. Short courses of antibiotics improve compliance, lower cost, and lower the frequency of adverse reactions.

Follow-up: No follow-up is necessary if resolution of symptoms occurs following therapy. Recurrence of symptoms requires a repeat urine culture and sensitivity.

Sequelae: Of women who experience cystitis, 40% have a recurrence.

Prevention/prophylaxis: Contraceptive method that does not include the use of a diaphragm and spermicide.

Examination of urine has a long-standing tradition in health-care screening. Dipsticks have made assessment of bacteria in urine quick and inexpensive. Since urinary tract infections are known to be a signifi-

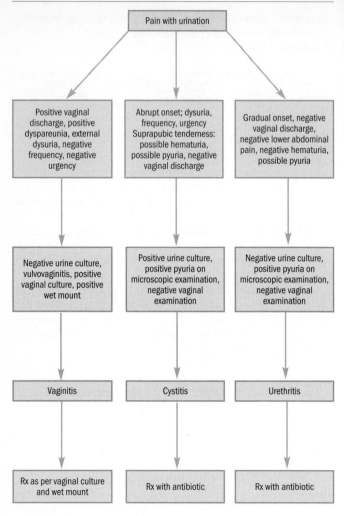

Figure 5–2. Cystitis.

cant source of morbidity for diabetic, pregnant, and older women, most authorities recommend screening of these populations.

Screening is also advocated to detect hematuria, an indication of urinary tract malignancy. These malignancies, which increase in occurrence after age 40, are more common in men than in women. The sensitivity of dipstick testing for hematuria is good (91%–100%).

Referral: Recurrent infections require referral.

Education: Increase fluid intake, void after intercourse, complete antibiotic regimen.

INTERSTITIAL CYSTITIS

SIGNAL SYMPTOMS▶   urinary frequency; pain with urination

Cystitis	ICD-9-CM: 595
Interstitial cystitis	ICD-9-CM: 595.1

Description: Interstitial cystitis is a symptom complex characterized by pelvic pain, urinary urgency, urinary frequency, and nocturia. Interstitial cystitis is a chronic inflammatory condition of the bladder wall. There is an absence of any definable cause for these symptoms. Onset is gradual.

Etiology: Unknown.

Occurrence: Between 44,000 and 45,000 diagnosed cases in the United States. Interstitial cystitis affects 0.5% of women. Female-to-male ratio is 9:1.

Age: Average age is 40–46 years.

Ethnicity: Predominantly Caucasians.

Contributing factors: Unknown.

Signs and Symptoms: Urinary frequency, bladder pain, and nocturia. Interstitial cystitis is a diagnosis of exclusion. Evaluation includes ruling out other disorders that produce similar symptoms.

Diagnostic Tests:

Test	Results Indicating Disorder	CPT Code
Cystoscopy	Inflammation of the bladder wall.	52204

Differential diagnosis:

- Urinary infection (positive culture)
- Carcinoma (positive cytology)
- Radiation- and medication-induced cystitis (history of radiation exposure, history of ingestion of medication that can cause cystitis)

Treatment: Until etiology and pathogenesis of interstitial cystitis are identified, specific therapy is not possible. However, symptomatic treatment is helpful and includes dimethyl sulfoxide, antihistamines, anti-inflammatories, intravesical silver nitrate, heparin, and surgery. Bladder training can be helpful to some women. Antibiotics offer no relief.

Follow-up: Unknown.

Sequelae: Unknown.

Prevention/prophylaxis: Unknown.

Referral: Interstitial cystitis requires referral.

Education: Symptoms increase with sexual intercourse and with menses. Bladder training to prolong voiding intervals should be attempted.

SYMPTOMATIC LOWER URINARY TRACT INFECTION

SIGNAL SYMPTOMS▶ pain with urination: urinary frequency; urinary urgency

Cystitis	ICD-9-CM: 595

Description: Symptomatic lower urinary tract infection (UTI), also called cystitis or bladder infection, occurs when microorganisms infiltrate the bladder and the urethra. Women commonly seek health care for these infections.

Bladder infections occur frequently, even though the lining of the bladder has antiadherent capacities that prevent the colonization of bacteria if they do enter the bladder, and the washing effect of the urine cleanses the bladder. The establishment of a bladder infection depends on the virulence of the organism, the number of organisms introduced, and the woman's defense mechanisms.

Etiology: Current evidence suggests that most episodes of lower UTI in adult women are secondary to ascending infection. Bacteria that reach the bladder through the urethra may ascend into the bladder and possibly the kidneys through the ureters. About 80% of lower UTIs are caused by *E. coli,* about 15% by *Staphylococcus saprophyticus,* and the rest by organisms such as *Klebsiella pneumoniae* and *Proteus mirabilis.* All of these organisms reside in the GI tract.

Occurrence: Between 20% and 30% of women have a lower UTI in their lifetime, and 40% of women with one episode of lower UTI will have a recurrence.

Age: Adult women.

Ethnicity: Not significant.

Contributing factors: Colonization of bacteria in the vagina has been shown to be an essential first step in the production of bacteriuria. The normal vaginal pH is 4, which decreases the ability of bacteria to colonize. However, several factors known to elevate the vaginal pH increase the likelihood of bacterial colonization and also increase the risk of lower UTI. These factors include a decrease in estrogen, spermicides, vaginal infection, and sexual activity. Milking of the urethra by the penis during intercourse can help transport bacteria from the urethra to the bladder.

Some women are more prone to infection from *E. coli,* an organism that normally resides in the healthy large intestine. *E. coli* has the ability to adhere to uroepithelial cells, attaching to host receptor sites. Susceptible women possess an increased density of these receptors, thus facilitating adherence. These women are not "less clean" than other women; they simply are more prone to this organism ascending and infecting the urinary tract. This tendency could be genetic.

The most consistent behavior associated with lower UTI is sexual intercourse. Coital frequency directly relates to occurrence and recurrence of lower UTIs. Symptoms often develop within 24 hours of coitus. Use of a diaphragm may be related to a decreased urge to void or to residual urine, possibly increasing the risk of developing a lower UTI.

Signs and symptoms: Women present with pelvic pressure, dysuria, urgency, frequency, and sometimes incontinence and hematuria. A low-grade fever (less than 101°F) may be present. Explore the symptoms by determining their onset, frequency, and duration and the presence of internal or external burning on urination. Most lower UTIs have an abrupt onset of symptoms of frequency and urgency of urination, internal burning, and, perhaps, cramping with urination. They are usually of short duration. Nocturia, suprapubic pain, and mild backache may also be present. Fever, malaise, and back pain probably indicate that the infection has extended beyond the lower urinary tract. Dysuria can indicate acute bacterial cystitis or acute urethritis or both. It can also be associated with gonorrhea, *Chlamydia,* herpes, or vaginitis. Pain with urination can also be related to an allergic reaction to an irritating substance.

Bladder tenderness indicates a lower UTI. The bladder should, therefore, be palpated on all women who present with possible lower UTI. Pelvic examination is essential, noting urethral discharge; vaginal erythema, discharge, or atrophy; and presence of vesicles, cervical discharge, or cervical tenderness with motion.

Urethral infection presents with similar symptoms to lower UTI; however, urinalysis reveals a lower-than-expected colony count and only a few WBCs present in the urine. These women are presenting before true bladder infection has occurred and should be treated as if a lower UTI were present.

Determine the patient's history of previous lower UTIs and recent urinary catheterizations. A UTI that recurs after less than 2 weeks is probably a relapsing infection or a persistent infection. History should reveal if a woman is pregnant, menopausal, or perimenopausal. She should also be asked about diabetes, immunocompromising diseases, and sickle cell trait or disease because these women are at higher risk for renal necrosis (see Figure 5-3).

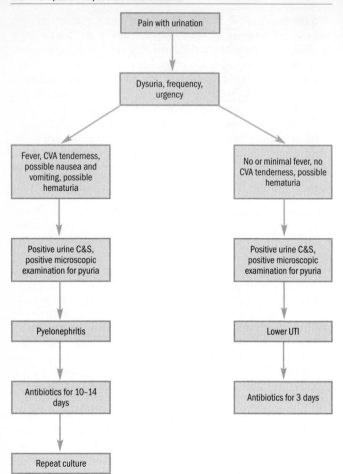

Figure 5–3. Urinary tract infection.

Diagnostic Tests:

Test	Results Indicating Disorder	CPT Code
Urine culture and sensitivity	This test shows greater than 5 WBCs per high-power field and the presence of bacteria without many squamous epithelial cells. The traditional criterion for infection is a colony count of more than 105 organisms per milliliter. However, as few as 10,000 colonies have been known to produce symptoms in women. Culture results will reveal the causative organism.	87088 (culture) 87181 (sensitivity)

Test	Results Indicating Disorder	CPT Code
Enzymatic (dipstick) testing	This is a less reliable but effective method of screening. Dipstick testing with reagent strips indicates hematuria, nitrites indicate presence of bacteria, and leukocyte esterase indicates presence of WBCs. After examination, urine should be sent for culture and sensitivity.	81000

Differential diagnosis:

- Sexually transmitted diseases (positive culture, history of exposure)
- Vaginitis (other organisms present, vaginal discharge, itching, irritation)
- Lack of estrogen can cause irritation of the perineum with symptoms suggesting UTI. In these cases, pain with urination is pain created by urine touching irritated external genitalia.
- Fungal infection of the urethra and bladder (positive fungal culture)
- Tuberculosis of the bladder
- Malignancy (positive cytology)
- Interstitial cystitis (positive for inflammation of the bladder during cystoscopy)
- Side effects of chemotherapy or radiation therapy (history of chemotherapy or radiation)
- High fever, restlessness, and marked costovertebral angle (CVA) tenderness suggest urinary obstruction or upper UTI.

Treatment: Treatment should be initiated when clinical evidence suggests lower UTI even before results of urine culture are available. Studies show that a 3-day treatment regimen for uncomplicated lower UTI is effective. A single-dose regimen is less effective. (See Table 5–1 for recommended antibiotics for therapy.) Treatment is chosen based upon cost, safety, side effects, effect on bowel and vaginal flora, and patient allergy. Treatment should also include the recommendation to increase intake of fluids. Intravaginal estrogen may be a recommendation for perimenopausal or postmenopausal women.

 Clinical Pearl: 80% of lower urinary tract infections are caused by *E. coli.*

Follow-up: Repeat urinalysis after completion of treatment if you suspect persistent lower UTI.

Sequelae: In approximately 30% of cases of sustained bladder infection, further extension of the infection through the ureters to the kidneys can occur.

Prevention/prophylaxis: Voiding after intercourse and decreased use of spermicide and diaphragm may be helpful in some women. Intravaginal estrogen in perimenopausal and postmenopausal women markedly reduces the incidence of UTIs.

The intake of cranberry juice on a regular basis may help prevent UTIs. In a study published in the *British Medical Journal*, 50 ml of cranberry juice five days per week for six months significantly decreased the incidence of UTI in women seen in a student health clinic.

Referral: Refer patients who experience relapse (a recurrence of symptoms of infection after a completed course of antibiotics); pregnant women; women who have a history of pyelonephritis or a chronic disease such as diabetes, suspected renal calculi, or interstitial cystitis; and women who frequently use catheters.

For patients who experience reinfection (infection that occurs weeks or months after treatment of previous lower UTI), referral is recommended only if infections are more frequent than three per year.

Education: Normal voiding eliminates some organisms; not voiding after intercourse may contribute to an increase in lower UTI in some women.

URINARY INCONTINENCE

SIGNAL SYMPTOMS▶   stress loss of urine; urge loss of urine

Bladder hyperactivity	ICD-9-CM: 596.51
Detrusor instability	ICD-9-CM: 596.59
Stress incontinence	ICD-9-CM: 625.6
Incontinence NOS	ICD-9-CM: 788.30
Urge incontinence	ICD-9-CM: 788.31
Mixed incontinence	ICD-9-CM: 788.33
Incontinence without sensory awareness	ICD-9-CM: 788.34
Continuous leakage	ICD-9-CM: 788.37

Description: Urinary incontinence (UI) is the involuntary loss of urine that results in a social or hygienic problem.

Etiology: Urinary incontinence is two to three times more likely to occur in women than in men owing to the difference in pelvic anatomy and the delivery of children. Neurologic and/or musculofascial damage can cause UI.

Occurrence: Approximately 20% of women between 25 and 64 years experience UI.

Age: Although UI primarily occurs in the elderly, it does affect younger populations as well. Of perimenopausal women, 31% report incontinent episodes at least once per month; 46% of women in the age group of 35–44 years; and 60% of women in the age group 45–54. Severity of stress incontinence increases with age.

Ethnicity: Not significant.

Contributing factors: White race, age, menopause, obesity, neurologic disease, smoking and chronic cough. Women who have delivered vaginally are 2.5 times more likely to report incontinence than women who have never been pregnant. The rate of reported incontinence increases with the number of vaginal deliveries; 38% of mothers report UI after one delivery, 57% after two vaginal births, and 73% after three vaginal births (Sampselle et al., 1997).

Medications that contribute to UI are diuretics, narcotics, hypnotics, and angiotensin-converting enzyme inhibitors.

Signs and Symptoms: There are **three** types of urinary incontinence:

Stress UI: Loss of urine during coughing, sneezing, laughing, or physical exercise

Urge UI: A strong desire to void that is sometimes associated with involuntary detrusor contraction

Mixed UI: A combination of stress and urge UI

Few women report pure symptoms of stress or urge associated urinary loss. 30% to 50% of women reporting symptoms have both stress and urge incontinence (Weidner, 2001)

Include in the history from the woman:

- Type of symptoms
- Duration of symptoms
- Factors that trigger incontinence
- Number of pads used and type of pads
- Pain with urination
- Hematuria
- Frequency of urination
- Urgency of urination
- Hesitancy with urination
- Nocturnal enuresis
- Dribbling post-urination
- Feelings of incomplete emptying after voiding
- Symptoms of prolapse

The history should also include consumption of bladder irritants such as caffeine and alcohol. Any history of previous therapies for incontinence should be solicited.

Diagnostic Tests:

Test	Results Indicating Disorder	CPT Code
Urinalysis	Negative	81001
Urine culture and sensitivity	Negative	87088 (culture) 87181 (sensitivity)

Differential diagnosis:

- UTI diagnosed by urine culture and sensitivity
- Atrophic vaginitis diagnosed by pelvic examination
- Urethritis determined by urinalysis, urine culture and sensitivity, and pelvic examination

---

Box 5-1
Pelvic Muscle Contractions or Kegel Exercise:

Ideal Pelvic Muscle Contractions Have the Following:
- Pelvic floor contracts upward and inward.
- Anus pulls inward and lifts upward.
- Contraction is of moderate to nearly maximum level of intensity.
- Bearing-down or straining-down effort is absent.
- Thigh muscle contraction is absent.
- Gluteal muscle contraction is absent.
- Contraction is held for at least 3 seconds, building to a hold of 10 seconds.
- At least 10 seconds of relaxation is allowed between contractions.

Treatment: The treatment of choice for UI includes bladder training and pelvic muscle exercise (see Figure 5–4). Bladder training consists of providing the woman with information about normal bladder function and use of a voiding schedule. The woman is asked to keep a 24-hour voiding schedule and from this a desired initial voiding schedule is established. The initial voiding schedule should match the average frequency (or leakage) of urine demonstrated in the diary. For example, if the average urinary frequency is every 60 minutes, the initial voiding schedule should be every 60 minutes. Systematic delay in voiding is accomplished through distraction and relaxation techniques. The interval between urination is gradually increased until voiding occurs, ideally, every 3–4 hours.

Pelvic muscle exercise, also called Kegel exercise in recognition of the physician who recommended its use, is a technique that strengthens the supportive pelvic floor muscles. Thirty contractions per day are recommended.

Bladder training and pelvic muscle exercises are effective in reducing stress incontinence in women with mild to moderate symptoms. The combination of these two therapies in no way jeopardizes future therapy if referral is necessary.

Estrogen cream applied to the atrophic vagina and external genitalia may reduce incontinence. One half an applicator of estrogen cream applied nightly at bedtime for seven nights followed by an applicator applied two times a week can be helpful in decreasing UI.

Medical therapy may include the use of imipramine, an anticholinergic that can inhibit bladder contractions and increase urethral tone, and/or tolterodine, an antagonist that decreases detrusor hyperactivity and therefore decreases urinary urgency. Oxybutynin, an anticholinergic agent that affects bladder smooth muscle, may also be utilized.

Follow-up: Several weeks are required before improvement can be expected. Follow-up visits can be scheduled at monthly intervals for 4 months to monitor progress.

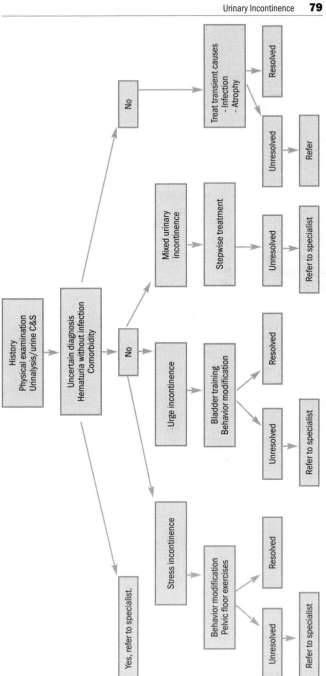

Figure 5—4. Urinary incontinence.

Sequelae: Of women who complete a 3-month pelvic exercise program, 56% had a greater than 50% reduction in the number of incontinent episodes.

Prevention/prophylaxis: Diuretics and caffeine can cause urgency, frequency, and incontinence. Anticholingerics can impair detrusor contractility, resulting in overflow incontinence. Alpha-adrenergic blockers can cause incontinence through lowering urethral tone.

Referral: Minimal or no improvement in symptoms following 16 weeks of therapy is an indication for referral. Refer any women with a positive history of any neurologic deficit, including multiple sclerosis, stroke, or spinal cord injury. Some women are unable to execute even a weak pelvic muscle contraction or cannot implement bladder training and will require referral.

Referral should be made to a health-care provider with specialized knowledge of incontinence. These providers are skilled in the use of supplemental equipment such as vaginal weights, biofeedback, and electrical stimulation. To find such health-care providers, call the National Association for Continence (800-252-3337).

Education: For additional information on UI, see the list of agencies in the Appendix.

VIRAL HEPATITIS

SIGNAL SYMPTOMS ▶ Fatigue; anorexia; nausea and vomiting; fever; pain

Hepatitis A	ICD-9: 070.1
Hepatitis B	ICD-9: 070.3
Chronic hepatitis C without mention of coma	ICD-9: 070.54

Description: Viral hepatitis is a contagious disease estimated to affect more than 500,000 people in the United States each year, according to the Centers for Disease Control (CDC). The majority of women infected are either asymptomatic or minimally symptomatic, but a number of women develop serious clinical illness and several thousand die from the disease each year.

Five distinct types of viral hepatitis have been identified: A, B, C, D, and E. Hepatitis A, transmitted by a fecal-oral route, is an uncommon complication of pregnancy and is not associated with perinatal transmission. In contrast, hepatitis B is more common and clearly poses a serious risk to household contacts and neonates of infected mothers. ALL pregnant women should be tested for hepatitis B. Universal vaccination of all neonates with hepatitis B is recommended. Infants delivered to hepatitis B–infected mothers should be vaccinated immediately after birth.

Hepatitis E is rare in the United States and is similar to hepatitis A. Hepatitis A and E do not exist in a chronic carrier state. Perinatal transmission does occur with E. Hepatitis B, C, and D, which are transmitted parenterally and by sexual contact, have been associated with vertical transmission. No immunoprophylaxis is currently available for neonates of mothers with hepatitis C or E. Immunization against hepatitis B protects against transmission of hepatitis D. Hepatitis B, C, and D occur in both acute and chronic forms. When they persist in a chronic form, they serve as reservoir for infection and can give rise to chronic hepatitis, cirrhosis, and hepatocellular carcinoma. Prevention of hepatitis requires an understanding of the modes of transmission, periods of communicability, and the use of globulins and vaccines (see Table 5–2).

Etiology: Hepatitis is a viral disease. Types A and E are transmitted by the fecal-oral route. Type B results from parenteral exposure and/or intimate contact. Type C is the predominant type occurring after transfusion. Type D requires coinfection with hepatitis B.

Occurrence: Hepatitis affects more than 500,000 people in the United States each year. The number of chronic carriers of hepatitis is unknown.

Age: In a study of 6,253 pregnant women infected with hepatitis B or C, the incidence of hepatitis B infection was significantly higher in women older than 30 years of age (Alvarez-Munoz et al., 1997).

Ethnicity: Not significant.

Contributing factors: Handling of infected blood or body fluids, risk of transmission by sexual contact, IV drug use, fecal-oral contamination.

- Family history of jaundice or anemia
- Detailed occupational review (contact with animals and exposure to toxins in particular)
- Travel habits
- Alcohol intake
- Contact with jaundiced persons
- History of injections

Hepatitis C occurs in as many as 33% of the patients with human immunodeficiency virus (HIV) infection. Coinfected women develop earlier and more severe liver disease. HIV coinfection in pregnant women increases the risk of perinatal transmission twofold (see Figure 5–5).

Signs and Symptoms: Acute viral hepatitis is usually a self-limiting illness; 85% of hospital patients and 95% of outpatients with the disease recover completely and uneventfully within 3 months. The majority of women with acute viral infection never become jaundiced. Symptoms include malaise, anorexia, nausea, vomiting, changes in taste and smell, low-grade fever, right upper quadrant discomfort, and fatigue. In 5%–10% of patients with acute hepatitis B, urticaria, arthralgia, fever, and polyarticular arthritis occur. Hepatitis A and E are the viruses most likely to produce cholestatic disease with jaundice and pruritus.

Table 5-2 Hepatitis

Type of Transmission		Chronicity	Susceptibility	Incubation	Facts for Women	Immunity
A	Fecal-Oral	No	Children and adolescents are most susceptible to infection.	30 days	More than 80% of women over age 60 test positive for the antibody to hep A.	Exposure to hep A creates an antibody that confers life-long immunity. Initially, the anti-hep A antibody is IgM; during convalescence it is IgG.
B	Parental, perinatal, and sexual contact. The virus has been found in women's saliva, vaginal secretions, and breast milk.	Yes; approx. 1%–2% of women with clinical disease develop chronic infections.	Spouses of people with hep B, women with multiple sexual partners, health-care personnel, infants by vertical transmission from their mothers. Handling infected blood or body fluid	12 wks	A large number of infected women never experience apparent illness, making the actual number of chronic cases unknown. Many women are asymptomatic carriers.	Hep B vaccine available
C	Parental, perinatal, vertical transmission rate 18%	Yes	IV drug abusers, intimate contact with infected persons, infants by vertical transmission from their mothers, infants via breast feeding, recipients of transfusions not screened for hep C. Handling infected blood or body fluid	Similar to hep B		Assays for antibodies turn positive during infection and remain so.
D	Coexists with hep B	Yes	IV drug abusers, intimate contact with infected persons, infants by vertical transmission from their mothers	Similar to Hep B		Vaccination for hep B eliminates Hep D.
E	Fecal-oral (found primarily in India and Asia)	?	Younger adults rather than children are affected.	40 days	Pregnant women with hep E have a high mortality rate.	Unknown

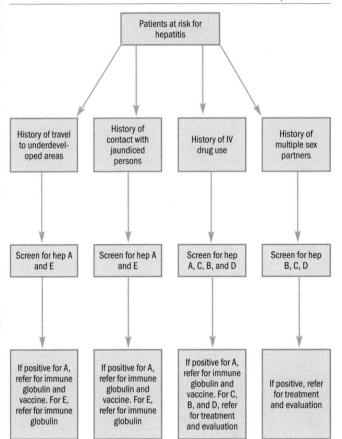

Figure 5–5. Screening for hepatitis.

Diagnostic Tests:

Tests	Results Indicating Disorder	CPT Code
Serum antibody for hepatitis A	Present	86709
Serum antibody for hepatitis B	Present	86704 (core) 86705 (IgM) 87340 (Surface) 86707 (Be)
Serum antibody for hepatitis C	Present	86803
Serum antibody for hepatitis D	Present	

Testing can determine chronic versus acute disease. Hepatitis panel includes all above (80074)

Differential diagnosis:

- Nonspecific viral syndrome
- Drug-induced hepatitis (history of hepatitis-inducing drug ingestion)
- Nonviral hepatitis (an autoimmune mechanism seen in women ages 20–40)

Treatment: Hepatitis is usually treated on an outpatient basis with diet and decreased activity levels. The diet consists of small, frequent meals; adequate calorie intake; and no alcohol. Activity is as tolerated, with increased rest. Hepatitis often affects previously active people. Prolonged malaise can lead to depression.

Alcohol should be forbidden.

Drugs utilized for therapy for hepatitis C include interferon and ribavirin.

Follow-up: After early diagnosis, office visits at 1- to 2-week intervals for evaluation of symptoms and laboratory work.

Sequelae: Acute disease can develop into overwhelming liver cell necrosis and liver failure. This result is most often seen in hepatitis B, but the incidence is also high in pregnant women with hepatitis E.

Chronic hepatitis (not with A or E) occurs with hepatitis infection. The likelihood is higher when acute infection occurs in an immunocompromised host or when the infection occurs at birth. Clinical manifestations of chronic disease usually are the persistence of mild symptoms. Chronic disease can lead to cirrhosis.

Pregnant women infected with hepatitis B or C pose a risk of infecting their newborns. Every year an estimated 20,000 infants are born to women in the United States with positive hepatitis B antigen. These infants are at risk for hepatitis B infection and chronic liver disease as adults.

Chronic infection with hepatitis B is a significant problem on a worldwide scale affecting over 300 million people. Hepatitis C virus infection is probably the most common cause of chronic viral hepatitis, end stage liver disease and hepatocellular carcinoma in the world.

Prevention/prophylaxis: Principles of prevention include minimizing exposure and the use of globulins and vaccines.

Administering immune globulin within 1–2 hours of exposure prevents hepatitis A infection. Immune globulin is 80% effective in preventing clinical disease in nonimmunized individuals. For household contacts and small groups experiencing a common source of outbreak, begin immune globulin prophylaxis and hepatitis A vaccine. Restrict intimate contact and encourage careful hand washing. Routine immunoprophylaxis is not necessary for casual contacts. The CDC recommends administering hepatitis A vaccine to users of illegal injected and noninjected drugs.

To prevent hepatitis B, provide a susceptible person with a protective antibody. Immune globulins containing anti–hepatitis B are given along with the hepatitis vaccine. Hepatitis B vaccine is recommended routinely prior to exposure. Screen for hepatitis B in all pregnant women. Administer the vaccine to all newborns and all women who have not been vaccinated.

Immune globulin and hepatitis B vaccine have not proved to be effective in preventing hepatitis C infection.

Prevention of hepatitis B infection also prevents hepatitis D infection. Hepatitis E has no immunoprophylaxis available.

Referral: A diagnosis of viral hepatitis requires referral to a medical provider.

Education: Teach the patient the following guidelines:

Hepatitis A and E

- Practice hand washing after the use of the toilet.
- Avoid intimate contact with infected people.
- Infected women should not handle or serve food to others.
- Give immune globulin and/or vaccine to household contacts and people traveling to areas known to have an increased incidence of the disease.

Hepatitis B, C, D

- Screen blood donors.
- Follow universal precautions for handling materials that may be infected with hepatitis.
- Use proper hand washing after direct contact with infected people.
- Avoid intimate contact with infected people.
- All three doses of the vaccine should be received—initial dose, followed by second dose at 1 month, and third dose at 6 months.
- Universal vaccination of all newborns.
- Globulin injection given to nonimmune individuals after exposure.

Hepatitis C

Hepatitis C precautions are the same as for hepatitis B, and vaccination against hepatitis B prevents hepatitis D.

REFERENCES

General

Goroll, A, et al: Primary Care Medicine. Lippincott, Philadelphia, 1995.
Havens, C, et al: Manual of Outpatient Gynecology. Little, Brown, Boston, 1988.
Ostergard, D, and Bent, A: Urogynecology and Urodynamics, Theory and Practice. Williams & Wilkins, Baltimore, 1996.

Acute Pyelonephritis

Miller, L, and Cox, S: Urinary tract infections complicating pregnancy. Infect Dis Clin North Am 11(3):13, 1997.

Asymptomatic Bacteriuria

Devereaux Melillo, K: Asymptomatic bacteriuria in older adults: When is it necessary to treat? Nurse Pract 20(8):50, 1995.

Patterson, T, and Andriole, V: Detection, significance, and therapy of bacteriuria in pregnancy. Infect Dis Clin North Am 11(3):593, 1997.

Cystitis

Freeman, S: Common genitourinary infections. JOGNN 24(8):735, 1995.

Hooton, T: Association of acute cystitis with the stage of the menstrual cycle in young women. Clin Infect Dis 23:635, 1996.

Kontiokari, T, et al: Randomized trial of cranberry juice and *Lactobacillus* drink for the prevention of urinary tract infections in women BMJ 322:1, 2001.

Pollen, J: Short term curse for uncomplicated cystitis. Contemp Nurse Pract 1(4):21, 1995.

Interstitial Cystitis

Department of Urology, Queens' University in Kingston, Ontario, Canada: Interstitial Cystitis. Canadian Fam Phys 46(12):2430, 2000.

Interstitial Cystitis Association: Interstitial cystitis. World J Urol 19(3):157, 2001.

Nigro, D, et al: Associations among cystoscopic and urodynamic findings for women enrolled in the Interstitial Cystitis Data Base Study. Urology 49(5A suppl):86–92, 1997.

Symptomatic Lower Urinary Tract Infection

Barger, M, and Woolner, B: Primary care for women: Assessment and management of genitourinary tract disorders. J Nurse Midwif 40(2):231, 1995.

Hooton, T, and Stamm, W: Diagnosis and treatment of uncomplicated urinary tract infection. Infect Dis Clin North Am 11(3):551, 1997.

Leiner, S: Recurrent urinary tract infection in otherwise healthy women. Nurse Pract 20(2):48–55, 1995.

Urinary Incontinence

Adam, R, and Preston, M: Urinary incontinence. Women's Health 2(4):218, 2002.

Maloney, C, and Cafiero, M: Achieving bladder control. Adv Nurse Practit 5:73, May 2002.

Sampselle, C, et al: Continence for women: Evidence based practice. JOGNN 26(4):375, 1997.

Weidner, A.C. et al: Which women with stress incontinence require urodynamic evaluation?, Am J Obstet Gynecol 184(2):20, 2001.

Viral Hepatitis

ACOG Educational Bulletin: Viral Hepatitis in Pregnancy, Number 248m, July, 1998.

Alvarez-Munoz, MT, et al: Infection of pregnant women with hepatitis B and C viruses and risks of vertical transmission. Arch Med Res 28(3):415, 1997.

Balayan, MS: Epidemiology of hepatitis E virus infection. J Viral Hepatitis 4(3):155, 1997.

Centers for Disease Control and Prevention: 2002 Guidelines for Treatment of Sexually Transmitted Disease. Centers for Disease Control and Prevention, Atlanta, 2002.

Freitag-Koontz, MJ: Prevention of hepatitis B and C transmission during pregnancy and the first year of life. J Perinat Neonat Nurs 10(2):40, 1996.

Hepatitis C Unit, Department of Medicine, National University of Ireland: The Irish paradigm on the natural progression of hepatitis C virus infection. Internat J Molec Med 92(2):179, 2002.

Hunt, CM: Hepatitis C in pregnancy. Obstet Gynecol 89:883, 1997.

Iv. interni klinika: Risk factors for the transmission of Hepatitis C. Casopos Lekaru Ceskych 141(6):185, 2002.

Keck School of Medicine, University of Southern California: Hepatitis C in patients with human immunodeficiency virus infection. Arch Intern Med 160(22):3365, 2000.

Memorial University, Cental Newfoundland Regional Health Centre: Epidemiology, prevention and treatment of viral hepatitis. Ethiopian Med J 38(2):131, 2000.

Muller, R: The natural history of hepatitis C: Clinical experiences. J Hepatol 24(2):52, 1996.

Chapter 6

MUSCULOSKELETAL DISORDERS

FIBROMYALGIA

SIGNAL SYMPTOMS ▶ pain, fatigue

Fibromyalgia	ICD-9-CM: 729.1

Description: Fibromyalgia syndrome is a clinically defined pain disorder. Fibromyalgia is a complex, chronic disease that causes widespread pain and fatigue.

Etiology: Unknown.

Occurrence: As many as 6 million people are diagnosed as having fibromyalgia. The overall prevalence is 2%. The condition is more common in women than in men. Of people with fibromyalgia, 80%–90% are women. Fibromyalgia occurs in 2%–5% of the female population.

Age: 90% of people with this disorder are women between the ages of 30 and 50. The peak incidence is at age 35.

Ethnicity: Not significant.

Contributing factors: Change in weather exacerbates symptoms of fibromyalgia.

Signs and symptoms: The most significant symptom is pain. Pain involves fibrous tissue, muscles, tendons, and ligaments. Typically, the woman has difficulty localizing her chief complaint. 90% of people with fibromyalgia complain of morning stiffness. There is an underlying sleep disorder in this disease. The woman complains of overwhelming daytime fatigue. Women have difficulty falling asleep and difficulty staying asleep. More than 75% of people with fibromyalgia report sleep disturbance. Women may also have symptoms of irritable bowel syndrome and cystitis in the absence of infection. Cold intolerance is common in people with fibromyalgia. Dysmenorrhea can accompany fibromyalgia. 20% of people with this syndrome have major depression. Tension or migraine headaches accompany this disorder. Examination reveals paired tender points. The points will be symmetric. Other than the tender points, the musculoskeletal examination will be normal. The diagnosis is made clinically, based on history and physical examination and exclusion of other disorders. Widespread pain in combination with tenderness at 11 or more specified tender points is the criterion for diagnosis (see Figure 6-1).

Diagnostic tests: No single test or combination of tests makes the diagnosis. Lab tests, x-rays and electromyography tend to be normal.

Differential diagnosis:

- Rheumatoid arthritis (positive rheumatoid factor, ANA test, elevated ESR)
- Lyme disease (history of exposure to ticks, red macular skin lesion, *B. burgdorferi* isolated from skin, blood, CSF. Elevated ESR, elevated titers)
- Overuse syndrome (history of repetitive actions)

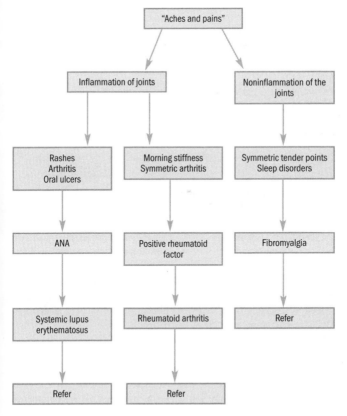

Figure 6–1. Multiple joint pain in women.

- Chronic fatigue syndrome (severe, prolonged fatigue)
- Hypothyroidism (fatigue, weight gain, dry skin, elevated TSH)
- Epstein-Barr (positive Epstein-Barr antibody test)
- HIV neuropathies (positive for HIV)
- Viral hepatitis (positive for hepatitis)
- Depression (altered mood, history of depression)

Treatment: Improve the underlying sleep disorder with medication. Cardiovascular fitness training, which raises the pain threshold, is an important part of the treatment program. Complementary therapies can be utilized to provide symptomatic relief. Tricyclic antidepressants and non-narcotic analgesics have been utilized as pharmacologic treatments.

Follow-up: Fibromyalgia is a chronic disease that requires a lifetime of close follow-up evaluation and care.

Sequelae: Fibromyalgia is a chronic disease. Symptoms increase and decrease based upon changes in the weather, degree of stress, and amount of rest. The number and location of tender points appear to be stable throughout time.

Prevention/prophylaxis: None.

Referral: Diagnosis and treatment should be under the direction of a physician.

Education: A program to improve physical fitness is important to the therapy. Such a program must be designed specific to the woman's lifestyle.

OSTEOPOROSIS

SIGNAL SYMPTOMS▶ frequent broken or fractured bones

Osteoporosis	ICD-9-CM: 733

Description: Osteoporosis is a systemic skeletal disorder characterized by low bone mass and structural deterioration of bone, resulting in bone fragility and an increased risk for fracture.

Etiology: Multifactorial, related to osteoclastic resorption of bone. When bone formation does not keep pace with bone resorption, osteopenia and osteoporosis result. Bone strength is directly proportional to its density.

Occurrence: Approximately 1 in 10 people in the United States has osteoporosis; 80% are women; 150,000–250,000 hip fractures occur annually in women over 65. More than 1 million fractures in women occur per year because of this disease.

Ethnicity: White or Asian women are at increased risk for osteoporosis.

Age: Women at age 50 have a 40% lifetime fracture risk. Risk increases with age. Skeletal mass begins to decline in women past age 40. The rate of decline is most rapid within 2 years after menopause.

Contributing factors:

- Family history
- Thin body mass
- Smoking
- Low calcium intake
- Anorexia or bulimia
- Physical inactivity
- Alcoholism
- Use of corticosteroids
- Early menopause
- Excessive exercise (i.e., sufficient to induce amenorrhea)

 Clinical Pearl: Medications that can induce osteoporosis are thyroid replacement therapy, barbiturates, anti-seizure medications, chemotherapeutic agents, methylprogesterone acetate injections, or gonadotropin-releasing hormone analogs.

Signs and symptoms: Osteoporosis is asymptomatic until fracture occurs. Fracture occurs with minor trauma. Spinal osteoporosis creates multiple compression fractures over time, thus creating the classic "dowager's hump" of osteoporosis.

 Clinical Pearl: Osteoporosis is asymptomatic until fracture occurs.

Diagnostic tests:

Tests	Results Indicating Disorder	CPT Code
Bone mineral density at several skeletal sites	Bone mass loss (Fracture risk)	76075 (hips, pelvis, spine) 76076 (radius, wrist, heel)
Standard radiograph	Osteopenia (reduced amount of bone)	76061 (limited) 76062 (complete)
Computed tomography (CT)	Osteopenia (reduced amount of bone)	76070

Differential diagnosis:

- Vitamin D deficiency (low blood levels for Vitamin D)
- Metastatic carcinoma (positive cytology, evidence on x-ray)
- Multiple myeloma (x-ray shows diffuse bone lesions)
- Effects of medication (history of meds that cause bone loss such as corticosteroids)
- Endocrine disorders (lab studies show endocrine disorders)
- Renal disease (decreased creatinine clearance, Hgb, and Hct; increased Mg)
- Osteoarthritis (stiffness, x-ray showing changes consistent with osteoarthritis)

- Primary hyperparathyroidism
- Collagen disorders (polyarteritis, SLE, rheumatic fever)

Treatment: The best treatment is prevention. The goal is to reduce the risk of fracture by reducing loss of bone mass. If fracture has occurred, symptomatic relief and aggressive therapy to prevent further bone loss are indicated.

Follow-up: Osteoporosis is a chronic disease that requires close follow-up throughout the woman's life.

Sequelae: Fractures necessitate prolonged hospitalization and surgery with the resulting risks. Of women with hip fractures, 15%–25% require long-term nursing home placement.

Prevention/prophylaxis (see Figure 6-2):

Calcium supplementation, in doses of 1–1.5 g daily, reduces bone loss. Calcium can be found in many food sources and can be supplemented with over-the-counter preparations. Calcium supplements should be consumed with meals to increase their absorption.

Hormone replacement therapy is the treatment of choice for postmenopausal osteoporosis. Estrogen reduces bone loss and decreases fractures. The dose required to reduce bone loss is 0.625 mg daily. (Estrogen must be given with progesterone if the woman's uterus is present. Progesterone does not alter the therapeutic effect of estrogen.) There are risks involved with prolonged administration of hormone therapy. Adverse effects of estrogen include migraine headaches, cholelithiasis, and thrombosis. Benefits of estrogen and progesterone or estrogen alone must be carefully weighed for each woman. It is unknown whether adding calcium to the estrogen regimen reduces the amount of estrogen needed for the desired result.

Exercise plays an important role in preventive therapy. Exercise and physical activity increase skeletal mass. Regular weight-bearing exercise can reduce bone loss. 30 to 45 minutes of a brisk activity that is weight-bearing, such as walking four or five times a week, is recommended.

Antiresorptive drugs bind to bone mineral and inhibit resorption. In this way, the drug acts to increase density and reduce fracture.

Referral: Fractures must be referred to a physician.

Education: There is no universal agreement regarding which women should consider estrogen replacement therapy for osteoporosis. Women who are at risk for osteoporosis must weigh all factors before deciding on estrogen therapy. Postmenopausal women should be taught how to reduce the risk of falling. The home environment should be evaluated for risk of falls.

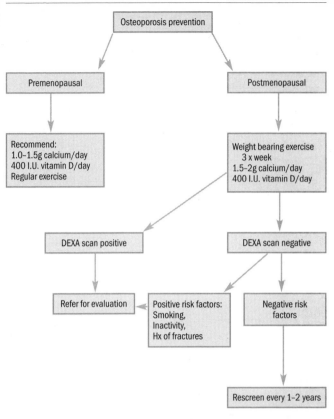

Figure 6–2. Osteoporosis prevention.

RHEUMATOID ARTHRITIS

SIGNAL SYMPTOMS ▶ joint stiffness; stiff feeling in the morning

| Rheumatoid arthritisl | CD 9-CM: 714.0 |

Description: Rheumatoid arthritis (RA) is a systemic, immunologically mediated, chronic, and potentially disabling disease.

Etiology: Unknown.

Occurrence: RA is an inflammatory systemic disease that manifests itself in joints. RA is probably the most common cause of chronic inflammatory arthritis, affecting 1%–2% of the general population. Women are affected 2.5 times more often than men.

Age: Prevalence increases with age. Incidence peaks in the fourth decade.

Ethnicity: Not significant.

Contributing factors: There is a genetic predisposition to RA.

Signs and symptoms: Joint stiffness after inactivity is the hallmark of the chronic inflammation associated with this disease. Stiffness occurs in the morning upon awakening and after sitting for long periods. The small joints of the feet and hands are involved. Eventually nearly every joint in the body becomes involved. Synovitis of the wrist joints is a nearly uniform feature of RA and may lead to limitation of movement.

On physical examination, the joints are "boggy" because of underlying synovitis. RA is a systemic disease and may involve multiple organ systems. The woman may experience low-grade fever, fatigue, and mild weight loss.

Diagnostic tests:

Test	Results Indicating Disorder	CPT Code
Serum rheumatoid factor	Positive in 70–85% of cases	86431 (Quantitative); 86430 (Qualitative)
Radiographs of the hands, wrists, and feet	Evidence of RA	73110 (wrist, 3 views) 73130 (hands, 3 views) 73630 (feet, 3 views)

Differential diagnoses:

- Osteoarthritis (stiffness, x-ray changes consistent with osteoarthritis)
- Spondyloarthropathies
- Gout (red, swollen tender joint)
- Lyme disease (rash, history of tick bite, elevated titer)
- Fibromyalgia (chronic muscle soft tissue pain, fatigue, depression may be present)
- Tendinitis (pain with movement of affected area, history of overuse)
- Bursitis (pain with direct pressure on bursa)

Treatment: Treating RA requires a multidisciplinary approach. Physical and occupational therapy are important. RA is treated with corticosteroids and nonsteroidal anti-inflammatory drugs (NSAIDs) or COX-2 inhibitors such as rofecoxib. Disease-modifying antirheumatic drugs (DMARDs) such as methotrexate are a standard of care. At times, surgery is required for treatment.

Follow-up: RA is a chronic disease that requires close follow-up throughout the woman's life. Several issues exist for women with RA who require surgery of any type. Pregnancy with RA requires close follow-up.

Sequelae: The clinical course is one of remissions and exacerbations. Approximately 40% of women diagnosed experience disability within 10 years. Some women experience a self-limiting disease and others suffer a chronic progressive illness.

Prevention/prophylaxis: None.

Referral: RA is a chronic systemic disease. Therapy must be designed and provided by a physician. A team of care providers that involves an NP, physical therapist, and occupational therapist is a preferable referral source.

Education: Patient education deals primarily with dismissing misconceptions while minimizing discomfort and preserving function.

SYSTEMIC LUPUS ERYTHEMATOSUS

SIGNAL SYMPTOMS▶   Fatigue; joint pain; butterfly rash

| Systemic lupus erythematosus | ICD-9-CM: 710.0 |

Description: Systemic lupus erythematosus (SLE) is a multisystem disease associated with the production of multiple autoantibodies.

Etiology: Unknown.

Occurrence: More common in women than in men, with a 9:1 ratio.

Ethnicity: More common in African-American and Asian women than in white or Hispanic women.

Age: SLE is most common in women of childbearing age.

Contributing factors: Genetic, environmental, and hormonal

Signs and symptoms:

- Arthritis occurs in 76%–88% of the cases (joint involvement similar to that of RA). Arthritis is systemic and inflammatory, involving multiple joints.
- Rashes, including the classic butterfly rash occurring across the nose and on the cheeks. Rashes come and go without scarring.
- Painless oral ulcerations.
- Alopecia.
- Fever, fatigue, weight loss.
- Symptoms increase during pregnancy.
- A combination of malaise, fatigue, weight loss, and fever are present in 73% of SLE patients.

Diagnostic tests:

Test	Results Indicating Disorder	CPT Code
Serum Antinuclear antibody (ANA)	Positive (greater than 95% sensitive for SLE)	86038

Differential diagnosis:

- ANA is positive in RA, thyroiditis, chronic infection, and malignancy.
- RA (joint deterioration present)
- Malignancy (progressive aching pain at rest; history of previous malignancy)
- Drug reaction (rash resolves when drug is discontinued)

Treatment: NSAIDs for arthritis, corticosteroids.

Follow-up: SLE is a chronic disease that requires close follow-up after diagnosis.

Sequelae: Ovarian failure related to steroids, renal disease, neuropsychiatric lupus, hypertension, leukopenia, hemolytic anemia, and thrombocytopenia.

Prevention/prophylaxis: None.

Referral: Refer for diagnosis and treatment.

Education: Avoidance of the sun and use of sunscreen should be advised.

REFERENCES

Fibromylagia

Clark, S and Odell, L: Fibromyalgia syndrome. Clin Rev 10(5):57, 2000.

Leake, N: Looks can be deceiving: the behind-the-scenes battle of fibromyalgia. Adv Nurse Practit 9(6):40, 2001.

Schaefer, K: Health patterns of women with fibromyalgia. J Adv Nurs 26(3): 565, 1997.

Osteoporosis

Davidson, M, and DeSimone M: Osteoporosis update. Clin Rev 12(4):75, 2002.

Fuller, V: Bone density testing, Adv Nurse Practit 9(10): October 2002.

Yonclas, P, et al: Osteoporosis: How much exercise is enough for bone health? Consultant 42(7):829, 2002.

Rheumatoid Arthritis

Belilios, E, and Carsons, S: Rheumatologic disorders in women. Med Clin North Am 81(1):77, 1998.

Callahan, L, et al: Arthritis and women's health prevalence, impact and prevention. Am J Prev Med 12(5):401, 1996.

Morbidity and Mortality Weekly Report: Prevalence and impact of arthritis among women—United States 1989–1991. Mortality Weekly Report 44(27):517, 1995.

Ruoff, G: Rheumatoid arhtritis. Consultant 42(3): March 2002.

Sherman, J: Rhematoid arthritis. Adv Nurse Practit 9(12): Dec. 2001.

Systemic Lupus Erythematosus

Barth, W: Office evaluation of the patient with musculoskeletal complaints. Am J Med 102(1A):3S, 1997.

Germillion, R: Update of systemic lupus erythematosus. Clin Adv Nurse Practit Feb 25, 2000.

Chapter 7

PERIPHERAL VASCULAR DISORDERS

SUPERFICIAL THROMBOPHLEBITIS

SIGNAL SYMPTOM▶   leg pain

Superficial thrombophlebitis, leg	ICD-9-CM: 451.0
Thrombophlebitis, deep leg	ICD-9-CM: 451.2

Description: Superficial thrombophlebitis occurs almost always in a varicose vein because of static blood flow. Deep venous thrombosis, an acute thrombus formation, varies in clinical presentation and is potentially life-threatening.

Etiology: The cause of acute thrombus formation in the venous system is unclear. In most instances, thrombus formation is related to damage, stasis, and hypercoagulability.

Occurrence: Venous thrombophlebitis can occur following gynecologic surgery. Studies report that 40% of deaths following pelvic surgery are attributable to venous thrombosis and pulmonary embolus.

Age: The frequency of venous thrombosis increases with age. Venous thrombosis is reported most often in women over 50 years of age.

Ethnicity: Not significant.

Contributing factors: Varicose veins, sedentary lifestyle, obesity, hypertension, diabetes, pelvic surgery, duration of pelvic surgery, prolonged immobilization, malignancy, hypercoagulable states, and estrogen therapy.

Signs and symptoms:

- Localized warmth, redness, tenderness, and swelling of the extremity
- Pain in the limb that increases with movement
- Positive Homan's sign (pain with dorsiflexion of the foot)
- Clinical findings for thrombus are not specific. When thrombosis is suspected, noninvasive testing should be performed. Diagnosis based on history and physical examination alone is reported to be correct only 50% of the time

All pulses should be palpated at every woman's health examination. (Include the radial, brachial, femoral, popliteal, dorsalis pedis, and posterior tibial arteries.)

- Note the temperature of the feet and legs.
- An important ominous clinical sign is edema of the legs. Compare one leg to the other, noting presence of edema (see Figure 7-1).
- Note the color of the extremities and the presence of ulcers or varicose veins.

Diagnostic Tests:

Test	Results Indicating Disorder	CPT Code
Doppler Ultrasound	Venous occlusion secondary to thrombosis or thrombophlebitis	93965

Differential diagnosis:

- Varicose veins (pain and/or tenderness aggravated by standing for long periods, dilated superficial vessels)
- Venous insufficiency (confirmed by venogram or Doppler ultrasound)

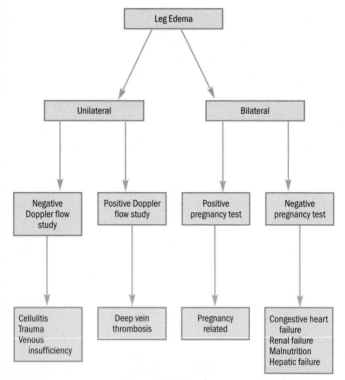

Figure 7–1. Leg edema.

Treatment: Prophylaxis is preferable to treatment. Thrombosis in a deep vein is treated with anticoagulants. Superficial thrombosis is treated with analgesics, anti-inflammatory medication, elevation, and rest.

Follow-up: Thrombus formation requires close follow-up for evaluation of underlying disorders. Prevention of further episodes is imperative.

Sequelae: Calf vein thrombosis is generally associated with a good prognosis. Thrombosis above the knee is associated with pulmonary embolism.

Prevention/prophylaxis: Thromboembolytic deterrent stockings (TEDS), heparin therapy prior to pelvic surgery.

Referral: Thrombus formation above the knee requires immediate referral and subsequent hospitalization. Deep vein thrombosis below the knee requires referral for evaluation, treatment, and close follow-up.

Education: The clinical symptom that most closely correlates with diagnosis of thrombosis is unilateral leg swelling. All women should be informed of the significance of this finding. Pain may or may not be present with the swelling.

REFERENCES

Brochier, M, and Arwidson, PA: Coronary heart disease risk factors in women. Eur Heart J 19(Suppl A):45, 1998.

Goodheart Institute, Rotterdam, the Netherlands: Exclusion and diagnosis of deep vein thrombosis. Clin Applied Thrombosis/Hemostasis, 5(3):171, 1999.

Goroll, A, et al: Primary Care Medicine. Lippincott, Philadelphia, 1995.

Seltzer, V, and Pearse, W: Women's Primary Health Care. McGraw-Hill, New York, 1995.

Chapter 8

ENDOCRINE, METABOLIC, AND NUTRITIONAL DISORDERS

AMENORRHEA, PRIMARY

SIGNAL SYMPTOM ▶ lack of menses

Amenorrhea, primary	ICD-9-CM: 626.0

Description: The mean age for appearance of menses, known as **menarche**, is 12 years. Girls who do not experience menses by age 16 or 17 **(primary amenorrhea)** require evaluation.

Etiology: The causes of primary amenorrhea are divided into two categories: those with the absence of secondary sex characteristics, and those with the presence of secondary sex characteristics. If secondary sex characteristics are absent, etiology includes absence of ovarian estrogen, hypothalamic disease, or pituitary disease. In the presence of secondary sex characteristics, amenorrhea is related to anatomic defects, androgen insensitivity syndrome, nutritional amenorrhea, systemic disease, or hyperprolactinemia. The most common reason for primary amenorrhea is polycystic ovarian syndrome, in which a self-perpetuating state of chronic anovulation occurs. This ovulatory dysfunction involves the hypothalamus, pituitary, ovaries, adrenals, and peripheral adipose tissue.

Occurrence: Unknown.

Age: Lack of onset of menses by age 16 or 17 years.

Ethnicity: Not significant.

Contributing factors: Amenorrhea can be exercise-induced. Body weight low enough to influence hypothalamic function is seen in middle- and long-distance runners, gymnasts, ballet dancers, and swimmers. It is also seen in women with anorexia.

Signs and symptoms: Lack of menses, hirsutism, lack of development of secondary sex characteristics, infertility, elevated follicle-stimulating

Table 8-1 Primary Amenorrhea

Diagnosis	Secondary Sex Characteristics	Serum FSH level
Delayed menarche	Yes	Normal
Anatomic defects	Yes	Normal
Gonadal dysgenesis	No	Elevated
Ovarian-hypothalamic-pituitary disease	No	Low
Nutritional amenorrhea	Yes	

hormone (FSH) and luteinizing hormone (LH) levels. Careful physical examination will reveal lack of secondary sex characteristics past age 13 (see Table 8–1).

Diagnostic tests:

Test	Results Indicating Disorder	CPT Code
Karyotype	Chromosomal abnormality	85130
FSH levels*	<25 mIU (elevated)	80426
LH levels*	<25 mIU (elevated)	80426
TSH	>0.2 u/mL (decreased)	84443
Serum prolactin levels	>25 ng/ml	84146

* Values vary according to the age of the woman and the day of the menstrual cycle.

Differential diagnoses:

- Delayed physiologic menarche (history)
- Sheehan syndrome (postpartum pituitary necrosis)
- Post-traumatic hypopituitarism (history of trauma, history of hypopituitarism post-trauma)
- Radiation-induced hypopituitarism (history of radiation exposure)
- Cushing's syndrome (fatigue, weakness, amenorrhea, polycystic ovaries, hirsutism)
- Menopause (night sweats, hot flashes)
- Thyroid disease (thyroid panel, may be hypothyroid)
- Central nervous system (CNS) lesions
- Ovarian tumor (radiologic evaluation)

Treatment: Estrogen replacement therapy is the most common treatment modality.

Follow-up: A reproductive endocrinologist should follow women with primary amenorrhea.

Sequelae: Loss of bone density can occur with primary amenorrhea.

Prevention/prophylaxis: None.

Referral: Girls should be referred to a reproductive endocrinologist if they have not experienced menses by age 16 or 17. Lack of secondary sex characteristics after the age of 13 requires referral.

Education: All women should be educated concerning puberty and menarche. Teach mothers when to refer their daughters for evaluation.

ANOREXIA AND BULIMIA

SIGNAL SYMPTOM▶   inability to maintain recommended weight

Anorexia	ICD-9: 307.1
Bulimia	ICD-9: 307.51

Description
Eating disorders have common features. These include weight loss, an irrational fear of gaining weight and abnormal physiologic functioning. Eating disorders are usually mild; a small minority are severe and complex.

 Clinical Pearl: Loss of menses is not essential for a diagnosis of anorexia.

Etiology: Anorexia is related to a body image distortion and a great fear of becoming obese. Anorexia is diagnosed via history of significant weight loss. Amenorrhea is not required for a diagnosis of anorexia. Bulimia is characterized by consuming large quantities of food over a short interval (bingeing) followed by vomiting and/or use of laxatives or diuretics and/or restricted eating. Purging is not required for the diagnosis. However, 80% of bulimics do purge. The remaining 20% compensate with exercise and food restriction.

Occurrence: Approximately 5% of young women meet the *DSM-IV-R* criteria for an eating disorder.

Age: The most common age group for anorexia is 12–30 years. The most common age group for bulimia is 17–25 years.

Ethnicity: Anorexia and bulimia occur more frequently in Caucasian females.

Contributing Factors: Emotional distress, depression, anxiety, conflicts within relationships, and social isolation. Current or past substance abuse has been associated with anorexia and bulimia. A history of sexual abuse has also been associated with anorexia and bulimia.

Signs and symptoms:

Anorexia
The anorectic woman usually denies that she is ill, but her thinness attracts the NP's attention. The woman usually does not complain of hunger, but may complain of difficulty sleeping, bloating after eating, constipation, or cold intolerance. Amenorrhea is common in anorectics. Most women with anorexia are restless, physically active, and some exercise to excess.

History will reveal an inability to maintain a recommended weight, secretive eating, frequent weighing, persistent feelings of dissatisfaction with weight, and mood changes associated with food.

Bulimia

Bingeing and purging are symptoms of bulimia.

Diagnostic tests:

A brief set of questions can alert the practitioner to a possible eating disorder (see also Table 8–2).

- Are you concerned about your weight?
- Are you trying to lose weight?
- Have you lost weight and, if so, how much?
- Do you experience out-of-control binge eating?
- Do you practice any form of purging such as vomiting or use of laxatives or diuretics?
- Do you exercise compulsively?
- Does your self-esteem depend excessively on your weight or shape?
- Are you preoccupied with fears of becoming fat or desires to be thinner?
- How much time each day do you think about your weight or shape?

(Courtesy of Arnold Andersen, MD)

Differential diagnoses:

- Malignancy (positive cytology)
- Chronic infection (elevated WBC, positive cultures)

Table 8–2 Eating Disorders

	Anorexia Nervosa	Bulimia	Obesity
Characteristics	Refusal to maintain normal weight, fear of gaining weight, amenorrhea	Binge eating, self-induced vomiting, use of laxatives or diuretics, fasting	Compulsive overeating not related to hunger
History	Cannot maintain weight, resists giving diet history, excessive exercise, amenorrhea	Binge/Purging patterns, weight fluctuations	History of unsuccessful diets, restricted social activities because of weight
Physical findings	Low weight, pale and emaciated, lanugo, atrophied or poorly developed breasts, arrhythmias, overuse muscular injuries, amenorrhea	Normal weight or slightly overweight, "chipmunk" appearance, conjunctival hemorrhage, dental enamel eroded, overuse muscular injuries, menstrual irregularities	Excessive body fat, hypertension, hirutism, varicosities, abdomen protuberant, arthritis, depression
Treatment	Medications, diet, exercise, psychotherapy	Medications, diet, counseling and therapy	Medications, diet, exercise, group therapy

- Intestinal disorders (history, diarrhea, constipation, abdominal pain)
- Endocrinopathies (laboratory studies)
- Tumors of the CNS (neurological symptoms, radiologic evaluation)
- Depression (history of depression)
- Anxiety (history of anxiety)
- Substance abuse (history)
- Obsessive compulsive disorders (history)

Treatment: Medical management, pharmacotherapy, nutrition therapy, behavioral therapy, cognitive therapy, and family therapy. Hospitalization is necessary if weight loss is severe and rapidly progressing or signs of complications such as cardiac arrhythmia or hypokalemia occur. Suicidal ideation requires hospitalization.

Follow-up: Treatment is a multidisciplinary team effort. Follow-up with the team will be necessary for long-term resolution.

Sequelae: Of women with anorexia, 9% do not survive. Amenorrhea of hypothalamic origin occurs with severe weight loss. Loss of bone density occurs with extreme weight loss. Outcome studies show that 60% of anorectics achieve normal weight and menstruation, 49% achieve normalized eating patterns, and 20% endure chronic symptoms. Bulimia can produce dental erosion, swollen salivary glands, gastrointestinal irritation, and electrolyte imbalance. Of all bulimics, 20% endure chronic symptoms.

 Clinical Pearl: There is no evidence of permanent damage from secondary amenorrhea due to weight loss.

Prevention/prophylaxis: Overall advice to prevent an eating disorder includes the following guidelines:

- Eat a variety of nutritious meals and snacks throughout the day.
- Eat favorite foods in moderation.
- Avoid skipping meals.
- Keep healthy foods on hand.
- Find alternatives for managing uncomfortable feelings.
- Avoid dieting.

Anorexia and bulimia are "culture bound" disorders that occur in societies that value thinness. Among young women in the northern hemisphere, thinness is highly valued. 40% of girls in the fourth and fifth grade think that they are too fat. By high school, 75% of girls think that they weigh too much.

Referral: The shortest time between onset of symptoms and the beginning of treatment is associated with a more favorable outcome. Refer to a multidisciplinary team that involves mental health professionals and nutrition specialists as soon as you suspect an eating disorder.

Education: NPs can educate all women about the importance of proper nutrition and the hazards of dieting.

DIABETES

SIGNAL SYMPTOMS polyuria; polydypsia; polyphagia; there may not be any symptoms

Diabetes mellitus, Type 1 uncontrolled	ICD-9: 250.1
Diabetes mellitus, Type 2, uncontrolled	ICD-9: 250.02
Diabetes mellitus, Type 2, controlled	ICD-9: 250.00

Description: Diabetes mellitus is a metabolic disorder characterized by abnormal metabolism of carbohydrates, fats, and proteins. Type 1 is insulin-dependent diabetes mellitus. Type 2 is non–insulin-dependent diabetes mellitus (NIDDM). Type 1 is generally diagnosed in childhood or early adulthood. Type 2 is generally diagnosed in adulthood.

Etiology: Type 2 is related to the destruction of the beta cells in the islets of Langerhans. Type 2 is related to a defect in insulin receptors or an altered state of response to insulin in the beta cells. Because this is a slowly evolving process, the harmful effects of insulin resistance may be present for some time—as much as ten years—before they are detected.

Occurrence: Diabetes occurs in 3%–7% of the U.S. population. Type 2 is 10 times more common than type 1. Similar rates of diabetes occur in men and women. Estimates from The American Diabetic Association indicate that some 8.1 million women have type 2 diabetes and one third of these women do not know they have the disease.

Age: The incidence of NIDDM, which increases with age, is usually diagnosed after age 40.

Ethnicity: NIDDM is ethnic group–related. The prevalence of the disease in Puma Indians is 35%, Native Americans 17%, Hispanics 12%, and African-Americans 5%. Mexican-Americans have a 1.6–1.9 times greater incidence of diabetes than Caucasians.

Contributing factors: A major risk factor for NIDDM is overnutrition with resulting obesity. Of diabetics, 80% are obese or have a history of obesity. Steroids reduce the receptor affinity for insulin. Other risk factors for NIDDM include family history of NIDDM, gestational diabetes, history of impaired glucose tolerance, history of coronary heart disease.

Signs and symptoms: The appearance of symptoms may be acute or subacute in type 1 diabetes. The deficiency of insulin leads to a breakdown of protein (an increase in amino acids), a breakdown in fats (increase in free fatty acids), and a breakdown in glycogen to glucose metabolism. These changes create hyperglycemia and metabolic ketoacidosis, which, if not treated, can lead to coma and death.

In type 2 diabetes, the disease may be insidious at the start. The classic symptoms of diabetes include polyuria, polydipsia, and polyphagia. Weight loss is another symptom of diabetes.

See Table 8–3 for a summary of characteristics of type 1 and type 2 diabetes.

Table 8–3 Characteristics of Type 1 and Type 2 Diabetes

	Type 1	Type 2
Age at onset	<20	>40
Incidence in patients diagnosed with diabetes	1 in 10	9 in 10
Symptoms	Acute or subacute	Slow onset
Obesity at onset	Uncommon	Common
Family history	Uncommon	Common
Ketoacidosis	Frequent	Rare
Insulin	Decreased	Variable
Treatment	Diet, insulin	Diet, oral hypoglycemic medication, insulin

Diagnostic Tests:

Test	Results Indicating Disorder	CPT Code
Fasting blood glucose	< 140–150 mg/dL on two separate occasions	82947
Random blood glucose	< 200 mg/dL	82947
Oral glucose tolerance tests		82951 + 82952 for each test beyond three
Fasting	<105mg/dL	See above
30 minutes	<160 mg/dL	Included in OGTT
One hour	<170 mg/dL	Included in OGTT
Two hours	< 125 mg/dL	Included in OGTT

Differential diagnosis: Hypoglycemia (low blood glucose).

Treatment: The goals of therapy for a diabetic include normalizing metabolism and preventing complications. Methods of therapy include education, meal planning, exercise, and the use of hypoglycemic agents or insulin.

Follow-up: Diabetes requires management throughout the woman's life.

Sequelae: Complications of untreated or undertreated diabetes include retinopathy, nephropathy, neuropathy, coronary heart disease (increased four times in women over men), cerebral vascular accident, and peripheral vascular disease. More than one half of the people with diabetes die from CVD. This risk is greater for women than for men. Women with diabetes are more likely to die from heart disease than women who do not have diabetes (Cooper and Caldwell, 1999).

Referral: Abnormal blood glucose levels require referral to an endocrinologist for evaluation.

Education: Management of diabetes requires in-depth education about the disease, diet management, risk factors, exercise management, and methods used to evaluate the disease process. Experts should provide education about diabetes.

HIRSUTISM

SIGNAL SYMPTOM▶ increased hair growth

Hirsutism	ICD-9: 704.1

Description: Hirsutism is excessive hair growth in women. Excessive hair is facial, pubic, axillary, abdominal, and chest. The hair is coarse and occurs in a male-like pattern.

Etiology: The majority of women with hirsutism have the idiopathic variety characterized by normal circulating androgens. There is a subset of women whose hirsutism indicates a hormonal abnormality. Increased androgenic activity causes the increased hair growth. The increase in androgen may indicate an underlying endocrine disease. The source of androgen may be the ovary, the adrenal gland, or both. Anabolic steroids can produce hirsutism, as can danazol, a drug used to treat endometriosis.

Occurrence: Excessive androgen action is the most common endocrinopathy of women, affecting 5% to 20% of U.S. women.

Age: Hirsutism usually begins after age 25.

Ethnicity: Hirsutism has familial, racial, and ethnic patterns. Eastern European women are more hirsute than Scandinavian women; white women are more hirsute than black women.

Contributing Factors:

- Insulin resistance can trigger excessive ovarian androgen production. A link between obesity and hirsutism exists.
- Hirsutism in conjunction with oligomenorrhea or amenorrhea may represent polycystic ovarian syndrome.
- Cushing's syndrome can produce hirsutism, as can congenital adrenal hyperplasia.

Signs and Symptoms: Increased hair growth. Acne and androgenic alopecia can occur with hirsutism. The ovaries may be normal in size, or enlarged and contain multiple cysts.

Diagnostic Tests:

Tests	Results Indicating Disorder	CPT Code
Free serum testosterone	>30-95 ng/dL (increased)	84402 (free); 84403 (total)
LH:FSH ratio	Depends on menstrual cycle	80426
17-hydroxycorticosteroids	<2.5 to >10 mg/24 hrs	83491
Urinary cortisol concentrations	>24–108 ug/24 hrs	82533

Clinical Pearl: A history of regular menses does not exclude ovulatory dysfunction.

Differential diagnosis: Virilization defined as temporary hair recession, acne, deepening voice, increased muscle mass, and clitoromegaly.

Treatment: Mild hirsutism not related to endocrine disease can be treated with hair bleaching, waxing, or electrolysis. Medical therapy is required for hirsutism related to endocrine disease. Give appropriate oral contraceptives or medications used to reduce androgen levels.

 Clinical Pearl: Eflornithine hydrochloride is a topical medication that can be utilized to treat hirsutism.

Follow-up: Hirsutism related to endocrine disease requires lifetime follow-up.

Sequelae: There is an increased incidence of type 2 diabetes in women with hirsutism as well as unfavorable lipid patterns.

Prevention/prophylaxis: Obesity is a modifiable risk factor.

Referral: Any woman with significant hirsutism should be referred to a reproductive endocrinologist for evaluation.

Education: Hirsutism can indicate a loss of femininity to women. After endocrine pathology has been ruled out or treated, referral for hair reduction, particularly in the facial area, is recommended.

HYPERLIPIDEMIA

SIGNAL SYMPTOMS none

Hyperlipidemia	ICD-9: 272.5

Description: Evidence has accumulated demonstrating that treating hyperlipidemia can reduce atherosclerosis and its resultant cardiovascular complications. The presence of hyperlipidemia does not guarantee the formation of plaques, nor does the absence of excessive lipids reassure against them. Multiple factors create an atherosclerotic condition. The presence of hyperlipidemia requires further evaluation for total cardiovascular risk assessment.

Etiology: Lipoproteins are combinations of lipids such as cholesterol and triglycerides combined with proteins that enable circulation. Lipoproteins can be either low- or high-density. Low-density lipoproteins (LDLs), the major carriers of cholesterol, are clearly present in atherosclerosis. High-density lipoproteins (HDLs) are believed to function in peripheral tissue as acceptors of cholesterol, which is then diffused out of cell membranes. The proportion of HDL to LDL is an important factor in evaluation of risk for atherosclerosis. Women with high HDL and low LDL have a reduced risk for developing cardiovascular disease.

Occurrence: Elevated or borderline cholesterol levels are present in 20%–30% of women.

Age: Cholesterol levels increase with age. Women carry a higher portion of HDL until menopause, after which the risk for cardiovascular disease rises to the same level as men.

Ethnicity: Not significant.

Contributing factors:

- Obesity
- Physical inactivity
- Genetic variations in lipoprotein structure, metabolic enzymes, and interaction between lipids and the cell wall
- Dietary fat and cholesterol intake have a substantial influence on serum cholesterol and LDL levels. Saturated fat in the diet is most noted to affect cholesterol and LDL levels

Diagnostic tests: A single measurement should never be used for diagnosis of hyperlipidemia.

Test	Results Indicating Disorder	CPT Code
Total Cholesterol	> 200	82465
LDL	> 130	83721
HDL	> 60	83718
Triglycerides	> 150–199	84478
Lipid profile	Includes all of the above except LDL	80061

Signs and symptoms: Hyperlipidemia causes no symptoms. Diagnosis is made through blood screening (see Figure 8–1).

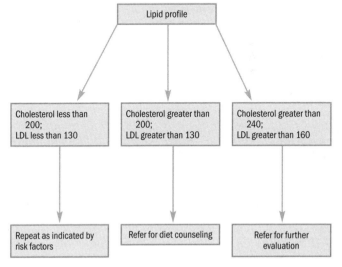

Figure 8–1. Hyperlipidemia.

Differential diagnosis:

- Hypothyroidism (thyroid panel, weight gain, dry skin, mental and physical lethargy)
- Nephrotic syndrome (lab studies)
- Diabetes secondarily leading to hyperlipidemia
- Certain drugs (e. g., beta blockers) can affect lipid levels as well

Treatment: Lipid abnormality is a component of total cardiovascular disease risk. Hyperlipidemia can be treated with dietary modifications, exercise, and weight reduction. Pharmacologic therapy is reserved for women in the highest overall risk category.

Follow-up: A diagnosis of hyperlipidemia requires at least annual follow-up. The total cardiovascular risk assessment may necessitate closer follow-up.

Prevention/prophylaxis: The goal is to reduce coronary morbidity and mortality by reducing the risk for the first coronary event.

Referral: Risk is evaluated based on hyperlipidemia plus blood pressure, smoking, diabetes, family history, age, and presence or absence of cardiovascular disease. Women with hyperlipidemia should be referred for evaluation of risk for cardiovascular disease.

Education: Treatment for hyperlipidemia requires a change in eating and exercise habits. Careful education and monitoring of behavior are required for successful intervention. (see also Tables 8-4 and 8–5).

OBESITY

SIGNAL SYMPTOM▶ excess weight

Obesity	ICD-9-CM: 278.00
Morbid obesity	ICD-9-CM: 278.01

Table 8–4 ATP III Classification of LDL, Total, and HDL Cholesterol (mg/dL)

LDL Cholesterol–Primary Target of Therapy	
<100	Optimal
100–129	Near optimal/better than average
130–159	Borderline high
160–189	High
≥190	Very high

Total Cholesterol	
<200	Desirable
200–239	Borderline high
≥240	High

HDL Cholesterol	
<40	Low
>60	High

Source: U.S. Department of Health and Human Services, Public Health Service, National Institutes of Health, National Heart, Lung, and Blood Institute, NIH Publication No. 01-3305, May, 2001.

Table 8–5 ATP III Classification of Serum Triglycerides (mg/dL)

Range	ATP Classification
<150	Normal
150-199	Borderline high
200-499	High
>500	Very high

Source: U.S. DEPARTMENT OF HEALTH AND HUMAN SERVICES, Public Health Service, National Institutes of Health, National Heart, Lung, and Blood Institute, NIH Publication No. 01-3305, May 2001

Description: Obesity is an excessive accumulation of body fat. Obesity is a multifactorial disease that involves genetics and biochemistry as well as environmental and cultural factors. The National Institute of Health defines obesity as body mass index (BMI) of 30 or greater.

Etiology: In the year 2000, the United States became the fattest nation in the world, with 55% of its citizens being overweight or obese. Obesity is increasingly becoming a major public health problem in the United States. Obesity can create a number of health-related problems for women including cardiovascular disease and joint disorders. Obesity is rarely the result of an endocrine disorder; rather, obesity is usually a disease of appetite regulation and metabolism.

Occurrence: Obesity is the most prevalent nutritional disorder of affluent nations, including the United States. Over the past decade, obesity and diabetes have become more prevalent in the United States. In a study by Mokdad (2001), 184,450 people were interviewed about their weight. The prevalence of obesity (BMI > 30 kg/m^2) was 19.8% (self-reports). This reflects a 61% increase since 1991. The self-reported prevalence of diabetes increased by 49% since 1990.

Age: Obesity can occur at any age.

Ethnicity: Obesity is more common in African-American and Mexican-American women than in Caucasian women. Of African-American and Mexican-American women, 50% are obese.

Contributing factors: Familial tendency, emotional problems.

Signs and symptoms: Mild obesity is defined as 20%–40% above the average weight for women of the same height and build. Moderate obesity is defined as 41%–100% above the average. Severe obesity is defined as more than 100% above the average.

Diagnostic tests:

These are no diagnostic tests. Check height and weight, diet history, physical examination.

Differential diagnosis:

- Cushing's syndrome (fatigue, weakness, amenorrhea, polycystic ovaries, hirsutism)
- Hypothyroidism (thyroid panel, weight gain, dry skin, mental and physical lethargy)

- Polycystic ovarian syndrome (amenorrhea, hirsutism, infertility, lack of ovulation)
- Hypothalamic injury
- Congestive heart failure (lab studies, ECG)
- Renal failure (lab studies, weight gain)

Treatment: Competently designed treatment programs tailored to individual needs have the greatest success rate. Therapy includes dietary approaches, behavior modification, and exercise. Therapy may include pharmacologic treatment. A multidisciplinary approach is recommended.

Follow-up: Motivation is a key factor to weight reduction. Long-term follow-up with a multidisciplinary team is needed for weight reduction and maintenance.

Sequelae: Obesity is associated with oligo-ovulation, polycystic ovarian syndrome, endometrial cancer, and, after menopause, breast cancer. (Obesity increases the production of estrogen, increases the free testosterone levels, and increases the androgen levels.) Obesity is associated with infertility.

Obesity increases the risk for morbidity and mortality in women. Pregnancy in obese women is handled as high risk. Coronary artery disease in middle-aged women, sleep apnea, surgical risk, osteoarthritis, and gallbladder disease have an increased incidence in obese women.

Referral: Refer obese women to a multidisciplinary team for weight loss. The team should include a registered dietitian. In the Mokdad study, 42.8% of the participants who reported that they were obese also reported that they were advised by their practitioner to lose weight. If the practitioner recommends weight loss, the woman may be more likely to pursue a weight loss goal.

Education: Realistic goals and expectations are critical. The woman must be willing to alter eating and exercise patterns permanently.

 Clinical Pearl: To find a BMI (body mass index) using the standard system

Weight (lbs)/ height (inches)^2 x 703 = BMI

PREMENSTRUAL SYNDROME

SIGNAL SYMPTOMS ▶ discomfort prior to menses including emotional lability, headache, breast tenderness

Premenstrual syndrome	ICD-9: 625.4
Premenstral dysphoric disorder	ICD-9: 625.4

Description: Premenstrual syndrome (PMS) is a cyclic recurrence in the luteal phase of the menstrual cycle of distressing symptoms (physical, psychologic, and/or behavioral) that interfere with normal activities.

Etiology: Unknown.

Occurrence: Most women (80%–90%) have some distressing symptoms prior to menses. Of these, 30% report severe temporary distress, with 3%–5% reporting disabling temporary symptoms. Less than 10% of menstruating women suffer from premenstrual dysphoric disorder, a severe form of PMS.

Age: PMS can occur at any age, but it is most common in later reproductive years.

Ethnicity: Not significant.

Contributing factors: Deficient diet, lack of exercise, chronic illness, stress

Signs and symptoms: A complex cluster of symptoms occurs 7 to 14 days prior to menses. Timing of the symptoms is a critical part of the diagnosis. The follicular phase should be symptom free. Symptoms can include any combination of the following: breast swelling and tenderness, lower abdominal bloating and constipation, loose stool or diarrhea 24 hours prior to menses; and for the first 1 to 2 days of menstrual bleeding, increase in appetite and cravings, fatigue, emotional lability and depression, irritability, insomnia, menopausal-like hot flashes, night sweats, and migraine-like headaches. Dysmenorrhea does not usually occur with PMS, although it may in adolescence (see Figure 8-2).

Reviewing a symptom calendar makes the diagnosis. Diagnosis is made by the nature, severity, and timing of the symptoms. Symptoms occur at the onset of or after ovulation and resolve 6–7 days following the onset of menses. There is at least 1 week without symptoms. Symptoms do not occur suddenly; they gradually increase over the years. The symptoms are consistent and predictable. The symptoms do not resolve without intervention.

Diagnostic Tests: There are no laboratory tests that help diagnose PMS. A CBC and thyroid screen can be used to rule out anemia and thyroid disease.

Test	Results Indicating Disorder	CPT Code
CBC	May show anemia	85025
Thyroid screen	May show hypothyroid or hyperthyroid disease	84443 (TSH) 84436 (T4) 84439 (free T4) 84479 (thyroid uptake) 84480 (T3)

Clinical Pearl: The follicular phase of the menstrual cycle should be symptom free.

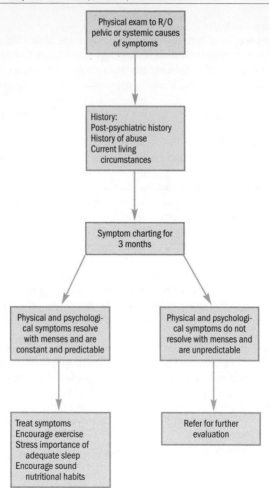

Figure 8–2. PMS.

Differential diagnosis:

- Depression (history of depression)
- Chronic pelvic pain (history)
- Post–tubal ligation syndrome (change in menses including menorrhagia and dysmenorrhea)
- Perimenopausal symptoms (irregular menstrual cycle, increase in FSH and LH levels; estrogen and androgen levels remain the same)

Treatment: Treatment of PMS should include counseling and reassurance. A decrease in salt and sugar intake can be helpful in relief of symptoms. Eliminating caffeine and increasing exercise can reduce symptoms. Stress management, a healthy diet, and regular aerobic exercise are helpful. Complementary therapies such as St. John's Wort purport to provide PMS relief. Women whose symptoms are not relieved by lifestyle change may require medication.

Medications can be utilized. Vitamin B_6, pyridoxine, 100–200 mg daily, may help relieve symptoms. Headache can be treated with medication. Oral contraceptives are not helpful for relief of this syndrome. Luteinizing hormone–releasing hormone (LHRH) agonists, gonadotropin-releasing hormone (GnRH) agonists, and continuous oral progesterone have been utilized to reduce PMS. Antidepressants can be utilized for severe PMS.

Recently selective serotonin reuptake inhibitors (SSRI) have been used to treat severe PMS.

Follow-up: After initiation of therapy, monthly visits for 3 months are recommended for evaluation.

Sequelae: None.

Prevention/prophylaxis: Normal physiologic changes in the menstrual cycle precipitate the symptoms. No prevention can be recommended.

Referral: Referral to a physician is appropriate if there is no relief of symptoms after 3 months. A mental health referral may be appropriate. A referral to a nutritionist may be helpful. Support groups for PMS have been helpful to some women.

Education: An understanding of the normal menstrual cycle may enhance understanding of PMS.

THYROID DISEASE

SIGNAL SYMPTOMS▶   Fatigue; weight gain or weight loss

Thyrotoxicosis with or without goiter	ICD-9: 242.0
Toxic uninodular goiter	ICD-9: 242.1
Toxic multinodular goiter	ICD-9: 242.2
Thyrotoxicosis from ectopic thyroid nodule	ICD-9: 242.4
Thyrotoxicosis of other specified origin	ICD-9: 242.8
Thyrotoxicosis without mention of goiter or other cause	ICD-9: 242.9
Hypothyroidism, congenital	ICD-9: 243
Hypothyroidism, postsurgical	ICD-9: 244
Hypothyroidism, postablative	ICD-9: 244.1
Hypothyroidism, iatrogenic	ICD-9: 244.3
Hypothyroidism, other acquired/secondary NEC	ICD-9: 244.8
Hypothyroidism, primary NOS	ICD-9: 244.9

Description: Disease of the thyroid can create hypothyroidism or hyperthyroidism. Thyroid nodules are also common. The thyroid gland is a possible site for malignant growth.

Etiology: The most common cause of hypothyroidism is an autoimmune disease that results in gradual destruction of the thyroid gland. The most common cause of hyperthyroidism is Graves' disease, also an autoimmune disease. Cancer of the thyroid is a relatively rare disease, with a low mortality rate.

Occurrence: All thyroid disorders, benign and malignant, are more common in women than in men. Hyperthyroidism is 5 times more common in women and hypothyroidism is 10 times more common. Thyroid tumors occur twice as frequently in women.

Age: The incidence of thyroid cancer has a bimodal and age-specific index with a peak in the 30s, increasing with age after the third decade.

Ethnicity: African-Americans are at a lower risk for thyroid cancer.

Contributing Factors: Radiation to the head and neck increases the probability of thyroid cancer.

Signs and Symptoms: Signs of hypothyroidism are fatigue, lethargy, weakness, cold intolerance, weight gain, and menorrhagia. The woman may also have bradycardia and/or loss of axillary, pubic, and scalp hair. The woman may experience menstrual disturbances, constipation, and/or muscle cramps and weakness. The thyroid gland may or may not be enlarged. TSH level will be elevated and T_4 level low.

Signs of hyperthyroidism include nervousness, increased sweating, heat intolerance, palpitations, fatigue, and weight loss. Symptoms can include change in appetite, decreased menstrual flow, irritability, sleep disturbance. The woman may also have a goiter, tremors, or tachycardia. The thyroid gland may or may not be enlarged. Exophthalmos may be present. T_4 level will be high and TSH level low.

Singular or multiple thyroid nodules may indicate thyroid cancer (see Table 8-6).

Diagnostic Tests

Tests	Results Indicating Disorder	CPT Code
TSH	< or > 10 μ/ml Hyperthyroidism (low TSH) Hypothyroidism (high TSH)	84443
Thyroid T 131 uptake test	Increased (or decreased) uptake Hypothyroidism (decreased uptake) Hyperthyroidism (increased uptake)	84479
Thyroid Ultrasound	Abnormal size, position, structure	76536

Table 8–6 Thyroid Disease

	Hypothyroid	Hyperthyroid
Symptoms	Nonspecific presentation; one third present with cold intolerance, weight gain, dry skin, fatigue, menstrual irregularity	Tremulousness, palpitations, heat intolerance, weight loss, amenorrhea
Laboratory results	High TSH, low T_4 level	Low TSH, elevated T_4 level
Treatment	Thyroid hormone replacement	Antithyroid drugs, beta blockers, radioactive iodine

Differential diagnoses:

- Euthyroid goiter (scintigram)
- Mild transient enlargement of the thyroid gland postpartum
- Benign adenoma

Treatment: Hypothyroidism treatment involves thyroid replacement therapy, usually for life. Hyperthyroidism is treated with medications that interfere with thyroid hormone synthesis, radioactive iodine, or surgery. Thyroid cancer requires surgery.

Follow-up: Thyroid disease requires lifelong medical management. Thyroid testing and medication adjustment occurs at regular intervals throughout the woman's life.

Sequelae: Extremes of thyroid dysfunction are associated with ovulatory and menstrual disturbances. Hypothyroidism can delay puberty and create a state of chronic anovulation. Hyperthyroidism can delay puberty and create amenorrhea and chronic anovulation.

Prevention/prophylaxis: None.

Referral: Endocrine disorders require medical management. Refer any suspected cases of thyroid disease to a physician.

Education: Emphasize the importance of long-term follow-up after diagnosis and referral.

REFERENCES

General

Carr, B, and Blackwell, R: Textbook of Reproductive Medicine. Appleton & Lange, Stamford, CT, 1998.

Goroll, A, et al: Primary Care Medicine. Lippincott, Philadelphia, 1995.

Amenorrhea, Primary

Department of Obstetrics and Gynecology, University of Milan, Italy: A practical guide to the diagnosis and management of amenorrhea. Drugs 52(5):671, 1996.

Marantides, D: Management of polycystic ovary syndrome. Nurse Pract 22(12): 34, 1997.

Redmond, G: Androgens and women's health. Int J Fertil Women's Med 43(2):91, 1998.

University of Michigan Medical School, Chelsea: Evaluation of amenorrhea. Am Fam Phys 53(4):1185, 1996.

Anorexia, Bulimia, and Obesity

Allen, K, and Phillips, J: Women's Health across the Lifespan. Lippincott, Philadelphia, 1997.

Anderson, A: Managing eating disorders in primary care practice. The Clinical Advisor June 2002, pp 31–45.

Bongain, A, et al: Obesity in obstetrics and gynecology. Eur J Obstet Gynecol Reprod Biol 77(2):217, 1998.

Department of Psychiatry, University of South Florida: Eating disorders. Primary Care 29(1): 81, 2002.

Department of Psychology, University of Toronto: Causes of eating disorders. Ann Rev Psychol 53:187, 2002.

McGilley, B, and Pryor, T: Assessment and treatment of bulimia nervosa. Am Fam Phys 57(11):2743, 1998.

Ricchini, W: For your patients: Recognizing eating disorders. Adv Nurse Pract 6(4):25, 1998.

Diabetes

Cooper, S, and Caldwell, J: Coronary artery disease in people with diabetes. Clin Diabetes 17(2):58, 1999.

Harris, M, et al: Prevalence of diabetes, impaired fasting glucose, and impaired glucose tolerance in U.S. adults. Diabetes Care 21(4):518, 1998.

Weiss, J and Scott, L: Stalking the #1 killer of women: detecting diabetes and heart disease, AWHONN Lifelines, Oct-Nov 2001, pp 28–34.

Hirsutism

Ambulatory Care Center, University of Rochester: Hirsutism: diagnosis and management. J Gender Specific Med 42(2):29, 2001.

Department of Obstetrics and Gynecology, The University of Alabama at Birmingham: Idopathic hirsutism. Endocrine Rev 21(4):347, 2000.

Division of Family Medicine, University of California: Approach to patients with hirsutism. West J Med 165(6):386, 1996.

Young, R, and Sinclair, R: Hirsutes I: Diagnosis. Aust J Dermatol 39(1):24, 1998.

Obesity, Hyperlipidemia

Foreyt, J, and Poston, W: Obesity: A never-ending cycle. Int J Fertil Women's Med 43(2):111, 1998.

Leake, N: The heart of the matter. Adv Nurse Practit Jan 2002, 1:42-48.

Martins, I, et al: Smoking, consumption of alcohol and sedentary life style in population grouping and their relationships with lipidemic disorders. Rev Saude Publica 29(1):38, 1995.

Mokdad, AH, et al: The continuing epidemics of obesity and diabetes in the United Sates. JAMA 286:1195, 2001.

Turner, J, et al: Nurse practitioner and client partnership in long term holistic weight management. Am J Nurse Practit 6(6):9, 2002.

U.S. Department of Health and Human Services Public Health Service, National Institutes of Health, National Heart, Lung, and Blood Institute: NIH Publication No. 01-3305, May, 2001.

Walsh, J, and Grady, D: Treatment of hyperlipidemia in women. JAMA 274(14):1152, 1995.

Premenstrual Syndrome

Community Support Program, VA Central Iowa Health Care System: PMS and PMDD in the domain of mental health nursing. J Psychosocial Nurs and Mental Health Services 39(1):16, 2002.

March, D, and Yonkers, K: Premenstrual disorders. Consultations in Primary Care 990: 2001.

Thyroid

Demester, N: Diseases of the thyroid. Clin Rev 11(7): July 2001.

School of Nursing, University of Conneticut: Thyroid disease. J Am Acad Nurse Practit 12(6):226, 2000.

Seltzer, V, and Pearse, W: Women's Primary Health Care. McGraw-Hill, New York, 1995.

Chapter 9
HEMATOLOGIC AND IMMUNE DISORDERS

ANEMIA

SIGNAL SYMPTOM ▶ fatigue

Anemia of chronic disease	ICD-9-CM: 280.0
Atypical (primary)	ICD-9-CM: 285.9
Pernicious anemia	ICD-9-CM: 281.1
Vitamin B_{12} deficiency	ICD-9-CM: 281.1
Folate Deficiency	ICD-9-CM: 281.2
Iron-deficiency anemia	ICD-9-CM: 280.9
Blood loss anemia	ICD-9-CM: 280.0
Hemolytic anemia	ICD-9-CM: 272.4
Sickle-cell anemia	ICD-9-CM: 282.60
Thalassemia	ICD-9-CM: 282.4
Anemia NOS	ICD-9-CM: 285.9
Low Hct	ICD-9-CM: 285.9

Description: Normal hemoglobin levels in women are 12–14 g/dL. The iron requirement increases in women at menarche from 0.7–0.9 to 2.2 mg daily. During pregnancy, blood volume increases beginning as early as the sixth week. Erythropoietin levels increase during pregnancy by 30%. Plasma volume also increases. Normal hemoglobin levels in women who are not pregnant differ from those of pregnant women. A hemoglobin level less than 11.5 g/dL in a woman who is not pregnant and less than 10 g/dL for a pregnant woman is considered low and reflective of anemia.

Etiology: The most common cause of anemia in women is iron deficiency.

Occurrence: Iron-deficiency anemia, an insufficient supply of iron and thus of hemoglobin in the red blood cells of the body, is the single most prevalent nutritional disorder in women. Iron-deficiency anemia affects millions of people worldwide. Of nutritional anemia cases, 85% are iron-deficiency anemia; the remaining 15% are the result of iron deficiency combined with folate and other nutritional deficiencies.

Clinical Pearl: The World Health Organization estimates that 48% of the world's pregnant women are anemic. The majority of these cases are related to iron deficiency.

Age: Infants, small children, adolescents, women of childbearing age, and pregnant women are the most vulnerable.

Ethnicity: Iron-deficiency anemia is seen more commonly in women of Caribbean, Latin American, Asian, Mediterranean, and African descent.

Contributing Factors: Low stores of iron in women are related to menses and pregnancy. It takes about 4 months for adult women to display a drop in hemoglobin after iron stores have been depleted.

Signs and symptoms: Fatigue may be a symptom. Pale skin and pallor of the conjunctivae may be present. Many women with low hemoglobin levels are asymptomatic. Anemia is discovered with screening (see Figure 9–1). The most common time for screening is during pregnancy.

Diagnostic tests:

Tests	Results Indicating Disorder	CPT Code
CBC	Hemoglobin < 12 Hematocrit < 38-47%	85031
Serum iron	<50 µg/dL	83540
Total iron-binding capacity (TIBC)	<300 µg/dL	83550

Differential diagnosis:

- Pernicious anemia (weakness, numbness, confirmed by lab)
- Chronic anemia related to HIV, diabetes, or chronic infection
- Chronic renal failure (creates serious anemia)
- Sickle cell anemia (anemia, reticulocytosis, sickling of anoxic erythrocytes hemogloblin, electrophoresis)

Treatment:

Mild iron deficiency can be treated with change in diet to increase iron intake. If medication is required:

- Give oral iron therapy at 60–180 mg daily.
- Recheck hemoglobin in 2–3 weeks. If no change, further investigation is required.
- Treat pernicious anemia with injections of vitamin B_{12}.
- Give folate, needed during pregnancy and periods of rapid growth, at 1–2 mg daily.

Follow-up: After initiating iron therapy, recheck the hemoglobin level in 2–3 weeks.

Sequelae: None for iron-deficiency anemia if diagnosed and treated.

Prevention/prophylaxis: Periodic screening of hemoglobin levels

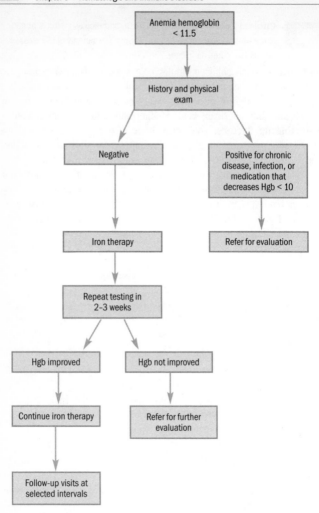

Figure 9–1. Anemia (nonpregnant females).

should be performed on all women with a history of excessive menstrual bleeding. Hemoglobin levels are screened on every prenatal client.

Referral: Women unresponsive to iron therapy should be referred for further evaluation. A common first-line referral is to a gastroenterologist for evaluation.

Education: Women are unlikely to consume via diet adequate amounts of iron. Women in industrialized countries tend to have low iron stores.

Adolescent girls may have a daily iron intake that is very low. These low iron stores set the stage for anemia during pregnancy.

Physiologic iron requirements are three times higher in pregnancy than they are in menstruating women. Folate is also needed during pregnancy for the health of both mother and baby. Establishment of early prenatal care allows for early supplementation of iron and folate.

HUMAN IMMUNODEFICIENCY VIRUS (HIV-1, HIV-2)

SIGNAL SYMPTOMS▶   fever, malaise, opportunistic infections

HIV infection with specified conditions (HIV-1, HIV-2)	ICD-9-CM: 042
HIV infection causing other specified conditions	ICD-9-CM: 043
Other HIV infection	ICD-9-CM: 044
Asymptomatic HIV	ICD-9-CM: V08
AIDS, unspecified	ICD-9-CM: 042.9

Description: Women represent the fastest-growing group of adults with AIDS (symptomatic HIV). Women account for an increasing percentage of all AIDS cases. In 1999, the CDC reported 18% of all cases of AIDS as female. Typically, the woman infected may not progress to the symptomatic stage of the disease for 10 years, although individual variation is wide and the range is 1–20 years.

Etiology: HIV is a viral disease. The CDC estimates that at least 54% of newly diagnosed cases of AIDS in women were acquired through heterosexual sex.

Occurrence: AIDS was first reported in women in 1981. In 1990, it was the sixth leading cause of death in women aged 25–44. The overall AIDS rate in women is lower than in men, at 9.3 per 100,000 woman compared to 32.4 per 100,000 men.

Age: Younger women are disproportionately at risk.

Ethnicity: AIDS is more prominent in African American and Latin American women than in Caucasian women. Of all reported AIDS cases in 1998, 61% of the women were black and 18% were Latina. Reported AIDS cases occur more in the southern part of the country.

Contributing Factors: Poverty, drug abuse (injection with a contaminated needle), victims of violence, sexual contact, contact with infected body secretions, receipt of infected blood. In the AIDS cases reported to the CDC is 1998, many women reported no identifiable risk factor. Heterosexual sex appears to be the method of transmission (see Figure 9–2).

Signs and Symptoms: Three phases of the disease exist:

Acute or primary: This phase lasts 2–12 weeks. Viral replication is high in this phase and viral load is high. Of people infected, 20%–70% report nonspecific symptoms such as fever, malaise,

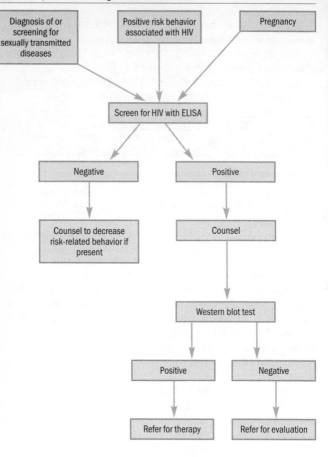

Figure 9–2. Screening for HIV in women.

lymphadenopathy, sore throat, and maculopapular rash on the upper thorax. Plasma is HIV-positive in this phase. Antibody screening is negative.

Clinical latency: This phase lasts for 1–20 years. Viral load decreases. Antibodies become detectable. Replication of the virus occurs primarily in the lymphoid tissue. The women are asymptomatic other than painless lymphadenopathy.

Symptomatic phase: This phase is commonly referred to as AIDS. Symptoms include opportunistic infections, neoplasms, neurologic complications, and severe wasting.

Diagnostic Tests:

Test*	Results Indicating Disorder	CPT Code
Enzyme-linked immunosorbent assay (ELISA)	Positive for infection or exposure	87390 HIV-1 87391 HIV-2
Western blot	Confirms infection with HIV*	86689
CD4 + T-Cell count	Low; count $<350/mm^3$ is one factor used to consider treatment	86360
Plasma HIV RNA (viral load)	High; count $>55,000$ copies/mL is one factor used to consider treatment	

* Informed consent must be obtained prior to HIV testing.

 Clinical Pearl: Women with undiagnosed HIV often present with a gynecologic infection or concern. Abnormal pap smears are present in 40% of HIV-infected women and 58% are infected with HPV. Many undiagnosed HIV-infected women enter the health care system with a sexually transmitted disease.

 Clinical Pearl: Prevalence and incidence of cervical squamous intraepithelial lesions, a precursor for cervical cancer, are strongly associated with HIV as well as HPV. In HIV-infected women, HPV infections are more prevalent and persistent.

Differential diagnosis:

- Epstein-Barr virus infection (positive for Epstein-Barr antibody test)
- Cytomegalovirus (CMV) infection (positive for CMV)
- Mononucleosis (positive monospot)

Treatment: HIV is treated with antiretroviral agents, including protease inhibitors and nucleoside reverse transcriptase inhibitors. A combination of agents is utilized because it is difficult for the virus to develop multiple mutations simultaneously. The goal of treatment is to slow the decline of the immune system.

 Clinical Pearl: Antiretroviral therapy has proven to be highly effective in women. However, women are less likely to use these therapies than men.

Follow-up: HIV infection is a chronic disease. Women infected with the virus are followed carefully throughout their lives.

Sequelae: Progressive immunosuppression results in opportunistic infections (see Table 9–1). Women with HIV have an increased incidence of genital tract neoplasms and a higher mortality rate than men with HIV. Access to care may account for the difference.

Prevention/prophylaxis: Reduction of risk factors. HIV-infected women have an increased susceptibility to sexually transmitted diseases. Sexually transmitted diseases increase susceptibility to HIV. A woman who

Table 9–1 Opportunistic Diseases

CD4 number	Condition
200–500 mm³	Thrush
	Kaposi's sarcoma
	Tuberculosis reactivation
	Herpes zoster
	Bacterial sinusitis/pneumonia
	Herpes simplex
100–200 mm³	*Pneumocystis carinii* pneumonia
	All of the above
50–100 mm³	Systemic fungal infections
	Primary tuberculosis
	Cryptosporidiosis
	Cerebral toxoplasmosis
	Progressive multifocal leukoencephalopathy
	Peripheral neuropathy
	Cervical carcinoma
0–50 mm³	Cytomegalovirus disease
	Disseminated *Mycobacterium avium* complex
	Non-Hodgkin's lymphoma
	Central nervous system lymphoma
	AIDS dementia complex

is diagnosed with any sexually transmitted disease should be counseled about HIV infection and screened for HIV.

Referral: Women diagnosed with HIV require referral to a team centered on the care of HIV-positive women. The team should include medical, nursing, and social services. Women with HIV require special care during pregnancy, during considerations for birth control, and during any infection, including sexually transmitted diseases and pelvic inflammatory disease.

Education: Teaching women to reduce risk-related behaviors including the risks present with heterosexual sex is very important. A partner's desire not to use a condom is a frequently reported reason for inconsistent use. Risk associated with this behavior should be clear at each clinical encounter.

Women should be taught about strategies to reduce heterosexual transmission beyond condom use via methods such as refusing or avoiding unsafe sex or using a female condom.

Early diagnosis and facilitation of care are critical in the care of women and children. Of those treated with combination drugs, 60%–90% have prolonged periods of undetectable levels of HIV RNA. Early identification of HIV-infected women can greatly reduce the number of infected infants. Of HIV infection in infants, 60%–70% occur at delivery; 30% of infections occur earlier in the prenatal course. Prenatal therapy for HIV can reduce transmission by 60%–70%. Pregnancy is a window of opportunity for prevention of vertical transmission. Counseling and referral for testing for all pregnant women is recommended. Breastfeeding, which contributes to the risk of transmission of HIV, accounts for one third to one half of vertical transmission worldwide.

REFERENCES

General
Seltzer, V, and Pearse, W: Women's Primary Health Care. McGraw-Hill, New York, 1995.

Anemia
Beard, J: Iron requirements in adolescent females. J Nutr 130(2S):440, 2000.

Dugdale, M: Anemia. Obstet Gynecol Clin North Am 28(2):363, 2001.

Tapiero, H, et al: Iron: deficiencies and requirements. Biomed Pharmacother 55(6):324, 2001.

Rasul, K: An approach to iron deficiency anemia. Can J Gastroenterol 15(110):739, 2001.

Viteri, F: A new concept in the control of iron deficiency. Biomed Environ Sci 1(1):46, 1998.

HIV/AIDS
Bulterys, M, and Lepage, P: Mother to child transmission of HIV. Curr Opin Pediatr 10(2):143, 1998.

Burger, H, and Weiser, B: Biology of HIV infection in men and women. Clin Obstet Gynecol 44(2):137, 2001.

Cohen, M: Natural history of HIV infection in women. Obstet Gynecol Clin North Am 24(4): 743, 1997.

Ehrhardt A, and Exner, T: Prevention of sexual risk behavior for the HIV infection with women. AIDS 14(Supp 2):s53, 2000.

Hader S, et al: HIV infection in women in the United States. JAMA 285(9):1186, 2001.

Hewitt, R. et al: Women's health. The role of gender in HIV progression. AIDS Reader, 11(1): 29, 2001.

Hoyt, L: HIV infection in women and children. Postgrad Med 102(4):165, 1997.

Korn, A, and Abercrombie, P: Gynecology and family planning care for women infected with HIV. Obstet Gynecol Clin North Am 24(4):855, 1997.

Kreiss, J: Breast feeding and vertical transmission of HIV-1. Acta Paediatr Suppl 421:113, 1997.

Levine, A: Evaluation and management of HIV infected women. Ann Intern Med 136(3):228, 2002.

McDonald, M, and Kessenich, C: HIV/AIDS and women. Lipincott's Primary Care Practice 4(1):66, 2000.

Norse, C, and Butler, K: Perinatal transmission of HIV and diagnosis of HIV infection in infants. Ir J Med Sci 167(1):28, 1998.

Phair, J, and Murphy, R: Contemporary Diagnosis and Management of HIV/AIDS Infections. Handbooks in Health Care, Newtown, PA, 1997.

Chapter 10

PSYCHOSOCIAL DISORDERS

ANXIETY

SIGNAL SYMPTOMS▶ excessive worrying, anxiety, hypervigilance

Anxiety disorder due to (indicate medical condition)	ICD-9-CM: 293.89
Anxiety disorder NOS	ICD-9-CM: 300.0
Panic disorder with agoraphobia	ICD-9-CM: 308.81
Generalized anxiety disorder	ICD-9-CM: 300.2
Panic attack	ICD-9-CM: 300.01
Social phobia	ICD-9-CM: 300.23
Specific phobia	ICD-9-CM: 308.81
Obsessive-compulsive disorder (OCD)	ICD-9-CM: 300.3
Acute stress disorder	ICD-9-CM: 308.3
Post-traumatic stress disorder (PTSD)	ICD-9-CM: 309.81

Definition: Generalized anxiety disorder (GAD) is a chronic and highly prevalent disorder in adult women. Second only to depression in women seeking mental health services, anxiety is two to three times more likely to occur in women than in men. Mild anxiety motivates people to perform well and serves a protective function. Severe anxiety can incapacitate and disable.

Etiology: Anxiety can be situational or general. Anxiety can occur in the form of panic attacks, phobias, or obsessions.

Occurrence: Anxiety is reported by 5% of the general population. The rate is as high as 10% among women 40 years of age and above.

Age: Prevalence for anxiety disorder is low in adolescents and young adults, but increases substantially with age.

Ethnicity: Not significant.

Contributing factors:

- Traumatic events, including domestic violence and sexual assault
- Unemployment
- Chronic medical illness
- Comorbidity with depression

Signs and symptoms: Apprehension, agitation, and heightened arousal are the classic symptoms of anxiety (see Box 10–1).

Somatic complaints occur with anxiety, including fatigue, insomnia, weakness, dizziness, tremulousness, restlessness, palpitations, chest pain, tachycardia, hyperventilation, dry mouth, diarrhea, nausea, and urinary frequency.

Situational anxiety is a normal reaction to an anxiety-provoking situation.

General anxiety is anxiety lasting more than 6 months. The woman does not report being worried about one specific thing. She is fearful and panicked with an impulse to flee. She has a feeling of impending doom.

Panic attacks are often associated with a positive family history. Of people experiencing panic attacks, 80% are women. Panic attacks affect 3% or 4% of women. During a panic attack, the woman experiences palpitations, diaphoresis, shakiness, chest pain, and dizziness. (The hypervigilance associated with panic attacks may mimic cardiac or neurologic disease.)

Phobia is an irrational fear of a specific stimulus. Women will seek to avoid the stimulus.

Obsessive-compulsive disorder (OCD) affects 3% of the population. Obsessions and compulsions impair the ability to function. Obsessions are unwanted thoughts. Compulsions are ritualized repetitive behaviors.

Post-traumatic stress disorder (PTSD) occurs after a traumatic event (outside the range of the normal human experience). PTSD occurs in 17%–30% of women who are exposed to trauma. The

Box 10–1
Symptoms of Anxiety

Tachycardia
Dyspnea
Diaphoresis
Sweating palms
Urinary urgency
Diarrhea
Decreased appetite
Dizziness
Tremulousness
Fatigue
Apprehension
Restlessness
Tension
Difficulty concentrating
Lack of interest
Insomnia

woman re-experiences the event through thoughts or dreams; she also has intrusive memories and flashbacks. She avoids behavior related to the event, and experiences states of hyperarousal (hypervigilance). She may experience panic attacks, and she may have difficulty sleeping. PTSD in women is most closely associated with loss of a loved one and a history of violence. Women are at higher risk for PTSD than men (see Box 10–2).

Diagnostic tests: Psychosocial history should be a part of all history taking, but it should be emphasized in women with somatic complaints that may be related to anxiety.

Differential diagnosis:

- Depression (history of depression)
- Psychosis (history of mental illness)
- Drug effect (history of drug ingestion)
- Diet-related (caffeine, monosodium glutamate [MSG])
- Hyperthyroidism (weight loss, tremor, palpitations, nervousness, thyroid function)

See Box 10–3 for a general summary of the types of anxiety disorders.

Treatment: A combination of psychotherapy, behavioral therapy, and education are indicated for anxiety disorders. Women seek treatment for

---

Box 10–2
Post-traumatic Stress Disorder

Physical harm occurs when something or someone assaults the body. Post-traumatic stress disorder (PTSD) occurs when the mind and emotions are assaulted. The American Psychiatric Association has recognized PTSD as a psychiatric diagnosis since 1980.

The cause of PTSD is defined as an event or series of events that involves actual or threatened death or serious injury or a threat to physical integrity. It might be a natural disaster, an accident, or a human action. Examples include fire, earthquakes, floods, assault, rape, child abuse, and torture. The immediate response to such an event is intense fear, helplessness, or horror. The event may be witnessed rather than directly experienced. The response may begin immediately or may emerge days, weeks, months, or even years later. The symptoms of PTSD include:

- Hyperalertness—defined as being irritable, easily startled, or constantly on guard. Victims sleep poorly, are agitated easily, and have difficulty concentrating.
- Involuntary re-experiencing of the event in the forms of memories, nightmares, and flashbacks. Re-experiencing can be triggered by anything that resembles or recalls the event.
- Emotional numbing—defined as a need to avoid feelings, thoughts, and situations reminiscent of the event.

The risk for the development of PTSD is high when the stress is sudden, unexpected, severe, prolonged, and repetitive, and when it causes physical harm, threatens life, humiliates the victim, or destroys the victim's community and social support system.

Nearly one half of the people with PTSD also suffer from major depression and more than one third from phobias and alcoholism.

Box 10–3
Anxiety Disorders

Generalized Anxiety
    Lasting > 6 months
    Concern over many issues
Panic Attacks
    Extreme anxiety episodically
    Avoidance behavior
Phobia
    Irrational fear of a specific stimulus
Obsessive-Compulsive Disorder
    Obsession, intrusive thoughts
    Compulsion, repetitive ritualistic behaviors
    Symptoms that impair functioning
Posttraumatic Stress Disorder
    History of trauma
    Re-experiencing of trauma
    Avoidance
    Increased arousal

---

anxiety more often than men. Women are most frequently treated with a combination of medication and psychotherapy.

Follow-up: Anxiety disorders require multiple visits for treatment.

Prevention/prophylaxis: Prevention of violence against women.

Sequelae: Substance abuse is a common sequela to anxiety in women. Women who abuse substances show high rates of PTSD (30%–59%).

Referral: Women experiencing anxiety that interferes with functioning should be referred to a source that deals with anxiety disorders.

Education: The use of illicit drugs, prescription drugs, and alcohol to reduce anxiety should be decreased. The source of the anxiety should be discovered in order to reach resolution of the symptoms.

DEPRESSION

SIGNAL SYMPTOMS▶   associated with guilt, anxiety, increased appetite and sleep, weight gain, and comorbid eating disorders.

Depressive disorder, not elsewhere classified	ICD-9-CM: 311
Major depressive disorder, single episode	ICD-9-CM: 262.2
Major depressive disorder, recurrent	ICD-9-CM: 296.3

Definition: Depression is the most common severe mental disorder in women; depression occurs in women twice as often as in men.

Etiology: Depression can be related to genetic, cognitive, social, or economic factors. The genetic factors include neurotransmitter and neuroendocrine functions. Cognitive factors include powerlessness, learned helplessness, and decreased self-concept. Social factors include trauma, abuse, and multiple roles.

Occurrence: Depression affects more than 1 million women in the United States. Approximately 2 million visits to a psychiatrist per year are made by depressed women. Approximately 1 woman in 10 of the women who are diagnosed is severely depressed.

Age: Mean onset of depression in women is 40 years. One half of women initially diagnosed with depression are between the ages of 20 and 50 years of age.

Depression in elderly women is an underdiagnosed and undertreated problem. Depression in the elderly population affects nutrition, activity, and medical treatment. Two thirds of depressed and hospitalized elderly persons are female. All elderly women, particularly those living alone, should be screened for signs of depression.

Depression during adolescence may lead to adverse outcomes later in life. Clinically significant depression should be suspected when adolescents withdraw from their friends and activities, do progressively poorer in school, begin to eat and sleep less or more, and are unable to enjoy things they enjoyed previously.

Ethnicity: Incidence of depression is higher in black women ages 18–24.

Contributing factors:

- Learned helplessness is related to decreased education, decreased socioeconomic level, unemployment, and young age.
- Lack of intimacy has been identified as an important provoking agent that increases the risk for depression in women.
- High levels of recent stress are also predictive of depressive symptoms. Life stress plays a larger role in the provocation of recurrent episodes of depression for women than men.
- Depression in girls ages 14–18 relates to lack of parental support, low self-esteem, and low levels of attachment.
- Depression in women can be related to violence and childhood sexual abuse.
- Depression in elderly women relates to loss of a spouse and lack of physical health.
- Depression can accompany borderline personality, dissociative disorders, eating disorders, substance abuse, and anxiety disorders.
- Depression may be related to infertility, recent surgery, or the postpartum period.

Signs and symptoms: Sadness is the number one symptom of depression, followed by irritability and loss of interest. Depressed women may be preoccupied with physical complaints, may have changes in memory or concentration, and may have disturbed sleep, disturbed appetite, or lack of energy.

Depression can be mild, moderate, or severe.

According to the *DSM-IV-R,* a diagnosis of major depression is made based upon the following (at least five of these symptoms must be present):

- Depressed mood
- Loss of interest in pleasure
- Sleep disturbances
- Significant weight loss
- Psychomotor retardation and agitation
- Decreased energy
- Feelings of worthlessness
- Impaired concentration
- Recurrent thoughts of dying

Diagnostic tests: Careful physical examination including a mental status exam.

Differential diagnosis:

- Chronic fatigue, Lyme disease, fibromyalgia, rheumatoid disease, endocrinopathies.
- Adjustment disorder in which mood is depressed following a significant life stressor. In adjustment disorder, coping mechanisms will develop and the woman will have a depressed mood for less than 6 months.
- Bereavement creates severe depression that persists for less than 6 months.

Treatment: Medications and psychotherapy (see Table 10–1).

Follow-up: Depression must be followed closely during treatment.

Sequelae: Suicide can be a consequence of depression. Every depressed woman must be asked directly about suicide. Does she have suicidal

Table 10–1 Classes of Antidepressants

Class	Generic Name	Brand Name
Tricyclic	Amitriptyline	Tryptizol
	Clomipramine	Anafranil
	Dothepin	Prothiaden
	Doxepin	Sinequan
	Imipramine	Tofranil
	Lofepramine	Gamanil
	Nortriptyline	Allegron
Tricyclic-related	Trazodone	Molipaxin
SSRI	Citalipram	Cipramil
	Fluoxetine	Prozac
	Paroxetine	Seroxat
	Reboxitine	Lustral
SNRI	Venlafaxine	Effexor

SSRI = Selective serotonin reuptake inhibitor—acts on the neurotransmitter serotonin

SNRI = Serotonin and noradrenaline reuptake inhibitor—acts on serotonin and noradrenaline

MAOI = Monoamine oxidase inhibitor—acts on both serotonin and norepinephrine

thoughts? Does she intend to commit suicide? Does she have any plans for suicide? A history of prior attempts and living alone increase the risk for suicide (see Boxes 10–4 and 10–5).

Prevention/prophylaxis: Early diagnosis and treatment of depression may prevent suicide.

Referral: Women who express intent and have a plan for suicide require immediate referral. Any women expressing feelings of complete failure, immobilization, or feeling trapped or paralyzed require immediate referral. All women with severe depression require referral for evaluation and treatment.

Women who are pregnant or wish to conceive and are taking antidepressant medication will require consultation with a medical doctor.

Education: Relief from the stigma of depression is an important goal for women suffering from depression. Women's health providers should encourage compliance with treatment.

INSOMNIA

SIGNAL SYMPTOMS difficulty falling asleep, and difficulty staying asleep

Insomnia	ICD-9-CM: 780.52
With sleep apnea	ICD-9-CM: 780.51
Subjective complaint	ICD-9-CM: 307.49

Definition: Insomnia is defined as difficulty falling or staying asleep that interferes with daytime functioning.

Etiology: Psychiatric disorders such as depression, anxiety, and character disorders account for one half of insomnia complaints. The remaining cases of insomnia, in the general population, are related to chronic pain, drug reactions, sleep apnea, and physical symptoms such as urinary

---

Box 10–4
Risk Factors for Suicide in Women

Age 55–65
History of prior attempts
Living alone
Depression
Unemployment
History of chronic pain, chronic illness
History of recent surgery or terminal illness
Substance abuse
Psychotic history
Positive family history of suicide
Specific plan for suicide formulated

From: Phillip Long, MD, www.mentalhealth.com

Box 10-5
Suicide Risk Assessment

Suicide is almost impossible to predict. There is no test sensitive enough to identify which people are going to kill themselves without intervention. Suicide is now the eighth leading cause of death in the United States. The actual number of suicides, however, is difficult to determine. Statistics are compiled from death certificates, but at times ruling out homicide gets more priority than does establishing suicide. When death is due to falls, automobile accidents, or drug or alcohol overdose, it is very difficult to establish suicide as the motive.

Factors that Contribute to Suicide

- Suicide rates are highest in old age; 40% of suicides are over age 60, and after age 75, the rate is three times higher than the average. The suicide rate in the elderly declined from 1950 to 1980, but has been rising since that time.
- The age group of 15 to 24 now accounts for 20% of male suicide and 14% of female suicide. The rate in this age group has quadrupled since 1950. Suicide attempts are a common reason for hospital admission in people under the age of 35.
- People who have never been married are twice as likely to take their own lives as are currently married people. The highest rate of all is among divorced or widowed people. Suicide is lower in rural areas than in cities. People with strong religious conviction have a lower suicide rate than average. Doctors have a higher rate of suicide and psychiatrists have a higher rate than any other medical specialty.
- The great majority of suicides are in people with mental or emotional disorders. The most common associated diagnosis is depression. One third of schizophrenic patients attempt suicide; 5%–10% succeed.
- Substance abuse can be an instigator of suicide. About 20% of suicides are in alcohol abusers. A drinking binge can lead to suicide, even in nonalcoholics. Illicit drug abusers have a high suicide rate.
- Rates of suicide are high in men who are abusers. Murderers commit suicide. Men who kill women are at particular risk. A "lovers' suicide pact" is often murder and suicide.
- Among the elderly who commit suicide, one half or more suffer from a chronic physical illness. Among adolescents who commit suicide, it is often associated with alcoholism, drug abuse, and family disorganization. Adolescents who commit suicide often suffer from child abuse and neglect. Separation, unemployment, imprisonment, and death are common in families of adolescents who attempt suicide.

Warning Signs of Suicide

- Eight out of 10 people who commit suicide give some sign of intention. People who talk about suicide, threaten to commit suicide, or call suicide hot lines are 30 times more likely to kill themselves than people who do not.
- Suicide attempts are by far the best indicator of a risk for suicide.
- No suicide threat or attempt should be treated casually.

Referral for People Threatening Suicide

Threatening suicide is an important sign. Failure to see the danger in a suicidal threat, failure to take preventive action, and incorrect treatment are bases for malpractice. Take all suicide threats seriously.

Adapted from: Philip Long M.D., Internet Mental Health, *www.mentalhealth.com*

frequency. The National Sleep Foundation reports that, in women, insomnia is largely a result of biological events such as menstruation, pregnancy, and menopause.

The hormonal change associated with sleep disturbance is decrease in estradiol level. Such decreases are associated with poor sleep particularly in women aged 45–49. Hot flashes are associated with poor sleep regardless of whether they occur during sleep.

In some women who report difficulty sleeping, menstrual cycles are regular. These patients report high anxiety, increased hot flashes, and increased depression.

Occurrence: Women are 50% more likely to experience insomnia than men.

Age: Insomnia can occur at any age.

Ethnicity: Black women are significantly more likely to report poor sleep than Caucasian women.

Signs and symptoms: Seventy-one percent (71%) of women report sleep disturbance in the first few and last few days of the menstrual cycle. Just prior to menses and at the beginning of menses, women report difficulty falling asleep, waking up in the middle of the night, and having trouble getting out of bed.

Seventy-nine percent (79%) of pregnant women report disturbed sleep related to heartburn, fetal kicks, and anxiety.

Fifty-six percent (56%) of menopausal women report disrupted sleep with hot flashes as the primary reason for sleep loss followed by the need to urinate. Menopausal and postmenopausal women report trouble falling asleep and waking in the middle of the night.

Diagnostic tests: A positive history is the most important diagnostic test for insomnia. Asking the woman to keep a sleep log may help make the diagnosis. Any history of pain, urinary frequency, and drug use should be explored in relationship to sleep loss.

Differential diagnosis:

- Endocrine disorders (lab evaluation)
- Psychiatric disorders (history)
- COPD (dyspnea, abnormal pulmonary functions studies, low O_2 Sat)
- CHF (history, ECG, lab studies)
- Caffeine withdrawal (history of significant intake of caffeine followed by abrupt removal of the caffeine-containing substances)
- History of panic attacks
- Restless leg syndrome

Treatment

Use medication to reduce insomnia only in severe sleep disorders. Avoid sedatives and hypnotics, especially in the elderly population.

Hormone replacement therapy may assist perimenopausal women with insomnia.

Special pregnancy pillows may assist pregnant women with interrupted sleep.

If anxiety or depression is the reason for insomnia, treatment of these underlying conditions will reduce sleep loss.

Follow-up: Follow-up visits for improvement of insomnia are important. Treatment of underlying conditions should improve insomnia. Pregnancy requires planned napping to "catch up" on lost sleep.

Sequelae: Interference with functioning in the daytime.

Referral: Women who report symptoms of sleep apnea—waking with air hunger—should be referred to a sleep specialist for evaluation.

Symptoms of sleep apnea include: chronic loud snoring, gasping or choking sounds during sleep, excessive daytime sleepiness, automobile- or work-related accidents, personality changes.

Education: Of women with insomnia, 20% use over-the-counter sleep aids, 13% use prescription drugs, and 8% use alcohol to induce sleep. Reduction of the use of alcohol and medications is preferable. Treatment of underlying conditions and counseling regarding good sleep habits is preferable to use of medication whenever possible.

SEXUAL DYSFUNCTION

SIGNAL SYMPTOMS▶   lack of desire, lack of arousal, lack of orgasm

Lack of desire	ICD-9-CM: 302.70
Lack of orgasm (organic)	ICD-9-CM: 607.84

Definition: Interruption or absence of any stage in the sexual response cycle (desire, arousal, orgasm, resolution) can result in sexual dysfunction. Dissatisfaction with a sexual relationship is a common complaint of women. Discomfort with intercourse may have a physical or a psychologic origin (see Figure 10–1 and Box 10–6).

Etiology: Prior negative sexual experiences, fear of sexual failure, interpersonal issues, situational stress, and anxiety.

Women may experience performance anxiety concerning sex.

The *DSM-IV-R* lists six female sexual dysfunctions. These are:

- Hypoactive sexual desire disorder
- Sexual aversion disorder
- Female sexual arousal disorder
- Female orgasmic disorder
- Dyspareunia
- Vaginismus

Occurrence: Unknown.

Age: Sexual dysfunction can occur in any sexually active female.

Ethnicity: Not significant.

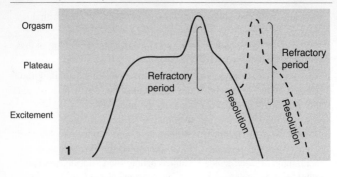

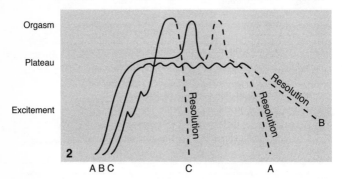

Figure 10–1. Human female sexual response cycle (see Box 10–6 for explanation).

Signs and symptoms:

- Lack of desire related to negative experiences, fear of failure, or interpersonal reasons
- Lack of arousal related to insufficient foreplay, distraction, or undesirable forms of stimulation
- Lack of orgasm related to lack of arousal or inability to achieve an orgasm (may be symptomatic of an underlying problem)
- Vaginismus (may occur following a major trauma such as rape or sexual abuse)
- Lack of vaginal lubrication related to menopause (can make intercourse uncomfortable)

Diagnostic tests:

History of the sexual dysfunction is needed for diagnosis.

Every basic history should include a sexual history. Without a brief and succinct sexual history, it is unlikely the women will reveal information about sexual activity.

Box 10–6
The Female Sexual Response Cycle.

Excitement Phase

This phase begins with sexual stimulation of some sort. As excitement heightens, blood pressure, pulse rate, and respirations increase. Nipples become erect, and breast size increases. A maculopapular rash appears late in the excitement phase. This rash begins in the epigastric region and spreads to include the breasts. Both voluntary and involuntary muscle contraction occurs. The clitoris becomes tumescent and extends out from under the hood. The vagina lubricates, expands and distends; vaginal wall color becomes darker because of the vasocongestion. The uterus partially elevates. The labia majora become vasocongested and move slightly laterally away from the midline.

Plateau Phase

If the excitement phase is not interrupted, sexual tension increases. The nipples become increasingly turgid, and breast size increases. The skin develops a widespread "flush." There is further increase in voluntary and involuntary muscular contraction, and voluntary contraction of the rectal sphincter. Hyperventilation can occur late in the phase. Pulse and blood pressure both increase. The clitoris retracts. There is further increase in the width and depth of the vagina as well as full uterine elevation with cervical elevation. The labia majora become more engorged, and there is vivid color change in the labia minora.

Orgasmic Phase

Involuntary muscle contractions are concentrated in the clitoris, vagina, and uterus. Skin "flush" continues. There is loss of voluntary control. Involuntary contractions of the rectal sphincter occur. Respiration rate increases as high as 40 per minute, heart rate can range from 110 to 180 beats per minute, blood pressure rises; systolic pressure may rise by increments of 30 to 80 mm Hg and diastolic by increments of 20 to 40 mm Hg. Vaginal contractions and uterine contractions occur.

Resolution Phase

After orgasm, sexual tension is dissipated. Breasts detumescence occurs rapidly. The flush disappears. Respiration, blood pressure, and pulse return to normal. A widespread film of perspiration appears. The clitoris returns to normal position. There is rapid detumescence of the vagina, and the uterus returns to its normal position. The cervical os gaps for up to 30 minutes in the resolution phase. Vasocongestion of the labia resolves.

Sample questions include:

- Are you currently in a sexual relationship?
- Are you currently sexual with men, women or both?
- Are you having any sexual problems or concerns?

A detailed account of discomfort with intercourse, lack of desire, or lack of orgasm must be obtained. History of sexual abuse must be obtained.

Current and recent stressors may be related to sexual dysfunction and therefore should be noted.

Complete pelvic examination must be performed.

Differential diagnosis:

- Vaginal infection (positive culture)
- Atrophic vaginitis (dysuria, vulvar and vaginal itching, urinary frequency, blood-tinged vaginal discharge, dyspareunia)
- Urinary tract infection (positive culture, pain on urination, frequency)

Treatment: Education about sexual functioning and the human sexual response cycle. Treatment of any underlying condition, such as anxiety, may be required.

Follow-up: Follow-up visits—including education, treatment, or referral—as necessary. In most cases, sexual dysfunction can be resolved.

Prevention/prophylaxis: Primary prevention of sexual abuse.

Sequelae: None.

Referral: Women with complex sexual problems of a psychologic nature require referral to a sex therapist. Sexual dysfunction that involves both partners requires referral.

Education: Teaching about normal sexual responses and taking the opportunity to answer questions and address concerns often resolves sexual dysfunction.

SUBSTANCE ABUSE AND DEPENDENCE

SIGNAL SYMPTOMS▶   overuse of a substance; change in behavior

Alcohol dependence	ICD-9-CM: 303.90
Alcohol abuse	ICD-9-CM: 305.00
Alcohol intoxication	ICD-9-CM: 303.00
Alcohol withdrawal	ICD-9-CM: 291.8
Drug dependence	ICD-9-CM: 304
Opioid dependence	ICD-9-CM: 304.00
Sedative, hypnotic, or anxiolytic dependence	ICD-9-CM: 304.10
Cocaine dependence	ICD-9-CM: 304.20
Cannabis abuse	ICD-9-CM: 305.20
Sedative, hypnotic, or anxiolytic abuse	ICD-9-CM: 305.40
Opioid abuse	ICD-9-CM: 305.50
Cocaine abuse	ICD-9-CM: 305.60

Definition: Substance abuse is the use of a psychoactive substance not consistent with medical guidelines, or non-medical use of prescription medications. Dependence is the need for repeated doses to avoid feeling "bad," both physically and psychologically.

Despite the fact that the rate of substance abuse and dependence is higher in men than in women, a diagnosis of substance abuse is not gender-specific. Male and female substance abusers are not the same. Women typically begin using substances later than men and they are strongly influenced by spouses or boyfriends to use the abused substance. Women enter treatment earlier than men do. Women have a significantly higher prevalence for comorbid psychiatric diagnoses, such as depression and anxiety.

A critical review of addiction specialty journals conducted in 1995 concluded that researchers commonly use male populations and generalize the findings to both genders. Recent research demonstrates that women become intoxicated after drinking half as much as men, metabolize alcohol differently, develop cirrhosis more rapidly, and have a greater risk of dying from alcohol-related accidents.

Etiology: Genetic, biologic, biochemical, sociocultural, psychologic, and learned behaviors are all components of substance abuse.

Occurrence: Three to five percent of American women have problems with alcohol. A National Health Interview Survey found that 4.3% of women interviewed were alcohol-dependent. A Gallup Poll found that among 26,000 women interviewed, 50% were nondrinkers, 45% were light drinkers, 3% were moderate drinkers, and 2% were heavy drinkers. Of the women who drank, 21% were "binge" drinkers and 4% drank during pregnancy.

In women, alcohol is still the most widely abused drug. Tobacco is the second most frequently used drug. In women, marijuana is the most commonly utilized illicit drug, followed by cocaine. Use of a prescription drug for non-medical reasons frequently occurs in women. Up to 70% of all prescription drugs in the United States are used without a prescription.

Age: Alcoholism can affect women at any age. Little is known about alcohol abuse in women older than 65. Drugs are prescribed disproportionately for older women (2.5 times more often than for older men). Elderly women are approximately 7% of the population, but 17% of psychoactive drug prescriptions are given to them, as are 20% of all prescribed sedatives and hypnotics.

Ethnicity: American Indian women are more susceptible to alcohol-related health problems. Alcohol mortality rates are significantly higher for women who are Native American.

Contributing factors: Alcohol abuse is seen 10% less in women than in men. Smoking rates appear to be about the same in women as in men. There is a minimal difference between men and women in the use of illicit drugs. Men drink more beer in a negative emotional state, particularly loneliness. Women drink more beer and wine when experiencing positive emotions. Women most frequently begin using cocaine in a social situation. Women often begin illicit drug use with their partners.

Signs and symptoms: Withdrawal creates agitation, anxiety, restlessness, tremors, anorexia, and insomnia. Symptoms of alcohol abuse may include excessive use of mouthwash or perfume, frequent complaints of not feeling well, elimination of or change in social interactions, protection of places in the home where alcohol may be hidden, changes in physical appearance, and a positive response to the CAGE questionnaire for screening (see Box 10–7).

Box 10–7
The Cage Questionnaire

Have you ever felt the need to **C**ut down on drinking?
Have you ever felt **A**nnoyed by criticism of drinking?
have you ever had **G**uilty feelings about drinking?
Have you ever taken a morning **E**ye opener?

Women are twice as likely as men to receive prescriptions for tranquilizers, analgesics, barbiturates, and amphetamines. Direct questions related to drug use are required to evaluate drug misuse appropriately.
Diagnostic tests: Careful history of drugs used and amount, frequency, and duration of use. Direct questions such as the following should be asked:

- In the past three months, have you consumed more than five drinks containing alcohol on a single occasion?
- Do you use drugs for recreation?

Alcoholics Anonymous interviews tell us that the disease process of alcoholism progresses in 2.8 years for men, but only 1.1 for women. The number of years from onset to problem drinking is 11 for men and only 3.6 for women. Early diagnosis and referral reduce complications. There appears to be less time to formulate early diagnosis in women.

Screen each woman who abuses substances for anemia, hypertension, diabetes, cancer, liver disease, eating disorders, and dental problems. All women should be screened for smoking. At every opportunity, ask women about their smoking habits.

Test	Results Indicating Disorder	CPT Code
Urine drug screen	Positive for drug tested	80100 (for each drug tested) 80102 (for each drug confirmed)
Breathalyzer or blood alcohol level	Positive for alcohol	82075 (breath) 82055 (BAT)

Differential diagnosis:

- Use of cocaine, marijuana, or opiates must be considered in women with amenorrhea, anovulation, or spontaneous abortion
- Cocaine and opiates can be related to hyperprolactinemia
- Alcohol can affect estrogen and progesterone levels, but the relationship is not well understood
- Bipolar disorder (patient has both manic and depressive episodes)
- Eating disorders (includes anorexia and/or bulimia)

Treatment: Offering brief but specific advice can motivate women to reduce their alcohol intake or reduce their use of drugs. One third of Alcoholics Anonymous participants are women.

Follow-up: Family planning must be discussed with every woman who abuses substances. Carefully follow women who identify themselves as having the ability to quit smoking or drinking or drug use "on their own." Carefully monitor their progress in quitting.

Prevention/prophylaxis: Identification of women with drug and alcohol problems leads to intervention. Complications can be prevented with early intervention.

Women reporting alcohol dependency also report receiving prescriptions for hypnotics and sedatives. Use of alcohol should be questioned prior to prescribing medication. Prescription drugs can be abused and should therefore be prescribed with caution.

Advise all smokers to stop. Supply self-help quitting materials to every woman smoker.

Sequelae: Alcohol abuse takes a great physical toll on women. Female alcoholics have death rates 50% higher than those of men. Causes of death for female alcoholics are suicide, alcohol-related accidents, cardiovascular disease, and cirrhosis of the liver.

Alcohol abuse is associated with hepatitis B infection, gastrointestinal bleeding, malnutrition, and pancreatitis.

Fetal alcohol syndrome is caused by alcohol abuse during pregnancy.

Alcohol impairs judgment and increases risky behavior that can lead to unwanted outcomes.

Cocaine causes abruptio placentae, preterm labor, fetal distress, and stillbirth. Babies are born in withdrawal. Cocaine causes hypertension, respiratory distress, arrhythmias, seizures, psychiatric problems, hyperprolactinemia, menstrual irregularities, and infertility.

Heroin is associated with human immunodeficiency virus (HIV), hepatitis, subacute bacterial endocarditis (SBE), tuberculosis (TB), accidents, suicide, and homicide. Heroin causes central nervous system (CNS) damage, respiratory depression, constipation, and anorexia. Heroin creates the risk of death from overdose. Withdrawal of heroin creates, in 9–15 hours, sweating, increased respiratory rate, increased blood pressure, insomnia, nausea and diarrhea, pain, and drug craving. Of women with AIDS, 27% are intravenous (IV) drug users.

Cigarettes are the leading cause of preventable death in the United States. Cigarettes kill more women than alcohol, drugs, auto accidents, homicides, suicides, and HIV combined. Cigarettes kill through cancer, coronary heart disease (CHD), peripheral vascular disease (PVD), chronic obstructive pulmonary disease (COPD), and intrauterine growth retardation (IUGR). Lung cancer is the most fatal cancer in women. (The lung cancer mortality rate exceeds that of breast cancer.) Cigarettes are related to infertility, peptic ulcers, and skin wrinkling.

Referral: If the patient is pregnant and is abusing a substance, treat the pregnancy as high-risk. Case management and social services are required.

Alcohol and drug dependency can be treated on an inpatient or outpatient basis.

If women cannot stop smoking without assistance, refer to a smoking cessation program. Women who are pregnant and/or raising children require referral to stop smoking.

Education: Women who abuse substances should be educated about HIV, sexually transmitted diseases (STDs), prenatal care, childhood safety and injury prevention, nutrition, and general health.

The following is a list of classes of over-the-counter drugs in order of most frequent sales:

- Vitamins
- Analgesics
- Antacids
- Laxatives
- Agents used to promote sleep

Women use a high proportion of these medications. Careful drug history should reveal inappropriate use of these substances. Education about nonpharmacologic approaches to common discomforts may reduce the intake of these medications.

VIOLENCE AGAINST WOMEN

SIGNAL SYMPTOMS physical and/or mental mistreatment

| Violence against women | ICD-9-CM: 995.81 |

Definition: Violence against women encompasses physical, emotional, and sexual abuse. Perpetrators of these acts may be known to the woman or they may be strangers. Violence against women occurs in all ages, races, socioeconomic groups, educational levels, and occupations.

A recent study demonstrated that homicide is the leading cause of death of women during and after pregnancy. U.S. authors looked at death certificates of reproductive age women and found deaths occurring during pregnancy or within one year after delivery had homicide as the leading cause of death. Integrating violence prevention into every clinical practice is one of the challenges of the twenty-first century.

Etiology: Theories about violence against women arise from sociology, psychology, and feminism. Sociology describes violence as learned behavior. The perpetrator learns to be violent in the family of origin. Psychology discusses pathology related to the abuser. Feminism believes that violence arises in a culture that tolerates such behavior.

Occurrence: Crimes of rape, sexual assault, and physical assault by a perpetrator known to the victim are frequently not reported to law enforcement. Crime surveys conducted by the Justice Department tell us that violent crimes against women are experienced by 2.5 million women annually. The number of women who report these crimes to law enforcement is much lower than 2.5 million. The number of women who seek health care for their injuries is even lower. For example, according to the Justice Department, reporting of rape to the police followed by emergency room examination takes place just 17% of the time.

Women are more frequently victimized by offenders they know than by strangers. Two out of three women who respond to Justice Department surveys report knowing the offender.

Any women can be a victim of violence. Violence against women occurs in all ages and in all socioeconomic groups.

Age: Younger women are at greater risk for sexual assault and domestic violence. Although sexual assault can and does occur against children and elderly persons, it is most likely to occur in women aged 14–24 years.

Ethnicity: International research studies are beginning to appear that address the unique experience of ethnically diverse women who experience intimate partner violence.

Contributing factors: There are many theories as to violence against women as explained previously in the Etiology section. Decreased self-esteem may also be seen in women with abuse in their history. Alcohol and drug abuse may contribute.

Signs and symptoms: Women who are victims of violence do not display particular physical symptomatology. Violence against women by intimate partners is so underreported that little is known about "typical" responses.

Women who have been raped or sexually assaulted may report to law enforcement and may then be escorted to an emergency facility that houses a sexual assault response team. As the number of sexual assault response teams grows throughout America, more information about responses to rape and sexual assault in both the immediate aftermath and in the long term is being collected.

Victims of domestic violence may or may not report their physical abuse to health-care providers. Domestic violence always includes emotional abuse with physical abuse. Sexual abuse occurs with physical and emotional abuse 50% of the time. The woman may be fearful of reporting. She may be fearful of how the abuser will respond to reporting, and she may be fearful of what action the abuser will take when she reports.

Every woman should be screened for domestic violence at every health-care encounter. Direct questions are appropriate. The first question should be a question that frames the question(s) to follow; for example: "So many women are victims of violence that I am now asking all my patients about their safety at home." The second question is more direct. It may be, for example, "Are you safe at home?" or "Does anyone hit you or slap you?" Develop the questions to suit your interview style,

> **Box 10–8**
> *Domestic Violence Screening Questions**
>
> Do you feel safe in your home?
>   Do arguments in your home sometimes get physical?
>   Are you presently in a relationship with a person who threatens you or physically hurts you?
>   Did someone cause these injuries?

*Screening must take place in the absence of the person accompanying the woman.

but ask each woman at every encounter about domestic violence (see Box 10–8).

The woman who has been victimized may display some of the following symptoms:

- Expressions of helplessness and powerlessness
- Symptoms of depression
- Inappropriate affect
- Unclear history of injury
- Multiple injury sites
- Incongruent explanation and examination

Diagnostic tests:

Test	Results Indicating Disorder	CPT Code
Careful history and physical exam	Show indices as described above	General exam code based on documentation
X-ray	Confirm injuries	70000 series, dependent on area affected
CT scan	Confirm injuries	70000 series dependent on area affected
MRI	Confirm injuries	70000 series dependent on area affected

Differential diagnosis:

- Depression (history of depressive disorder)
- Psychiatric disease (history of mental disorder)
- Substance abuse (history of drug or alcohol abuse)

Treatment: Physical injuries are treated as appropriate. Individual and/or group counseling is necessary after victimization.

Follow-up: Keep careful records and photographs of all women when abuse is suspected or reported. Counseling or therapy after victimization requires multiple visits and long-term follow-up.

Prevention/prophylaxis: Primary prevention is accomplished through education. Prevention of violence can be discussed individually or in groups. For example, teaching about dating violence and sexual assault to college and high school populations increases awareness and leads to a decreased incidence of becoming victims of these crimes. High-risk behaviors that may lead to victimization should be discussed at clinical encounters with women. Secondary prevention reduces the incidence of violence in at-risk populations, such as people unable to give consent for sexual activity. Examples include teaching people who work in nursing homes about violence and the elderly.

Tertiary prevention reduces the consequences of adverse effects after violence. Examples include domestic violence shelters and sexual response teams.

Sequelae: One third of all women murdered are murdered by their spouses, former spouses, or boyfriends. Injuries in both domestic violence and sexual assault are usually in the form of contusions, abrasions, and lacerations. More severe episodes can result in fractures, head injuries, and death. Long-term somatic complaints that arise from violence against women include chronic pelvic pain, gastrointestinal symptoms, back pain, and headache.

Psychologic sequelae of violent victimization are PTSD, major depression, alcohol or drug abuse, anxiety disorders, and eating disorders. Sexual abuse among women is associated with depression, anxiety, suicidal ideation, suicide attempts, and PTSD. Physical abuse is associated with depression, anxiety, suicidal ideation, and PTSD.

Referral: In cases of domestic violence, carefully evaluate the woman's strengths, support systems, and safety in her home. Refer all victims of domestic violence to resource centers specializing in domestic violence. All victims of recent sexual assault or rape should be referred to a sexual assault response team. This team will take a history of the event, treat and detect injuries, collect forensic evidence, prevent sexually transmitted diseases and pregnancy, and provide referral resources for follow-up. Victims of rape or sexual assault in the past should be referred to a sexual assault advocacy center.

Education: See Prevention/prophylaxis.

REFERENCES

Anxiety

Breslau, N, et al: Sex differences in posttraumatic stress disorder. Arch Gen Psychiatry 54(110):1104, 1997.

Brown, C: Depression and anxiety disorders. Obstet Gynecol Clin North Am 28(2):241, 2001.

Foa, E: Trauma and women: Course, predictors and treatment. J Clin Psychiatry 58 (Suppl. (9):25, 1997.

Hutchings, P, and Dutton, S: Symptom severity and diagnoses related to sexual assault history. J Anxiety Disorders 11(6):607, 1997.

Najavitis, L, Weiss, R, and Shaw, S: The link between substance abuse, posttraumatic stress disorder in women. Am J Addict 6(4):273, 1997.

Wittchen H, and Hoyer, J: Generalized anxiety disorder: nature and course. J Psychiatry 62(Suppl. 11):15, 2001.

Yonkers, K, et al: Is the course of panic disorder the same in women and men? Am J Psychiatry 155(5):596, 1998.

Depression

Bhatia, S, and Bhatia, S: Depression in women: Diagnostic and treatment considerations. Am Fam Physician 60(1):225, 1999.

Fergusson, D, and Woodward, I: Mental health, education, and social role outcomes of adolescents with depression. Arch Gen Psychiatry 59:225, 2002.

Frank, J, et al: Women's mental health in primary care. Depression, anxiety, somatization, eating disorders and substance abuse. Med Clin North Am 82(2):359, 1997.

Gil-Rivas, V, et al: Sexual and physical abuse: Do they compromise drug treatment outcomes? J Substance Abuse Treatment 14(4):351, 1997.

Koenig, H, and Kuchibhatla, M: Use of health services by hospitalized medically ill and depressed patients. Am J Psychiatry 155:871, 1998.

Kornstein, S: Gender differences in depression. J Clin Psychiatry 58 Suppl (15):12, 1997.

Little, J, et al: How common is resistance to treatment in recurrent, nonpsychotic geriatric depression? Am J Psychiatry 155:1035, 1998.

West, M., et al: Anxious attachment and self reported depressive symptomatology in women. Can J Psychiatry 43(3):294, 1998.

Wyshak, G, and Modest, G: Violence, mental health, and substance abuse in patients who are seen in primary care settings. Arch Fam Med 5(8):441, 1996.

Insomnia

Baker, A, et al: Sleep disruption and mood changes associated with menopause. J Psychosom Res 43(4):359, 1997.

Hall, M, et al: Intrusive thoughts and avoidance behaviors are associated with sleep disturbances in bereavement-related depression. Depression Anxiety 6(3):106, 1997.

Hollander, L, et al: Sleep quality, estradiol levels, and behavioral factors in late reproductive age women. Obstet Gynecol 98(3):39, 2001.

National Sleep Foundation: Sleep Tips for Women. National Sleep Foundation, Washington, DC, 1998.

Prettyman, A: Obstructive sleep apnea: diagnosis and management. Am J Nurse Practit Sept 2001.

Sexual Dysfunction

Allen, K, and Phillips, J: Women's Health across the Life Span. Lippincott, Philadelphia, 1997.

American College of Obstetricians and Gynecologists: Guidelines for Women's Health Care. The American College of Obstetricians and Gynecologists, Washington, DC, 1996.

American College of Obstetricians and Gynecologists: Sexual Dysfunction. ACOG Technical Bulletin. ACOG, Washington, DC, 1995.

Peck, S: The importance of the sexual health history in the primary care setting. JOGN 30(3), 2001.

Substance Abuse and Dependency

Brady, K, and Randall, C: Gender differences in substance use disorders. Psychiat Clin North Am 22(2), 1999.

Greenfield, S: Women and alcohol use disorders. Harvard Rev Psychiatry 10(2): 2002.

Humphries, J, et al: Intimate partner violence against women. Ann Rev Nurs Res 19, 2001.

Stein, M, and Cyr, M: Women and substance abuse. Med Clin North Am 81(4):979, 1997.

Taj, N, et al: Screening for problem drinking: Does a single question work? J Fam Pract 46(4):328, 1998.

Violence against Women

Browne, A: Violence against women by male partners. Am Psychologist 48(10):1077, 1993.

Campbell, J, and Lewandowski, L: Mental and physical effects of intimate partner violence on women and children. Psychiat Clin North Am 20(20):353, 1997.

Horon, I: Enhances surveillance for pregnancy associated mortality, JAMA 285, 2001.

Kroenke, K, and Spitzer, R: Gender differences in the reporting of physical and somatoform symptoms. Psychosom Med 60(2):150, 1998.

Martin, S, et al. Physical abuse of women before during and after pregnancy. JAMA 285(12), 2001.

NPWH: Strategies for enhancing midlife sexuality. Patient Care for Nurse Practitioners, Spring 2002.

Richardson, J, and Feder, G: Domestic violence: a hidden problem for general practice. Brit J Fam Pract 46(405): 1996.

Skinner, C, et al: The coexistence of physical and sexual assault. Am J Obstet Gynecol 172(5):1644, 1995.

Sutherland, C, et al: The long-term effects of battering on women's health. Women's Health 4(1):4170, 1998.

Williams, L: Failure to pursue indications of spousal abuse could lead to tragedy. Can Med Assoc J 152(9):1488, 1995.

Chapter *11*
CONTRACEPTION

BARRIER METHODS

Contraceptive Spermicides and Condoms

Description: The use of a condom and spermicide is a barrier method of preventing pregnancy. Condoms are thin sheaths, most commonly made of latex, that prevent the transmission of sperm from the penis to the vagina. Condoms can vary in texture and color. They are available lubricated or nonlubricated, and can also contain spermicide. Spermicides contain nonoxynol in various bases such as cream, jelly, foam, or suppositories.

The Food and Drug Administration (FDA) has approved a female condom. The female condom is a polyurethane pouch with a ring that, when inserted like a diaphragm, covers the cervix, and another ring that fits over the labia. The condom can be inserted several minutes or several hours prior to intercourse.

Effectiveness: Approximately 70%–94%. Effectiveness is influenced greatly by the skill of the users. The use of spermicide with condoms, provided that both methods are used correctly, has an effectiveness rate in the high 90% range. Latex condoms can be considered effective protection against HIV infection.

Method of action: Condoms, whether male or female, prevent semen from entering the vagina. Spermicide serves as a backup.

Risks and benefits:

- Some women are allergic to latex and therefore cannot use this method.
- Some women are allergic or sensitive to spermicide.
- The use of condoms necessitates interruption of the love-making process.
- Condoms may decrease tactile sensation.
- Condoms and spermicides decrease the risk for sexually transmitted diseases.

- Neither condoms nor spermicide require a prescription or fitting from a provider.
- The retail cost is low; condoms may be purchased at family planning programs at very low cost.

Contraindications: Allergy to spermicide or latex. (Condoms can be purchased that are not made of latex. However, these condoms do not prevent sexually transmitted diseases or HIV.)

Assessment: None required.

Instructions for Use:

- The base in which the spermicide is contained determines the method of use. Manufacturer's instructions should be followed.
- The condom must be applied to an erect penis prior to intercourse. About an inch of the condom should not be applied to the penis, to act as a reservoir for ejaculatory fluid and to prevent breakage. The open end of the condom should be held tightly during withdrawal to prevent spilling the ejaculatory fluid.
- If the condom has torn or slipped off, immediately insert contraceptive foam or gel into the vagina. Postcoital contraception can be used (two combined estrogen and progesterone pills [50 mg] as soon as possible, and two more 12 hours later).
- Store condoms in a cold, dry, and dark place. Condoms can be stored in a wallet for up to 1 month.
- Condoms should be used only once.
- Oil-based preparations such as mineral oil, baby oil, etc., should not be used with condoms, since these preparations damage the latex (see Patient Instructions for Contraceptive Spermicides and Condoms in Appendix B).

Follow-up: None is required or recommended unless the woman has expressed difficulty with use of this method.

Referral: None.

Cervical Cap

Description: The cervical cap is a barrier method of contraception in which a latex or silicone dome fits over the cervix. The cap comes in various sizes.

Effectiveness: The cervical cap, when used consistently, is very effective in preventing pregnancy. It is as effective as a diaphragm and in some users more effective.

Method of action: The dome fits tightly over the cervix and prevents the entry of sperm into the os.

Risks and benefits:

- Can be used with or without spermicide.
- Can be left in place for several days (user should wait at least 6 to 8 hours after last intercourse before removing cap). Cervical caps are comfortable and create less chance of bladder infection.

- Not all women can be fitted with a cap.
- Not all women can be taught to insert and remove the cap.
- There is a lack of practitioners trained to fit cervical caps.
- Latex cervical caps are imported from England and are issued in sizes 22, 25, 28, and 31.
- Silicone cervical caps are thinner than latex, non-allergenic, and come in two sizes.

Contraindications: Abnormal Pap smear, cap cannot be fitted, abnormal appearance of the cervix.

Assessment for appropriateness:

- The cervical cap should be fitted when the woman does not have menses. (CPT code: 57170)
- The woman must have a history of normal Pap smears, with the most recent Pap smear done on the date of cap fitting according to the FDA. (CPT code: 88142 – Pap Smear)
- A history of toxic shock should be ruled out prior to fitting.
- Previous cervical surgery may interfere with fitting.
- Caps should not be fitted until 6 weeks after vaginal delivery.
- Pelvic examination should include observations for cervical abnormalities and infection.
- The size, shape, position, and length of the cervix should be observed.
- The presence of uterine prolapse, cystocele, or rectocele should be noted on bimanual examination. The presence of pelvic relaxation may interfere with fitting.

Instructions for Use

1. During fitting, place the appropriate cap on the woman's cervix.
2. Evaluate the suction of the cap.
3. Re-evaluate the suction after at least 5 minutes.
4. Assess the coverage of the cap over the cervix.

The woman must practice inserting and removing the cap until she is confident in her ability to do so without the provider (see *Using a Cervical Cap* in Appendix B).

Follow-up: A visit for questions and comments after the cap has been used is encouraged.

Referral: Abnormal pelvic exam or Pap smear requires referral.

Diaphragm

Description: The diaphragm is a barrier contraceptive device made of latex and rubber that, when placed in the vagina, prevents pregnancy by covering the cervix. Diaphragms are made with various types of springs within a flexible rim and are available in various sizes and styles.

Effectiveness: Greatly affected by the woman's ability to use the diaphragm correctly, but the range is 80%–95%.

Method of Action: A diaphragm is held in place by the symphysis pubis and the posterior vaginal fornix. The diaphragm is used with spermicidal cream or jelly. The diaphragm covers the cervix and prevents sperm from entering the os. The spermicide acts as a backup for any penetration of sperm beyond the barrier.

Risks and benefits:

- Barrier methods have minimal side effects.
- Some women cannot be fitted well with a diaphragm, and some cannot be taught to correctly insert and remove the diaphragm.
- Diaphragms are associated with an increased incidence of bladder infection because of the pressure of the rim against the urethra.
- Toxic shock syndrome has been reported in women using the diaphragm during menses.
- Women can be sensitive or allergic to spermicide used with a diaphragm.
- A diaphragm is used until signs of wear indicate a need for replacement, or the woman gains or loses 20 lb., or delivers a child vaginally.
- Diaphragms are an economical means of birth control. After the initial investment in the diaphragm and the fitting, maintenance involves the purchase of spermicide.

Contraindications: Some women cannot be properly fitted with a diaphragm. Some women are uncomfortable with the idea of insertion and removal of a diaphragm.

Assessment for appropriateness:

- A diaphragm should fit snugly between the posterior fornix, the pubic symphysis, and the lateral vaginal walls. (CPT code: 57170)
- It should not create pressure or discomfort.
- The woman should be able to demonstrate proper insertion and removal.
- A diaphragm must be fitted with the assistance of a health-care provider.
- A diaphragm should be fitted after confirmation of a normal pelvic examination and Pap smear (CPT code: 88142).

Instructions for Use:

1. Insert prior to intercourse and remove no sooner than 6–8 hours after intercourse.
2. The diaphragm should be used with a spermicide designed for use with a diaphragm.
3. The diaphragm should be resized if significant weight loss or gain— more than 20 lb—or vaginal delivery occurs.
4. The diaphragm should be cleaned with soap and water, dried, and kept in a designated container between uses.
5. A new application of spermicide should be used prior to repeated intercourse.
6. The diaphragm should not be left in place more than 24 hours.

See *Using a Diaphragm* in Appendix B.

Follow-up: A follow-up visit after the woman has used the diaphragm is advised for questions or concerns.

Referral: Abnormal pelvic examination or Pap smear would require referral.

Today's Sponge

Description: The sponge is an over-the-counter, non-hormonal, woman-controlled contraceptive. It is a doughnut-shaped cervical barrier that prevents pregnancy by releasing the spermicide nonoxynol-9.

Effectiveness: The effectiveness reported by the manufacturer is 90%. It is as effective in preventing pregnancy as the condom but less effective than birth control pills.

Method of action: The sponge acts as a barrier over the cervix, and releases nonoxynol-9.

Risks and benefits:

- Sold over-the-counter
- Can be inserted as long as 24 hours before intercourse
- Can be left in place for multiple acts of intercourse
- Effective for 24 hours
- Minimal side effects

Assessment for appropriateness:

- Any woman who is not sensitive to nonoxynol-9 can use the sponge.
- The sponge does not protect against sexually transmitted diseases.

Instructions for use:

- The sponge is moistened and inserted into the vagina and over the cervix prior to intercourse.
- The sponge may be inserted up to 24 hours prior to intercourse.
- The sponge is effective for up to 24 hours.
- The sponge is removed after intercourse and discarded.

Follow-up: None required.

Referral: None required.

INTRAUTERINE DEVICES

Description: An intrauterine device (IUD) is a foreign body placed in the uterus to prevent pregnancy by causing a change in the cellular makeup of the endometrium.

Effectiveness: Rate of failure is 0.5%–2.9%.

Method of action: Exactly how an IUD prevents pregnancy is unknown. Hormonal surveillance for early pregnancy loss has not supported the hypothesis that IUDs act as abortifacients. A scarcity of viable sperm in the fallopian tubes has been noted in IUD users. Non-medicated IUDs produce a sterile inflammatory action that prevents sperm from reaching the fallopian tube.

One of the current IUDs available releases progesterone at a rate of 65 mg per day. The device is designed from a vinyl acetate copolymer with barium sulfate that makes it radiopaque. This progesterone-releasing IUD has a first-year failure rate of 2.9% and must be replaced annually because of depletion of the hormone reserve.

The most recently developed copper IUD is the Paraguard Cu 380A, the only available copper IUD. This device, with a first-year failure rate of 0.5%, has been approved by the FDA for 10 years of use. Other types of IUDs are being investigated including a levo-norgesterol releasing IUD.

Risks and benefits:

- Ease of compliance.
- Increased incidence of PID in users of IUDs.
- Uterine perforation at the time of the insertion.
- Increased incidence of second-trimester abortion in women conceiving with an IUD in place.
- Risk of premature delivery, low-birth-weight babies, and stillbirth increases when an IUD is not removed during the first trimester of pregnancy.
- Iron supplementation may be required for women who experience heavy menses.
- The risk of expulsion is 1.2%–7.1%. Most expulsions occur within the first three menstrual cycles.
- Increase in dysmenorrhea associated with the use of an IUD.
- Less expensive per year than hormonal methods.

Absolute Contraindications:

- Acute pelvic infection
- Known or suspected pregnancy
- Malignant disease of the cervix or uterus
- Undiagnosed vaginal bleeding

Relative Contraindications:

- Multiple sex partners
- History of PID
- History of ectopic pregnancy
- Abnormal uterine bleeding
- Abnormal Pap smear
- Impaired response to infection
- Impaired coagulation response
- Emergency treatment not readily available
- Heart disease (susceptible to bacterial endocarditis)
- Endometriosis
- Fibroids or bicornate uterus
- History of dysmenorrhea or menorrhagia
- Allergy to copper
- Anemia

Assessment for appropriateness:

- An IUD should be inserted during menses (CPT code: 58300).
- Complete physical exam is necessary prior to insertion.
- Negative Pap smear is required (CPT code: 88142).
- Negative cervical cultures of gonococci and *Chlamydia trachomatis* are required (CPT codes: 87850 and 87110).
- Hemoglobin and hematocrit levels must be within normal range (CPT code: 85025).
- The woman must be at least 6 weeks postpartum.

Instructions for use:

Insertion technique:

1. Bimanual exam is performed to determine position and size of uterus.
2. The vagina and cervix are cleansed with a povidone-iodine (Betadine) solution.
3. The uterus is sounded (must be 6 cm or more).
4. The IUD is inserted per manufacturer's instructions.
5. After insertion, the woman is observed for hypotension and syncope.
6. If the woman has mild cramping, any prostaglandin inhibitor in a dosage from 400–800 mg can be prescribed.
7. The woman is instructed not to have intercourse or use tampons for 7 days after insertion.
8. The woman must learn to feel the string that protrudes into the vagina. She must check for placement of the string frequently in the first few months of use and thereafter, after each menses (see *Intrauterine Devices* in Appendix B).

Warning Signs:

P Period late
A Abdominal pain or pain with intercourse
I Infection exposure or abnormal discharge
N Not feeling well, particularly fever and chills
S String missing

Follow-up: A follow-up appointment is made for 6 weeks after one menstrual cycle to rule out complications and to verify placement of the IUD.

Complications:

- During insertion, a severe vasovagal response can occur. A physician must be immediately available. Blood pressure and pulse must be monitored after insertion until the woman is stable. Oxygen can be given as needed. Use of atropine as per physician protocols
- Excessive bleeding or cramping may indicate perforation. Physician consultation is required for management.
- Missed menses requires elimination of pregnancy as a cause. The IUD must be removed when pregnancy is diagnosed.

- Breakthrough bleeding can occur. The IUD is removed only if hematocrit is less than 30 and/or the IUD is partially expelled, or the woman desires its removal.
- Cramping and pelvic pain can occur. If the IUD is partially expelled, it must be removed.
- PID must be ruled out as a reason for cramping and bleeding. If the woman is infected, she must be treated, cultured, and the IUD removed. The IUD is not to be reinserted for at least 3 months after treatment of infection.
- Spontaneous abortion must be ruled out when cramping and pelvic pain occur.
- Expulsion of the IUD has occurred if it is seen in the cervical os or vagina; if the string is lengthened, indicating partial expulsion; or the string is absent. If the IUD is partially expelled, it can be removed and replaced if the woman desires. Lost IUDs or no visualization of the device or the string requires physician consultation. If the IUD cannot be visualized at all, a physician consultation is required before an IUD can be reinserted.

Referral: Physician availability during insertion is required. Physician consultation for IUD complications is recommended.

ORAL CONTRACEPTION AND CONTRACEPTIVE VAGINAL RING

Description: Oral contraceptives (OCs) combine synthetic estrogen and progesterone to be taken orally to prevent conception. The tablets are consumed daily for 21 days, after which there is withdrawal menstrual bleeding. Women can choose to take an inert pill for the 7 days that the combination of estrogen and progesterone is not taken. There are a few progesterone-only contraceptive pills available.

One of the most promising new contraceptives is the combination ethinyl estradiol and norethindrone vaginal ring. Contraceptives are released continuously through a small Silastic ring at a rate of 20 µg per day of estrogen and one mg per day of progesterone.

Effectiveness: If taken as directed, oral contraceptives are almost 100% effective. If taken correctly, only 1 in 1000 women become pregnant.

Method of Action: Suppression of ovulation is the major method of action. Additional factors include altering the endometrium to make it unreceptive to implantation and altering cervical mucus to make penetration by sperm more difficult.

Benefits and risks of oral contraceptives:

There are numerous research-based noncontraceptive benefits of oral contraceptives (OCs):

- OCs protect against both ovarian and endometrial cancer. A protective effect (40% reduction) has been observed with as little as 3–6 months of use. Further declines in risk are accompanied by longer periods of use. The protective effect can last up to 15 years after consuming the last pill.

- OCs have a protective effect against benign breast disease, salpingitis, ectopic pregnancy, dysmenorrhea, and iron deficiency anemia.
- Fewer menstrual disorders, for example, menorrhagia, irregular menstrual bleeding, or intermenstrual bleeding, occur in OC users. OCs also improve primary dysmenorrhea.
- OCs can decrease acne by lowering serum testosterone levels.
- Risk of venous thrombosis in OC users is age- and weight-related. The WHO found age (over 35) and weight (obesity) to be the significant risk factors for venous thrombosis in OC users.
- OCs confer little or no risk of cardiovascular disease, particularly among women who are nonsmokers.
- The risk for MI in women OC users is related to age (over 40) as well as cigarette smoking and diabetes.
- There is a small increased risk of the development of breast cancer in OC users. This small risk continues for approximately 10 years after discontinuing the OCs.
- The cost of OCs varies greatly by manufacturer and distributor. The high cost of OCs in many pharmacies may prompt some women to discontinue the method.
- Depression (sometimes severe) and other mood changes may occur in women on OCs.

Risks and benefits of vaginal ring delivery:

- The ring is easily placed by the wearer into the upper vagina.
- The ring is worn for three weeks and removed for one week during which menses will occur. Breakthrough bleeding is reported to be minimal.
- The ring can be removed during sexual relations and replaced afterward if desired.
- Transient nausea associated with the ring can be reduced by overnight soaking of the ring before insertion.
- Vaginal discharge occurs in a small portion of users.

Contraindications: Personal history—not a family history—of:

- Thrombus or embolus
- Cerebrovascular accident
- Coronary artery disease
- Known or suspected carcinoma of the breast, uterus, cervix, or ovaries
- Disease of the liver (normal liver function studies for at least 1 year after disease process, prior to use of OCs)
- Pregnancy

Relative Contraindications:

- Migraine headaches
- Hypertension
- Mononucleosis

- Undiagnosed vaginal bleeding
- Elective surgery planned within first OC cycle
- Major injury to lower extremities
- 40 years of age or older coupled with another risk factor
- 35 years of age coupled with heavy smoking
- Diabetes
- Gallbladder disease
- Sickle cell disease
- Delivery within the past 10–14 days
- Cardiac or renal disease
- Lactation
- Smoking
- Elevated cholesterol

Assessment for appropriateness:

Test	CPT code
Pap smear	88142
General health panel	80050
Lipid panel	80061
Fasting blood sugar	Included in General Health Panel if done first thing in morning
Liver profile	80076

The woman should have a complete physical exam and Pap smear within 1 year of the prescription. In 1993, the FDA voted in favor of giving women an option to delay pelvic examination without being denied a prescription for OCs. Pelvic examination may be performed at follow-up examination.

1. Complete personal and family medical history.
2. Laboratory profile should include a lipid screen in women who have an immediate family member with hypertension under age 40 on medication, or with a family history of vascular disease or myocardial infarction (MI).
3. Fasting blood sugar should be considered if a family member is diabetic.
4. Liver profile should be considered if the woman has a history of hepatitis or other liver disease or she has a history of drug or alcohol abuse.

Instructions for use:

1. Begin oral contraceptives at onset of menses. One tablet is taken daily for 21 days at approximately the same time of day. Following the 21 days, no tablets or one inert tablet daily is consumed for 7 days. OCs are resumed on a daily basis after the 7 days of rest or inert tablets.
2. A backup method should be utilized if the woman runs out of pills, forgets to take a pill, discontinues the pill, and/or desires protection from sexually transmitted diseases.

3. There is a high rate of discontinuation of OCs. No more than 50%–75% of women who start using OCs are still using them after 1 year. Many women become pregnant after discontinuing OCs. Women who discontinue usually do so for non-medical reasons. For this reason, teaching a second method of birth control at the time of teaching about OCs is recommended.

4. If the patient misses one pill, she should take the tablet as soon as remembered. If two or three pills are missed, a backup method must be employed.

5. If the woman smokes, she should stop smoking.

Early Warning Signs:

A Abdominal pain—severe

C Chest pain

H Severe headache

E Eye problems

S Severe leg pain

Follow-up: After two or three cycles of OCs, blood pressure and weight should be taken and side effects and symptoms reviewed with the patient. Menstrual history on OCs should be reviewed.

Complications:

- Amenorrhea can occur with the use of OCs. If this occurs, pregnancy should be ruled out. When pregnancy is ruled out, reassurance can be provided or a change of OCs considered.
- Breakthrough bleeding on the first or second package of OCs is a common occurrence. If the bleeding persists longer than the first or second package or the breakthrough bleeding is significant in amount and frequency, a change in OCs is indicated. Breakthrough bleeding should be diagnosed after infection and pregnancy have been ruled out.

Referral: Physician consultation is required for the following:

- Change in vision
- Numbness
- Chest pain
- Possible phlebitis
- Severe recurrent headaches or new headaches
- Increase in blood pressure with a diastolic pressure of more than 90 mmHg
- Severe fluid retention
- Depression
- Scheduled surgery
- Development of any of the contraindications to taking the OC

Trends: Today, the most widely used preparations are low-dose pills containing 35 mg of estrogen or less combined with lower doses of progestins. The FDA recommends that women use pills containing the lowest effective amount of estrogen. Most recent clinical trials of 20 mg of estrogen OCs show a pregnancy rate that is no different than with 35-mg pills. This is because of the synergistic effect of estrogen with progesterone. Using 20-mg pills requires diligence in taking OCs at the same time each day. Benefits of 20-mg pills and incidence and management of side effects are under investigation.

Myths:

- Weight gain. Studies show that as many young women lose weight as gain weight on OCs.
- Taking a rest. There is no evidence to support the idea that women need a "rest" from OCs. "Taking a break" may lead to unwanted pregnancy and an increase in side effects.
- Infertility. There is no evidence that OCs cause permanent infertility. There may be a temporary delay in conception after the use of oral contraceptives.

Drug Interaction: Drugs that may reduce OC efficacy are antituberculosis medications, antifungals, anticonvulsants, and antibiotics. Drugs whose activities may be modified by OC use include analgesics, anticoagulants, antidepressants, tranquilizers, anti-inflammatories, bronchodilators, antihypertensives, and antibiotics. If a woman is on any of these medications concurrently with OCs, consultation is suggested.

INJECTABLE CONTRACEPTION

Description: Depo-medroxyprogesterone (DMPA) is progesterone that prevents ovulation by suppressing FSH and LH levels and eliminating the LH surge. This drug must be injected every 3 months IM. Women in whom estrogen is contraindicated can use DMPA, approved for contraception by the FDA in 1992.

Lunelle is marketed in the United States as a single-use ampule containing progesterone and estradiol. Lunelle is injected IM monthly.

Effectiveness: Failure rate is up to 0.7% for DepoProvera and up to 0.1% for Lunelle. These are extremely low failure rates compared to other highly effective contraceptives.

Method of Action: DMPA, a long-acting, injectable contraceptive progesterone, is delivered in microcrystals suspended in an aqueous solution that slowly dissolves and releases the drug into the body. Contraceptive levels of progesterone are maintained for up to 4 months following injection. In women using DMPA, circulating levels of progestogen block the LH surge; thus, the method works by suppressing ovulation. Secondary mechanisms of action include thickening of the cervical mucus and altering of the endometrium.

Lunelle suppresses ovulation with the estrogen component creating bleeding patterns that are similar to those in women not using hormonal methods of contraception.

Benefits and risks:

- Return to fertility may be delayed with DMPA regardless of the duration of use. In contrast, return to fertility occurs rapidly after discontinuation of Lunelle.
- Menstrual changes are reported with both injections. Almost one half of users of DMPA report amenorrhea, with most of the remaining reporting irregular bleeding and spotting. The majority of Lunelle users report regular menses. However, users of Lunelle report more bleeding and spotting days than users of OCs.
- Small weight gain may occur with both of these medications. Most weight gain reported is less than 1 kg.
- No increase in depression has been reported with these injections.
- Decreased libido has been reported.
- There appears to be no increased risk for breast cancer among users.
- These medications help prevent endometrial cancer, iron deficiency anemia, and ectopic pregnancy.
- No alteration in coagulation has been reported.
- No unfavorable impact on blood pressure has been reported.
- Because these injections suppress ovarian production of estradiol, bone density may be affected.
- No increased risk of stroke, MI, or venous thrombosis has been reported.
- An office visit is required for injection every month or 3 months.
- Cost of DMPA equals that of oral contraceptives.
- No demonstrated drug interaction between DMPA and antibiotics
- No adverse effect on lactation
- Can be started 1–4 days post-partum

Contraindications:

- Known or suspected pregnancy
- Unexplained vaginal bleeding

Relative contraindications:

- Pregnancy planned in the near future (for DMPA)
- Concern over weight gain
- Concern over irregular menstrual flow

Assessment for appropriateness:

- Pap (CPT code: 88142) and pelvic examination should be completed prior to injection of DMPA.
- Pregnancy must be ruled out prior to administration (CPT code: 84702 serum pregnancy test).
- DMPA can be administered after delivery.

See also Box 11–1.

Instructions for Use: A 150-mg dose of DMPA is administered IM every 12 weeks. There is a two-week grace period, according to the manufacturer. The first dose is given during the first 5 days of a menstrual cycle.

> **Box 11–1**
> ### Clinical Situations in Which DMPA Should Be Considered
>
> Lactation (begin with 6 weeks)
> Smokers
> Diabetes
> Lipid disorder
> Migraine headache

Lunelle is given every 28 days. The manufacturer gives a grace period of five days. These medications should be given IM with a 1 to 1.5 inch 21- to 23- gauge needle in the gluteus or deltoid. The anterior thigh is also suitable for Lunelle.

Warning signs:

- Weight gain
- Headaches
- Heavy bleeding

Follow-up: Every 1 to 3 months for injection and evaluation of side effects

Complications:

- Amenorrhea
- Weight gain, breast tenderness, and menstrual irregularity can occur during use of DMPA. These symptoms may persist for 6–8 months after discontinuing the medication.
- Return to fertility may be delayed for 6 months to 1 year after discontinuing DMPA.
- Almost all women using DMPA will experience spotting or irregular or prolonged bleeding, particularly during the first few months of use.

Table 11–1 Timing of First and Subsequent Injections

First Injection	DMPA	MPA/E$_2$C
• Spontaneous menses • Elective abortion • Delivery	• Within 5 days • Within 7 days • Within 3 weeks if not lactat- ing, within 6 weeks if lactating	• Within 5 days • Within 7 days • 21–28 days PP non- lactating
Switching from OCs	While taking active pills or within 7 days	While taking active pills or within 7 days
Switching from Norplant	Any time within 5 years	Any time within 5 years
Switching from DMPA	—	Within 13 weeks of last injection
Switching from MPA/E$_2$C	Within 35 days of last injection	—
Subsequent Injections		
Intersol	Every 12 weeks	Every 28 days
Grace period	2 weeks (pregnancy test prior to giving if more than one week)	Plus or minus 5 days

Referral: Management strategies for irregular bleeding can vary from simple reassurance to the use of estrogen. One or two cycles of OCs or a nonsteroidal anti-inflammatory drug other than aspirin can help stabilize the endometrium and stop the bleeding. Ibuprofen 800 mg three times daily for 5 days has been demonstrated to help reduce bleeding in some women. Anaphylactic reactions to DMPA are rare but have occurred immediately following injection. Emergency support measures such as epinephrine, steroids, and diphenhydramine should be available.

SUBDERMAL IMPLANTS

Description: A subdermal implant is progesterone (levonorgestrel) contained within nonbiodegradable silicone rubber capsules, designed to be placed under the skin of the arm, that release a progestin at a constant rate over 5 years.

Effectiveness: 99% effective for 5 years.

Method of action: The capsules that make up the system release progestin on an average of 30 mg daily into the bloodstream. The progesterone suppresses ovulation, thickens the cervical mucus, and alters endometrial proliferation. Norplant 11 has been approved by the FDA. Norplant 11 involves only two rods which are slightly longer but of the same diameter. Norplant 11 provides contraception for three years.

Risks and Benefits:

- Menstrual irregularities, including prolonged bleeding, spotting, and amenorrhea, can occur. These changes in menses are seen predominantly in the first year of use.
- Weight gain or loss, nausea, and depression have been reported.
- Infection at the implant site is uncommon, as is expulsion of the capsules.
- Fertility promptly returns to preinsertion levels once implants are removed.
- Women users must desire long-term contraception.
- A health-care provider must insert and remove the capsules.
- Initial economic investment is high. The cost over a 5-year period equals other hormonal contraceptives; 76%–90% of women continue to use the method after the first year; 33%–78% complete the 5 years.
- Subdermal implants are immediately reversible.
- Subdermal implants do not affect lactation.

Contraindications:

- Thromboembolic disease
- Acute liver disease
- Breast cancer
- Undiagnosed vaginal bleeding
- Pregnancy
- Cardiovascular disease
- Diabetes
- Heavy smoking

Assessment:

- History to rule out contraindications
- Physical examination including Pap smear (CPT code: 88142)
- Review of risks and benefits
- Explanation of insertion and removal techniques

Instructions for use: Clinical instruction is required for insertion of subdermal implants. The implants are inserted in the upper arm about 8–10 cm above the elbow.

Insertion (CPT code: 11975)

1. An insertion graph is used to guide cleansing with antiseptic solution.
2. The area is anesthetized.
3. Small incisions are made with a scalpel.
4. A trocar is inserted at a shallow angle.
5. The obturator is removed and loaded with a capsule.
6. After all capsules are loaded, the incisions are closed with Steri-Strips.
7. The insertion site is covered with dry compresses and gauze is wrapped around the arm.

Removal (CPT code: 11976)

1. Local anesthetic is applied to the area.
2. One small incision is needed to remove all of the implants.
3. Removal takes up to 30 minutes.
4. New implants may be inserted at this time.
5. Women who are susceptible to scarring may have a scar after removal.

After subdermal implants have been in for five years (or less) they must be removed, because they become ineffective. Removal requires local anesthesia and one or more small incisions.

The insertion site should be kept dry for 3–5 days. Implants become effective within 24 hours of insertion. Implants do not protect against STDs. Implants must be replaced every 5 years. See Patient Instructions for Subdermal Implants in Appendix B.

Warning signs:

- Severe lower abdominal pain
- Heavy vaginal bleeding
- Arm pain
- Pus or bleeding at the insertion site
- Delayed menstrual periods after an interval of regular menses
- Migraine headache

Follow-up: A follow-up visit for evaluation is scheduled for approximately 2 weeks after insertion. A repeat visit is scheduled at 3 months after insertion for evaluation of side effects and problems.

Complications:

- Inability to insert or remove implants correctly
- Hypermenorrhea

- Headaches
- Mastalgia
- Galactorrhea
- Acne

Referral: Women diagnosed with the following require consultation prior to insertion: hyperlipidemia, hypertension, migraine headaches, or use of anticonvulsants.

Drug Interaction: Anticonvulsants increase the failure rate of subdermal implants.

STERILIZATION

Description: Sterilization is surgical intervention to permanently prevent pregnancy. Sterilization can be performed on a man or a woman (see Table 11–2). For female sterilization, the most common method is access to the tubes by laparoscopy and application of bands or clips to each tube. This method is indicated for women who desire irreversible contraception.

Effectiveness: Failure rate is 1.9%.

Method of action: Surgical prevention of conception.

Risks and benefits: In the United States, sterilization is the leading method of contraception chosen by married individuals (both female and male); 26% of American women rely on sterilization for birth control, and 33% of women between ages 35 and 44 use sterilization as their method of birth control.

- Highly effective, permanent method of birth control.
- Menstrual dysfunction may occur after sterilization, and may be related either to discontinuing oral contraceptives or to the sterilization process itself. Research has proposed that changes in menstruation can be related to tissue destruction during tubal ligation.
- Of pregnancies that occur following sterilization, 33% are ectopic.
- Postpartum sterilization is not performed laparoscopically because of the presence of a large uterine fundus and vascular edematous adnexa. A surgical incision is required for postpartum sterilization. Postpartum sterilization must be discussed at length during pregnancy. Consent

Table 11–2 Comparison of Male and Female Sterilization

Characteristic	Male	Female
Effectiveness	Highly effective	Highly effective
Safety	Safest	Very safe
Location	Doctor's office	Hospital or outpatient surgery
Anesthesia	Local	General
Typical cost	450–700	1000–3000
Recovery time	2–3 days	2–3 days
Number in United States each year	500,000 (est)	640,000 (est), 34% of married couples

forms should be signed during pregnancy. Desire for sterilization should be confirmed with the woman after delivery. Sterilization should be performed only if mother and baby are healthy.

- Regret after sterilization is primarily associated with the age of the woman at the time of sterilization. Women under 30 are twice as likely to regret sterilization versus those over 40. Regret can also be linked to changes in marital status, death of a child, socioeconomic status, and emotional factors.
- Sterilization does not prevent sexually transmitted diseases (STDs).
- Sterilization is cost effective when cost is spread out over time.

See *Voluntary Sterilization* in Appendix B.

Contraindications: Desire for pregnancy in the future. Medical conditions that prohibit anesthesia and surgery

Assessment for Appropriateness:

- Physical and pelvic examinations are required prior to surgery, including Pap smear (CPT code: 88142) and serum pregnancy test (CPT code: 84702).
- Laboratory testing, as required by the physician, must be performed prior to the procedure to rule out abnormalities or contraindications for surgery (General Health Panel: CPT code: 80050)
- Counseling for the procedure must include explanation of the permanence of the procedure.
- Decision-making should occur well in advance of the operation, with both partners included in discussion and the decision. Sterilization should be discussed in the context of all other forms of contraception. Failure rate and risk of ectopic pregnancy should be discussed.

Complications: Anesthesia complications, surgical complications such as infection and bleeding, ectopic pregnancy, menstrual dysfunction, and post-sterilization regret.

Follow-up: Surgical intervention requires careful follow-up. Sterilization requires a short-term stay and follow-up for signs of bleeding and reversal of anesthesia. The incision should be examined within 1 week of surgery for signs of infection or bleeding. A pelvic exam to assess healing should be performed 4 to 6 weeks after the surgery.

Referral: Refer women for sterilization after careful discussion of the risks and benefits with the woman and her partner.

POSTCOITAL CONTRACEPTION

Description: Postcoital contraception prevents pregnancy after sexual intercourse. In the United States, methods available include oral contraceptives, progestin-only pills, and a copper IUD. RU-486, the French abortion pill, is completely different from the drugs used for postcoital contraception.

Effectiveness: Oral postcoital contraception reduces the risk of pregnancy by at least 75%. Plan B, progestin-only postcoital contraception, reduces the risk of pregnancy by 89%. Insertion of a copper IUD reduces the risk of pregnancy by 99%.

Method of action: Postcoital contraception prevents pregnancy by delaying or inhibiting ovulation, inhibiting fertilization, or preventing implantation.

Risks and benefits: According to the WHO, almost all women can use postcoital contraception. Even women who should not use oral contraceptives for their regular method of birth control can take postcoital contraception.

- There are no serious side effects to postcoital contraception. Temporary effects may be nausea, vomiting, and breast tenderness. Plan B has a lower incidence of nausea and vomiting than the estrogen and progestin combination.
- All methods of postcoital contraception require a prescription.
- Treatment may not be appropriate for women with active migraine.

Contraindications: Pregnancy

Assessment for Appropriateness: Approximately one half of the unintended pregnancies in the United States are related to contraceptive failure. Postcoital contraception can be utilized by any woman who has unprotected sex but does not want to be pregnant. One of the most compelling reasons for postcoital contraception is rape. Postcoital contraception is more effective the sooner it is initiated.

Instructions for Use:

Yuzpe regimen:

- Ovral two tablets within 72 hours of unprotected sex and two more tablets 12 hours later.

  or

- Lo/Ovral, Nordette, Levlen, Triphasil, Tri-Levlen, 4 tablets within 72 hours of unprotected sex and 4 more tablets 12 hours later

Plan B

- One tablet of levonorgestrel 75 mg within 72 hours of unprotected sex and one tablet 75 mg 12 hours later

Copper IUD

A copper IUD can be inserted up to seven days post–unprotected sex.

See *Emergency Contraception* in Appendix B, Chapter 11 Handouts.

Follow-up: Postcoital contraceptives are not 100% effective. Follow-up pregnancy test and pelvic examination are recommended.

Referral: Information about emergency contraception can be obtained by calling a toll free hotline, answered 24 hours per day, at 1-888-NOT-2-LATE. English and Spanish are available on the telephone.

See also Tables 11–3 and 11–4 for a summary of the main issues surrounding the use of contraception.

Table 11–3 Contraception: Risks and Benefits

Method	Desired Characteristic	Dangers	Side Effects	Benefits (non-contraceptive)
Oral contraceptives Vaginal ring	High efficiency	Cardiovascular complications	Nausea, bleeding, headaches, breast tenderness	Protective against some cancers and ovarian cysts; decreased's menstrual loss and dysmenorrhea
IUDs	High efficiency	PID, anemia	Increased vaginal bleeding	None
Implants	High efficiency	Infection at site	Menstrual changes	Lactation not disturbed; decreased's menstrual loss and dysmenorrhea
Injections	High efficiency	None	Menstrual changes, weight gain	Lactation not disturbed
Sterilization	High efficiency	Infection, anesthesia risk	Subsequent regret	None
Condoms	Limited or no side effects	None	Decreased sensation, allergy	Protects against STDs
Diaphragms	Limited or no side effects	Toxic shock syndrome	Pelvic pressure	Protects somewhat against STDs

Table 11–4 Contraceptive Options: Advantages and Disadvantages

Method	Advantage	Disadvantages	Effectiveness
Female sterilization	Continuous protection No need to remember daily	Permanent Surgery required	99%
Male sterilization	Continuous protection No need to remember daily Some health benefits	Permanent Surgery required	99%
Birth control pills Vaginal ring	Continuous protection Reversible	Need to remember daily Risks, esp. for smokers Side effects	99%
Subdermal implants	Protection for 3–5 years Reversible No need to remember daily	Minor surgery required Some side effects	99%
DMPA, Lunelle	Protection for 1–3 months No need to remember daily	Quarterly injections Some side effects Delayed return to fertility	99%
IUD	Protection for up to 10 years No need to remember daily	Expulsion possible Increased risk of infection	99%

**Table 11–4 Contraceptive Options: Advantages
and Disadvantages** (Continued)

Method	Advantage	Disadvantages	Effectiveness
Condom	STD prevented Easy to obtain Best used with spermicide	Less spontaneity Reduction in sensation possible Breakage possible	88%–99%
Diaphragm with spermicide	Insertion upto 6 hours before intercourse	Insertion required Increased risk of bladder infection	82%–94%
Cervical cap	Insertion prior to inter-course	Insertion required	82%–94%

Periodic abstinence	No intervention	Planning and motivation
		  required
		Method not for women
		  with irregular cycles
			80%–99%

Spermicide	Easy to obtain
	Good results when used
	  with condom or
	  diaphragm
		Insertion necessary
		Messy
		Reapplication with each
		  intercourse needed
			79%–97%

Withdrawal	No other intervention	Control required Sperm leaks prior to ejac-ulation	72%

DMPA = Depo-medroxyprogesterone acetate; IUD = intrauterine device.

REFERENCES

Archer, D: New Contraceptive Options. Clin Obstet Gynecol 44(1), 2001.

Burkman, R: Oral contraceptives: Current status. Clin Obstet Gynecol 44(1), 2001.

Cook, L, et al.: Diaphragm versus diaphragm with spermicides. Cochrane Database of Systematic Reviews 93 CD002031, 2002.

Curtis, K: Safety of implantable contraceptives for women. Contraception 65(1), 2002.

Gould, D: Contraception: the changing needs of women throughout the reproductive years. Nursing Standard 14(38), 2000.

Grimes, D, and Wallach, M (eds): Modern Contraception. Emron, Totawa, NJ, 1997.

Grow D, and Ahmed S: New contraceptive methods, Obstet Gynecol Clin North Am 27(4), 2000.

Hatcher, RA, et al: Contraceptive Technology, ed 16. Irvington Publishers, New York, 1994.

Kaunitz, A: Injectable long acting contraceptives. Clin Obstet Gynecol 44(1), 2001.

Schwartz, JL: Release of progestin only emergency contraception. Current Women's Health Reports 1(3), 2001.

Sucato G, and Gold, MA. New options in contraception for adolescents. Current Women's Health Reports 1(2), 2001.

United Nations Development Programme: Long term reversible contraception: Twelve years of experience with the TCu380A and the TCu220C. Contraception 56:341, 1997.

Chapter 12

ANTENATAL CARE

PRECONCEPTION

Preconception Care

Prior to pregnancy, medical or social conditions that may put the mother and/or fetus at risk should be identified. Preconception care is a term used to describe this process. In the US Public Health Service's Healthy People 2010, preconception care is recommended.
(www.health.gov/healthypeople)

Preconception History

Any medications or chemicals consumed that are potentially teratogenic should be identified before conception, and their use should be discouraged. All current prescriptions and nonprescription medications, including vitamins and herbs, should be reviewed. Every NP should have access to a reference, such as *Drugs in Pregnancy and Lactation* by Briggs et al., that includes reviews of reproductive literature relevant to drugs. The FDA categories of risk for drugs utilized during pregnancy—A,B,C,D and X—are explained in such a text (see also Box 12–1). The American College of Obstetricians and Gynecologists (ACOG) also provide recommendations related to medications during pregnancy.

Exposure to potential teratogenic toxins should be determined prior to pregnancy. A detailed history that includes occupational history and also household and hobby activities can reveal possible teratogenic exposure. Women planning a pregnancy should minimize the use of paint and paint removal products, bleaches, lye, and oven cleaners.

The woman's family history, including ethnicity, should be reviewed for genetic disorders such as cystic fibrosis, sickle cell anemia, Tay-Sachs disease, and neural tube defects. The age of the woman should be considered for genetic risk.

Any woman considering pregnancy should be screened for hepatitis B and HIV.

Box 12-1
Food and Drug Administration (FDA) Categories
Intended to Guide the Prescribing of Medication
During Pregnancy

Category A represents no risk during pregnancy.
Category B represents no risk identified in animal studies or studies with people, but there are not adequate studies to demonstrate safety.
Category C represents adverse effects in animal studies with no available studies with people, or there are no studies in animals or people.
Category D represents studies demonstrating birth defects in people, but the benefit outweighs the risk.
Category X represents contraindication during pregnancy with risks outweighing benefits.

Toxoplasma gondii is a teratogen that can cause anomalies. Screening is controversial, but all women who are considering pregnancy can reduce the risk of infection by avoiding raw and uncooked meats and delegating the chore of changing the cat litter to someone else in the household.

Daycare workers are at increased risk for cytomegalovirus (CMV) infection. Caring for children older than 36 months reduces the risk. Daycare workers planning a pregnancy may want to care for older children.

The NP should evaluate and update adult immunizations for women contemplating pregnancy. Update the vaccinations for tetanus, rubella, hepatitis, and varicella. ACOG recommended in November, 2002 that rubella vaccination may be given up to one month before becoming pregnant. (The previous recommendation was three months.) Recommendations for flu vary with the season. Current recommendations for flu vaccinations for women contemplating pregnancy should be sought at *www.cdc.gov/mmwr*

A woman's mental health can affect her pregnancy. The use of alcohol, tobacco, and illicit drugs should be reviewed at a preconception visit and the users counseled regarding risks to themselves and their fetuses.

A preconception visit is an ideal time to screen for domestic violence.

A balanced diet along with achievement or maintenance of ideal body weight improves pregnancy outcome. Women with eating disorders should be treated prior to pregnancy. Lactovegtarians (who eat no eggs) and vegans who eat only plants will require supplementation with calcium, zinc, iron, and B and D vitamins. Daily folic acid consumption of 0.4 mg should begin at least one month prior to pregnancy. For women who have had a child with a neural tube defect, 4.0 mg daily is recommended. The FDA recommends that pregnant women or women planning a pregnancy not consume fish that contain mercury. Fish to avoid include swordfish, mackerel, and tuna steaks.

Both mother and fetus benefit when the mother exercises during pregnancy. Initiation or continuation of an exercise regimen is recommended at preconception visits.

Chronic medical problems should be identified at a preconception visit and referral given for consultation with an obstetrician/gynecologist. Chronic medical problems requiring referral include: asthma, chronic hypertension, cardiac disease, thromboembolic disease, seizure disorders, chronic renal disease, autoimmune disorders, diabetes mellitus.

Every preconception visit should encourage women to seek early prenatal care. Encourage women at preconception visits to enhance the probability of pregnancy with midcycle coitus and over-the-counter ovulation monitoring.

PRENATAL CARE

The objective of prenatal care is to ensure that every wanted pregnancy culminates in the delivery of a healthy baby without jeopardizing the health of the mother. Creative strategies are necessary for reaching this objective and simultaneously meeting the requests of the prenatal client. Reaching the objective and creating an experience that the woman perceives as positive is best accomplished with a team approach. A balance between technology and sensitivity is also best achieved through a team approach, with the team consisting of the pregnant woman, advanced practice nurses specializing in women's health, obstetricians, perinatologists, nurses, social workers, and dietitians. Each of these team members contributes a unique perspective to the case management of each prenatal client. Each team member will represent a segment of the entire clinical picture. In a well-functioning team, plans for care can be devised that meet the health needs of the prenatal client and her fetus in a manner that is acceptable to the woman.

Twizer et al. (2001) report that the lack of prenatal care is an independent contributor to perinatal mortality and low birth weight. Women who do not receive prenatal care have statistically significantly higher rates of antepartum fetal deaths. Prenatal care is therefore significant. The structure of such care remains under discussion. Frequency and type of prenatal visits that create positive outcomes requires exploration. Nurse midwife Morrison (2000) reports that highly individualized care designed to help women become self-reliant and self-confident should be the goal of prenatal care. Morrison suggests that the three aspects of prenatal care, according to the American College of Nurse Midwives, are: spending time, developing relationships, and providing or receiving information. Klerman et al. (2001) report that increased prenatal visits for African-American women in a high risk clinic increased maternal weight gain and reduced the rate of preterm births. McCormick et al. (2000) report an association between a higher number of clinic appointments attended and greater gestational age and birth weight in a high-risk prenatal care program. Encouraging women to make and keep prenatal care appointments is a challenge for all nurses who are on a prenatal care team.

Effective strategies for prenatal care programs include: community based planning and implementation; case management; use of outreach workers and special services for mental health counseling, smoking cessation, and for substance-abusing women. Access to prenatal care can be improved via convenient hours, carefully selected locations (include transportation considerations) and culturally competent staff.

PRENATAL ASSESSMENT

The purpose of prenatal assessment is to evaluate the status of the woman and her fetus during pregnancy, to identify risks, and to plan for early intervention. Initial evaluation of the prenatal patient should include a comprehensive history, a physical assessment, diagnostic testing, and an overall risk assessment. A plan of care is formulated at the first visit, reviewed with the patient, and updated as needed throughout her prenatal course.

Health History

Health history should be obtained at the first prenatal visit and updated at each prenatal visit. The history should include general health, obstetrical status, and psychosocial status. The history should include at least the following information. Additional information should be obtained based on the health-related characteristics of the patient population.

- Name
- Age
- Race
- Gravida and para status
- Date of last normal menses and frequency of menses
- Contraceptive use prior to last menstrual period
- Obstetric history, starting with the first pregnancy and including all pregnancies up to the current pregnancy (including health of the children)
- Past illnesses and/or surgeries
- History of chronic illness
- Gynecologic history, including past or present genital infections and sexually transmitted diseases, previous Pap smears, history of fibroids, exposure to diethylstilbestrol (DES)
- Endocrine disorders
- Systems review
- Exposure to viruses during this pregnancy
- Medication use during this pregnancy

- Symptoms during this pregnancy, including bleeding, nausea, and vomiting
- Allergies and/or drug sensitivities
- Immunization history
- Human immunodeficiency virus (HIV) risk assessment
- Work history, including exposure to hazardous agents
- Substance abuse history, including past or present use of alcohol, caffeine, tobacco, prescription drug use, over-the-counter drug use, and illicit drug use
- Dietary habits before and during pregnancy
- Weight, current and before pregnancy
- Exercise patterns
- Elimination patterns
- Sleep patterns
- Significant stress
- Relationship with the father of the baby
- Support persons
- Domestic violence screening
- Socioeconomic status
- Cultural background and network
- Educational level
- Age, occupation, and race of father of the baby
- Family history, including allergies, cardiovascular disease, endocrine disorders, genetic or chromosomal disorders, hematologic disorders, mental retardation, multiple gestations, neurologic problems, psychiatric illnesses, renal disease, and child abuse

Physical Examination

Physical examination is performed during the first prenatal visit. This complete exam is essential for formulation of risk assessment.

- Weight and blood pressure must be obtained.
- Ears: Test for hearing ability; perform otoscopic examination.
- Nose: Note edema, ulcerations, perforation of the septum.
- Lips: Note pallor, cyanosis, presence of lesions or inflammation.
- Gums: Note gingivitis, bleeding.
- Oral mucosa: Note erythema, lesions, or ulcerations.
- Tongue: Note lesions, thrush, leukoplakia.
- Teeth: Note decay, condition of dental repairs, and quality of hygiene.
- Posterior pharynx: Note edema, exudate, presence of tonsils.
- Thyroid: Note size and position.
- Thorax and lungs: Note respiratory rate and listen to breath sounds.
- Heart: Note rate and rhythm, presence of murmurs.
- Breasts: Note masses, areola pigment changes, striae, nipple inversion.
- Back: Note costovertebral angle (CVA), tenderness, scoliosis, or lordosis.

- Abdomen: Note bowel sounds, striae; measure uterine height if appropriate; and listen to fetal heart tones if 10 weeks of gestation or more; determine fetal presentation if appropriate.
- Musculoskeletal: Note limitation of movement, swollen joints, or abnormal gait.
- Extremities: Note edema or varicosities (see Appendix B).
- Neurologic: Note affect and orientation; perform cranial nerve examination.
- Pelvic examination, including external genitalia: Note presence of warts, lesions, varicosities, edema, erythema, or presence of discharge; examine vagina, noting discharge, lesions; examine cervix, noting color, surface characteristics, discharge, tenderness, lesions; examine uterus, noting size, position, mobility, tenderness, masses; examine adnexa, noting size, mobility, and tenderness.
- Clinical pelvimetry: Note ischial spines, transverse diameter, and diagonal conjugate measurements.
- Rectal examination: Note hemorrhoids or masses.

Laboratory Data

Laboratory information assists in formulating a plan of care for each pre-natal client. The following are recommendations for laboratory screening for low-risk prenatal clients:

- Complete blood count at 15–16 weeks' gestation, repeated at 26–28 weeks' gestation (CPT code: 85025)
- Urinalysis (CPT code: 81002) and urine culture (CPT code: 87088) and sensitivity (CPT code: 87181) at 15–16 weeks' gestation, repeated as necessary throughout the pregnancy to rule out asymptomatic bacteriuria
- Blood group and Rh type drawn at 15–16 weeks' gestation (CPT codes: 86900 and 86901)
- Antibody screen at 15–16 weeks' gestation (CPT code: 86850)
- Rubella titer at 15–16 weeks' gestation (CPT code: 86762)
- Syphilis screen at 15–16 weeks' gestation (CPT code: 86592)
- Pap smear if last screening was more than 6 months prior to first prenatal visit (CPT code: 88142)
- Culture for gonorrhea and *Chlamydia* at first visit with repeat at 36 weeks' gestation (CPT codes: 87850 and 87110)
- Screen for HIV at 15–16 weeks' gestation (CPT code: 86689)
- Hepatitis B screen at 15–16 weeks' gestation (CPT code: 87340)
- Serum pregnancy test if indicated at first visit (CPT code: 84702)
- One-hour post 50-g Glucola drawn at 26–28 weeks' gestation (CPT code: 82950)
- Culture for group B streptococci at 34–36 weeks' gestation. The American College of Obstetrics and Gynecology in November 2002

recommended universal screening of all pregnant women for B streptococci. (CPT code: 87802)

- Additional testing may include screening for rubeola (CPT code: 86765) and cytomegalovirus (CMV) (CPT code: 86644); urine culture (CPT code: 87088), sickle cell screen (CPT code: 83020), and toxoplasmosis titer (CPT code: 86777) can be ordered.

Assessment of the prenatal population at the practice site will determine the laboratory profile. Plans for laboratory testing are altered according to patient's risk assessment.

Test	Results Indicating Disorder	CPT code
Alpha-fetoprotein (AFP)	Decreased level may indicate Down's syndrome Increased level may indicate neural tube defects	82105
Serum hCG	If it does not correspond to weeks' gestation	84702
Estriol	Lower than expected for gestation	82677
Ultrasound	Significant for neural tube defects	76801 (less than 14 weeks) 76805 (less than or equal to 14 weeks) 76815 (limited) 76816 (follow-up scan)
Amniocentesis	Significant for Down's syndrome or neural tube defects	59000
Chorionic villous sampling	Significant for chromosomal or genetic disorders	59015

Genetic screening should be discussed with each woman. Alpha-fetoprotein (AFP) or triple screen (combination of AFP, hCG, and estriol) (see Figure 12–1) should be offered to each patient. Additional testing for genetic disorders may be indicated based upon the woman's age and risk factors. AFP or triple screen should be done at 15 weeks' gestation, and thus the recommendation that other testing be coupled with this drawing of blood. If the patient does not desire AFP or triple screen, specimens for complete blood count (CBC), blood type and antibody screen, rubella, syphilis, hepatitis, and HIV can be drawn at any time. AFP is interpreted by multiple of the mean (MOM), compared to the mean, and is adjusted by gestational age, weight, and presence or absence of diabetes. A low maternal serum AFP level may be an indicator of Down's syndrome. A high serum maternal AFP level may be an indicator for neural tube defects. The sensitivity of the screening requires further testing to determine if Down's syndrome or a neural tube defect is actually present. Triple screen is defined as AFP plus human chorionic gonadotropin (hCG) levels and estriol measurement. Ordering a triple screen enhances the sensitivity and predictive value of the AFP screen. Abnormal triple

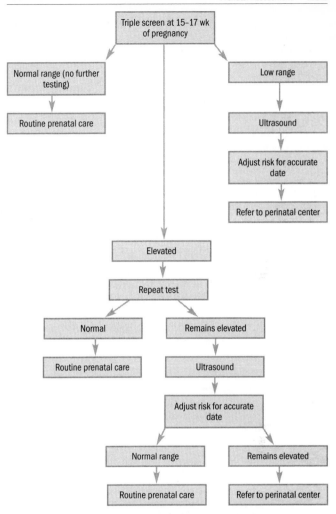

Figure 12–1. Triple screening for genetic disorders.

screen values require ultrasound (to confirm gestational age) and repetition of the test. A second abnormal screening requires amniocentesis to rule out Down's syndrome, or ultrasound to rule out neural tube defects.

Prenatal genetic testing may be recommended. It has long been established that as maternal age advances the risk for having a child with a chromosomal disorder increases. Women 35 years of age and older should seek genetic counseling. In addition, couples at risk for a genetic disorder should seek genetic counseling. For example, women who have a child with cystic fibrosis or women who have a close relative with cystic fibrosis (or the father of the baby has a close relative with cystic fibrosis) should seek genetic counseling.

Chorionic villous sampling and amniocentesis are the most reliable means for the detection of a chromosomal or genetic disorder in the fetus.

Risk Factor Assessment

The first prenatal visit includes history taking, physical examination, consideration of laboratory testing, and risk assessment. Significant risk factors are determined by history and confirmed by physical examination and/or laboratory or radiologic evidence. Risk factors must be noted on the woman's chart and discussed within a reasonable amount of time with a team of health-care providers that includes an obstetrician. Risk assessment is an important component in the formation of the prenatal care plan for a client. Significant risk factors that can be detected at the first prenatal visit include:

- Previous cesarean delivery, including type of uterine incision. (Medical records are required to validate type of incision.)
- Expected date of confinement (EDC) less than 12 months from previous delivery
- Parity of 7 or more
- Previous tubal pregnancy
- Previous cone biopsy
- Previous placental abruption or placenta praevia
- Severe hypertensive disorder during previous pregnancy
- Previous postpartum hemorrhage
- Previous abdominal or pelvic surgery
- Uterine anomalies
- DES exposure
- Previous preterm labor, birth, or ruptured membranes
- History of prolonged labor
- Two or more spontaneous abortions, second-trimester abortions, or multiple first-trimester terminations
- A newborn that was small or large for gestational age
- History of newborn with positive β-*Streptococcus*
- Multiple gestation
- History, including neonatal morbidity or congenital abnormalities
- Previous fetal or neonatal death
- Previous breast surgery
- Nutritional disorders, including anorexia and bulimia
- History of anesthesia complications
- Isoimmunization
- HIV-positive status
- Current drug addiction

- Current alcoholism
- Severe psychiatric illness
- History of infertility
- Maternal age less than 15 years or more than 40 years
- History of sexually transmitted diseases
- Severe psychosocial stress
- Chronic disease including cardiac disease, tuberculosis, asthma, renal disease, hepatic conditions, endocrine disorders, hematologic disorders, neurologic disorders, essential hypertension, malignancy, diabetes

CARE PLAN

A prenatal care plan is formulated after the initial visit and consultation with the team. The prenatal care plan includes:

- Diagnoses
- Anticipated problems
- Plan of management including rationale
- Predicted outcome for plan of management
- Alternative(s) to plan of management including rationale

Ongoing Assessment

During each prenatal visit following the initial visit, history is updated, a physical exam is performed that includes maternal and fetal assessment, and risk assessment is re-evaluated. Ongoing assessment at each visit will include:

- Updating health history
- Updating psychosocial health
- Physical assessment including weight and vital signs. Explanations for the necessity of weighing should be incorporated into the weighing procedure (Warriner, 2000).
- Performing microscopic evaluations of urine at each visit, performing a dipstick urine, and examining vaginal and cervical secretions as indicated
- Obtaining and interpreting laboratory tests
- Pap smear and follow-up as indicated
- Evaluating fetal well-being
- Prescribing medications as indicated
- Nutritional and diet counseling
- Health education
- Ongoing risk assessment
- Assessing and treating prenatal complication(s)
- Counseling as indicated, including social work counseling
- Implementing emergency procedures, if necessary

Ongoing Risk Assessment

The following risk factors, which can be revealed at any prenatal visit, require consultation with an obstetrician either by telephone or in person. Consultation should be performed during the prenatal visit whenever possible.

- Threatened or spontaneous abortion
- Positive antibody titer
- Gestation more than 28 weeks at first visit
- Clinical evidence of myoma or pelvic or abdominal masses
- Suspected polyhydramnios or oligohydramnios
- Suspected cardiac murmur
- Hematocrit (Hct) less than 28%
- Anemia not responsive to therapy
- Sickle cell (SS) hemoglobin
- Positive HIV test
- Abnormal Pap smear
- Multiple gestation confirmed by ultrasound
- Abnormal ultrasound findings
- Evidence of fetal chromosomal disorder
- Hypertension during pregnancy
- Deep venous thrombosis (DVT)
- Evidence of intrauterine growth retardation confirmed by ultrasound
- Gestational diabetes confirmed by glucose tolerance test
- Cardiovascular disease, including thrombophlebitis, chronic hypertension, heart disease, and pulmonary embolus
- Urinary tract disorders, including renal disease and pyelonephritis
- Metabolic or endocrine diseases, including diabetes mellitus and/or gestational diabetes, thyroid disease, and use of thyroid medications
- Chronic pulmonary disease, including asthma and chronic bronchitis
- Unexplained vaginal bleeding
- Abnormal weight gain (less than 12 lb or greater than 50 lb)
- Nonvertex presentation past 37 weeks' gestation
- Nondelivery at 41 weeks' gestation
- Lack of obstetric follow-up after 28 weeks of gestation
- Consistent nonattendance at office visits
- Evidence of nutritional disorders, such as anorexia or bulimia
- Evidence of maternal use of illicit drugs
- Neurologic disorders, including history of seizures, use of anticonvulsant drugs, and severe recurring migraines
- Psychiatric disorders, including previous psychotic episode, current mental health problem judged to be significant by psychiatric evaluation, or drug addiction
- Active infection, including tuberculosis (TB)
- Autoimmune diseases, including systemic lupus erythematosus (SLE)

PHYSIOLOGIC ADAPTATIONS OF PREGNANCY

Understanding the physiology of pregnancy is crucial to the development of a care plan for prenatal clients. The following is a review of the adaptations mandated by pregnancy, presented with a systems approach.

Reproductive Tract

Uterus increases in size from a 10-mL cavity weighing 70 g to a cavity enlarged to hold 5000 mL and weighing 1100 g. The uterus throughout pregnancy becomes increasingly elastic and fibrous. Growth is in response to estrogen and progesterone and in response to the products of conception. The cervix becomes cyanotic and soft because of increased vascularity and hyperplasia. Pregnancy produces more cervical mucus with more tenacious consistency. Corpus luteum forms in an ovary and must be maintained during the first 6–7 weeks of pregnancy. The vagina produces increased discharge that is acidic in nature. The vaginal mucosa becomes increasingly thick to allow for distention.

Skin

Striae, also called stretch marks, occur in approximately one half of all pregnant women. Increased pigmentation occurs in the linea nigra because of the presence of melanocyte-stimulating hormone.

Breasts

Nipple enlargement and increased pigmentation occur during pregnancy. Alveolar growth is induced as pregnancy progresses. Hypertrophy of the sebaceous glands embedded in the areola may be seen around the nipples.

A richer blood supply dilates the vessels beneath the skin. Venous congestion is obvious. Striae may appear on the outer aspect of the breasts.

During the second and third trimesters, growth of the mammary glands accounts for the progressive increase in breast size. The high levels of hormones in pregnancy promote proliferation of the lactiferous ducts and the tissue so that palpation of the breast reveals a coarse nodularity. Although development of the mammary glands is complete by mid-pregnancy, lactation is inhibited until a drop in estrogen occurs after delivery.

Cardiovascular System

Blood volume increases up to 32 weeks and then levels off. Blood volume increases 40%–50% during pregnancy. An increase in the plasma component is greater than the increase in the red blood cell (RBC) component, causing a physiologic anemia of pregnancy. A small decrease in systolic blood pressure occurs during pregnancy. A decrease in diastolic blood pressure becomes pronounced in mid-pregnancy. Blood pressure varies according to position. Blood pressure will be different in sitting position, left lateral position, and supine position because of vena caval compression and decreased venous return. Venous blood pressure increases in the lower extremities because of uterine growth. There is an increased tendency toward stasis, varicosities, and edema during pregnancy. The heart is displaced anteriorly and upward, causing an increased anteroposterior (AP) diameter and cardiothoracic ratio as well as a left axis deviation. Heart sounds change, with the first heart sound becoming louder and more greatly split. Systolic ejection murmurs are not uncommon in pregnancy. The cardiac output in lateral recumbent position increases by 30%–50%, peaking at 20–24 weeks. The uterus receives the largest increase of cardiac output, with increased blood flow from 50–500 mL/min. Renal blood flow increases by 30%. Increased blood flow to the skin during pregnancy may explain heat intolerance.

Hematologic

Red blood cell (RBC) production increases by 33%. Mean corpuscular volume (MCV) increases because of an increased number of reticulocytes. Serum iron level decreases in pregnancy. Iron requirements of 4 mg/day are needed to meet maternal and fetal needs (450 mg to increase RBCs, 350 mg to fetus, and 200 mg lost in delivery). White blood cell (WBC) total count is increased. The WBC value peaks at 30 weeks. Total lymphocyte count decreases, with the vast majority seen in decreased T-helper lymphocytes. All coagulation factors increase except factors XI and XIII. Platelets decrease in the third trimester.

Endocrine

Prolactin level increases during pregnancy, up to 150 ng/mL. The pituitary enlarges, as does the thyroid gland, owing to increased vascularity and hyperplasia. T_3 uptake decreases and T_4 values increase.

Pulmonary

Increased abdominal pressure causes the transverse diameter of the chest to increase by 2 cm. The costal angles widen, and diaphragmatic motion is increased. Total lung capacity is unchanged in the first half of pregnancy, but decreases in the second half because of decreased residual volume related to elevation of the diaphragm. Tidal volume is increased, probably mediated by progesterone. There is a 30% to 40% rise in nonpregnant value in the volume of air breathed each minute. Respiratory alkalosis is caused by increased ventilation. Diffusion capacity is increased in early pregnancy as a result of increased pulmonary blood flow. In later pregnancy, diffusion capacity decreases because of increases in hemoglobin concentration.

Renal

During pregnancy the kidneys enlarge by approximately 1 cm and weigh approximately 50 g more than in the nonpregnant state because of increased blood and water content. There is dilation of the entire collecting system because of a growing dextrorotated uterus, progesterone influence, and increased volumes of urine.

Renal blood flow and glomerular filtration increase during the first trimester and plateau into the second trimester by increments of 30%–50%. Renal blood flow increases to 500 mL/min from 100 mL/min. Glomerular filtration rate (GFR) increases to 150 mL/min from 100 mL/min. Glucose is filtered in the glomerulus and reabsorbed in the tubules. Glucosuria can occur during pregnancy because of GFR overwhelming the capacity for reabsorption. Physiologic proteinuria occurs at rates of up to 300 mg/24 hr because increased GFR overcomes the ability to reabsorb protein in the tubules. The reabsorption of HCO_3 has decreased, in compensation for respiratory alkalosis. The pregnant woman retains 1000 mEq of sodium, needed to expand the intravascular and extravascular compartments. She also retains 350 mEq of potassium, which compensates for the wasting of HCO_3. Serum osmolality decreases to 10 mOsm/kg, and there is an increase in urine volume of approximately 25%.

Digestive System

Gums become edematous and bleed more easily because of increased blood flow and increased mucopolysaccharide levels. The lower esophageal sphincter has increased pressure because of the enlarging uterus and increased progesterone. The stomach has decreased motility and tone because of progesterone. The small and large intestines have decreased motility, allowing for increased absorption. Production of liver proteins is increased, as is the production of alkaline phosphatase. The gallbladder increases to twice its size. Bile becomes more dilute and cholesterol is therefore less soluble, increasing the possibility of stone formation.

Metabolic Changes

Insulin levels are increased 2 to 10 times over those in the nonpregnant state, but glucose levels stay within 30–40 mg/dL. Fasting states show reduced fasting blood sugar by 5–10 mg/dL compared to the nonpregnant state. Peaks of glucose are delayed from 30–55 minutes as pregnancy progresses. Total caloric cost of pregnancy is 75,000 kcal. A wide range of weight gain is acceptable during pregnancy (20–45 lb). There is no correlation between prepregnant weight and weight gain during pregnancy. Weight gain in the first half of the pregnancy is related primarily to maternal components. During the second half of pregnancy, the largest growth is to the fetal placental unit, with the greatest growth noted between weeks 20 and 30. During the third trimester, maternal fat is stored as a caloric source for breastfeeding.

Medication during Pregnancy

Pregnancy can alter the absorption of oral drugs. Peristalsis is slowed, which increases the amount of exposure and absorption of any drug.

Excretion of medication is altered by increased renal plasma flow and increased storage into adipose tissue. Pregnancy can alter the distribution of any drug because of the change in intravascular and extravascular volume. Nausea and vomiting can affect the utilization and absorption of medication. There is no placental barrier to drugs. The fetus relies on the maternal circulation for detoxification and excretion.

ANTICIPATORY GUIDANCE DURING PREGNANCY

Danger Signs

The importance of the following symptoms should be explained to each woman upon diagnosis of pregnancy. Written information containing these symptoms should be distributed to each prenatal client.

- Pain with urination, frequency of urination, urgency of urination, fever, and backache (symptoms of urinary tract infection or pyelonephritis)
- Severe nausea and vomiting, particularly when fluid cannot be retained
- Persistent fever over 100 degrees Fahrenheit
- Lower abdominal pain in the first trimester that may or may not be accompanied by vaginal bleeding (symptoms of ectopic pregnancy)
- Vulvar pain or discomfort, change in vaginal discharge, swelling of the vulva, pelvic pain or tenderness (symptoms of vaginal infections and sexually transmitted diseases [STDs])
- Fluid gush from the vagina or leaking of fluid from the vagina. The fluid will not resemble urine (premature rupture of membranes)
- Uterine contractions in a regular pattern that are increasing in intensity prior to 36 weeks of pregnancy (premature labor)
- Rhythmic backache (premature labor or labor)
- Leg pain (thrombophlebitis)
- Absence of fetal movement for more than 24 hours
- Swelling of hands, feet, and face; visual disturbance; headache (pregnancy-induced hypertension)
- Vaginal bleeding during pregnancy

Alcohol

Consumption of alcohol during pregnancy can produce fetal alcohol syndrome. Safe advice to give pregnant women is to recommend complete abstention from the consumption of alcohol. Alcoholics Anonymous can be a very valuable resource for women with difficulty abstaining from alcohol.

Smoking

Smoking is related to low birth weight and premature delivery. The adverse effects increase with the number of cigarettes smoked daily.

Encourage women to stop smoking during pregnancy. Refer smokers to a support group that will assist them in reducing and eventually stopping smoking. Todd et al. (2001) encourages the incorporation of smoking cessation activities into routine nursing care in the prenatal period. Todd's recommendation is that all nurses involved in prenatal care obtain information on smoking assessment, cessation, and evaluation.

Drugs

Use of illegal drugs creates risk for prematurity and low birth weight as well as hepatitis B and HIV infection. Refer women using illegal drugs to a drug detoxification center specializing in the needs of pregnant women. Advise pregnant women to consult with a physician or nurse practitioner who specializes in women's health prior to consuming any over-the-counter medication. The use of prescription medication should be reviewed by a woman's health practitioner. Many prescription drugs can be harmful to the embryo or fetus, making review a wise consideration.

Radiation Exposure

There are recognized dangers to the fetus from diagnostic radiation, specifically chromosomal mutations and an increased risk for cancer in later life. Based upon animal experimentation, the only entirely safe dose of radiation is no dose of radiation. Pregnant women should therefore be advised to avoid radiation exposure. If radiation is necessary, shielding of the abdomen is essential. Radiation exposure during pregnancy can occur prior to the woman's knowledge that she is pregnant. The date of the last menstrual period should be elicited from every woman of child-bearing age prior to radiation exposure. Special attention should be given to women who work in environments that create exposure to radiation. These women must adjust their work patterns to reduce or eliminate radiation exposure during pregnancy.

Work

As the knowledge base about teratogens increases, pregnant women who work outside of the home should have accurate information. The Reproductive Toxicology Center in Washington, D.C., can be reached at 1-202-293-5137 or on the Web at *www.reprotox.org*

The Occupational Safety and Health Administration (OSHA) has also compiled information related to work, safety, and pregnancy. They can be reached at 1-800-356-4674 or on the Web at *www.osha.gov*

Women should be encouraged to reduce their exposure to chemicals during pregnancy. They should work in well-ventilated areas and wear protective gloves, clothing, and masks to reduce exposure to possible ter-atogenic agents. Lead pipes can be a source of lead contamination. Pregnant women, particularly those living or working in buildings constructed prior to 1980, should have their drinking water tested for lead. Neither food nor water should be stored in containers that may have lead contamination. Women should be encouraged to inform their employers of pregnancy as soon as possible. Work modifications should include:

- Reduction in hard physical labor, with lifting restricted
- Work days no longer than 8 hours
- Enforcement of at least two 10-minute breaks per day and 1 hour for lunch
- Availability to the pregnant woman of a bathroom and a place to rest and elevate her legs
- Provision of a short period of time every 1 or 2 hours to allow for walking for women who must stand or sit for long periods of time during work hours
- Avoidance of extremes in temperature, chemical exposure, and any activity that may threaten the pregnancy through trauma

Several medical diagnoses may inhibit a pregnant woman from working. Obstetrical diagnoses such as multiple pregnancy or cerclage may prohibit working. The type of work that a woman performs and the numbers of hours per day she works must be considered before restriction is implemented. Decisions concerning work safety and a pregnant woman must be made by a team consisting of the pregnant woman, the nurse practitioner (NP), the obstetrician, and the woman's employer.

Exercise

Exercise during pregnancy has multiple physical and psychologic benefits. Exercise patterns established prior to pregnancy can be maintained throughout the pregnancy with the following restrictions:

- Heart rate should be kept under 140 beats per minute, with elevated heart rate not exceeding 15–20 minutes per exercise session.
- The pregnant woman should not exercise in hot, humid conditions.
- Hydration must always be considered before, during, and after an exercise session.
- The woman should modify the exercise program as the physical demands of the pregnancy increase (as the weeks of pregnancy advance).
- The pregnant woman should stop exercising if she has pain, bleeding, prolonged dizziness, prolonged shortness of breath, or palpitations.

Women who have not exercised regularly prior to pregnancy should begin a program that gradually increases in length and intensity. New programs should be followed regularly, not sporadically, and should be supervised by a person familiar with exercise programs designed for pregnant women. Skiing, both snow and water; scuba diving; or any sport performed at elevated altitudes should be prohibited during pregnancy because of risks involved for both mother and fetus.

Saunas and hot tubs should be avoided during pregnancy. Blood being shunted to the skin because of the elevation in body temperature predisposes the woman to syncope.

Complications of pregnancy may inhibit exercise. These include incompetent cervix and premature labor. Medical diseases can also prohibit exercise during pregnancy. Any woman with an obstetric or medical complication of her pregnancy will require evaluation of her exercise program.

Sexual Activity

Sexual activity is not restricted during pregnancy unless a complication such as premature labor or placenta praevia develops. Pregnant women should be advised to assume their usual level of sexual activity throughout the pregnancy unless advised not to by a health-care provider. Assure pregnant women that the fetus is not injured by intercourse. Exploration of comfortable positions for intercourse during pregnancy may be suggested.

Prevention of STDs should be discussed with pregnant women. Advise the pregnant woman to use condoms if she has a new sexual partner or multiple partners, or if she is unsure about her partner's drug use or sexual activity.

Travel

Travel is best undertaken in the second trimester when risk for complication is lowest and comfort level during the pregnancy is highest. Advise the pregnant and traveling woman to discuss her travel plans with the nurse practitioner (NP). The NP should discuss with the woman plans for emergency care if it becomes necessary, and provide her with safety advice dependent upon her destination (drinking water, foods, etc.). Advise her to walk for a few minutes every one or two hours while traveling. She should keep herself well hydrated. Air travel is not restricted during pregnancy.

Seat belts should be used while traveling in a car. The lap portion of the seat belt should be placed below the abdomen and across the upper thighs. Both the lap and the shoulder straps should be utilized. Both belts should be worn snugly.

Traveling during the last month of pregnancy is discouraged. Labor initiating far from home places the woman in an anxiety-producing situation. Traveling in an automobile long distances while in early labor in an attempt to reach familiar providers is uncomfortable and potentially unsafe. Advise the pregnant woman to stay reasonably close to home in the last few weeks of pregnancy.

Nutrition

Throughout the pregnancy there is an increased need for all of the basic nutrients. Nutritional guidelines must be reviewed individually with each pregnant woman. Food preferences as well as activity level must be incorporated into the nutritional plan. A multiple pregnancy alters a nutritional plan. Pregnant adolescents have special nutritional needs. NPs caring for pregnant women should have access to a registered dietitian for patient consultation.

Calories must be sufficient to supply the increased energy and nutrient demands of pregnancy. An extra 300 calories per day is required throughout the pregnancy, a 10%–15% increase over the mother's prepregnancy need. The pregnant woman requires 60 g/day of protein, an increase of 10%–15%. Calcium needs increase 400 mg/day to 1200 mg. Iron needs increase 50% to 30 mg/day. The March of Dimes recommends folic acid in the amount of 0.4 mg/day, citing research indicating that this dose may help prevent neural tube defects. The Recommended Daily Allowance (RDA) standards suggest 70 mg/day of vitamin C, a 10-mg/day increase. The practice of providing vitamin supplementation prenatally has become routine for many health-care providers, even though there is no scientific evidence indicating that there is benefit to either mother or fetus. Extra nutritional requirements can be met with food, with the exception of iron and folic acid. Vitamin and mineral supplementation should not be regarded as a substitute for food.

Battering and Pregnancy

Although statistics vary widely, women do report battering during pregnancy. It is important for nurses who provide prenatal care to screen for domestic violence so that they can identify the nature and severity of the abuse, help plan intervention strategies, and provide referrals and follow-up visits. Battering during pregnancy can cause premature rupture of membranes, abruption, and low birth weight. Abdominal trauma during pregnancy can cause bruising, fractures, or even death of the fetus. Nurses should utilize direct questioning in order to identify victims of domestic violence. In addition, nurses should note a history of repeated assaults, injuries, delay in reporting injury, and inconsistency of injury findings with history given.

Victims of battering should be referred to a domestic violence advocate reached via a hotline. The advocate will develop and implement a safety plan for the victim and her family.

Trauma to the abdomen, in the case of pregnant women, requires careful history of the traumatic event(s), 30 minutes of continuous fetal heart monitoring, determination of Rh status in cases of bleeding, 24 hours of observation if the woman is contracting, bleeding, or complaining of uterine tenderness, and adequate documentation including photographs of any injury.

MANAGEMENT OF COMMON COMPLAINTS OF PREGNANCY

BACKACHE

SIGNAL SYMPTOM ▶ discomfort in the lower back

Backache (general)	ICD-9-CM: 724.5
Low back pain	ICD-9-CM: 724.2

Description: Backache is a common complaint of pregnancy, particularly during the third trimester.

Etiology: Backache arises from the shift in gravity related to the enlarging uterus, causing muscle strain.

Occurrence: Throughout the pregnancy, but particularly during the third trimester.

Contributing factors: Pre-existing back pain, excessive weight gain during pregnancy.

Signs and symptoms: The woman generally reports dull aching back pain that increases throughout the day.

Diagnostic tests:

Test	Results Indicating Disorder	CPT Code
Physical exam	Low back muscle spasm	Per extent of physical
Neurological exam	Decreased or hyper reflexes, decreased sensation or reaction	Included in physical assessment
Pelvic exam	Abnormal	57410
Urine culture and sensitivity	Presence of bacteria	87088 and 87181
Monitoring if contractions	Presence of contractions prior to expected due date	59020

Differential diagnosis:

- Uterine contractions
- Pelvic inflammatory disease (low bilateral abdominal/pelvic pain, vaginal discharge, dyspareunia, dysuria)
- Urinary tract infection (positive culture)
- Sciatica and herniated disk must be ruled out. The woman should not have CVA tenderness or pain with straight leg raises.

Treatment: The woman with backache related to pregnancy should be taught proper body mechanics and techniques for lifting. A regular back exercise program should be encouraged. She should avoid long periods of standing or sitting. A supportive mattress and sleeping in a lateral position may help relieve backache. Massage and relaxation techniques can help to relieve backache. Acetaminophen, 650 mg every 4 hours, may be taken for relief.

Follow-up: As indicated.

Sequelae: None.

Prevention/prophylaxis: Avoid excessive weight gain during pregnancy.

Referral: Radiologic studies are limited during pregnancy. If sciatica or herniated disk is suspected, referral into the primary care system for further evaluation may be necessary.

Education: Teach the woman to avoid wearing high-heeled shoes. Excessive weight gain during pregnancy should be avoided. Heavy lifting during pregnancy should be avoided. Proper body mechanics and lifting techniques should be reviewed.

BREAST CHANGES

SIGNAL SYMPTOM▶   tenderness in the breasts

Breast changes	ICD-9-CM: 611.71

Definition: A common complaint during pregnancy relates to the increase in breast size and tenderness.

Etiology: Increased levels of estrogen and progesterone cause the fatty layers of the breast to thicken and also cause the development of milk ducts and glands. As a result, the breasts increase in size and weight and feel tender.

Occurrence: Women frequently complain of breast tenderness in the first trimester of pregnancy.

Contributing factors: Caffeine.

Signs and symptoms: Breast enlargement and tenderness.

Diagnostic tests: Physical examination, including vital signs and breast examination. (CPT code included in general exam code).

Differential diagnosis: History during first trimester of pregnancy may include breast tenderness, but without pain, redness, fever, injury, masses, or bloody discharge. Physical examination and vital signs should be within normal limits, and there should not be any areas of inflammation, masses, dimpling, skin changes, enlarged nodes, or bloody discharge. Mastitis, breast cancer, and breast injury must be ruled out.

Treatment: Reduce caffeine intake. Wearing a supportive bra can be helpful in relieving tenderness.

Follow-up: As indicated.

Sequelae: None.

Prevention/prophylaxis: Reduce caffeine intake.

Referral: Breast tenderness related to infection or injury should be referred. Symptoms of breast cancer require medical referral.

Education: Explain to the woman that breast tenderness decreases in the second trimester. The woman may find wearing a supportive bra helpful. Caffeine increases breast tenderness and should be avoided. Breast self-examination should be conducted throughout pregnancy on a monthly basis.

CONSTIPATION

SIGNAL SYMPTOM▶ difficulty passing stool

Constipation	ICD-9-CM: 564.00

Definition: Constipation is inability to pass, or difficulty with passing, stool.

Etiology: Large amounts of circulating progesterone cause decreased contractility of the gastrointestinal tract, resulting in slow movement through the intestines and increased water reabsorption. The large bowel is also compressed by the growing uterus in the first trimester, and again in the third trimester. Iron taken by mouth during pregnancy increases the likelihood of constipation.

Occurrence: Constipation is a common complaint during pregnancy.

Contributing factors: Oral iron intake, low-fiber diet, decreased fluid consumption, decreased activity, constipation prior to pregnancy

Signs and symptoms: The woman will report difficulty with passing stools, and stools that are dry and hard.

Diagnostic tests: Physical examination including abdominal and rectal examination. (CPT code included in general exam code)

Differential diagnosis:

- Preterm labor
- Appendicitis (RLQ abdominal pain that decreases with flexing of the right thigh)
- Fecal impaction (history of constipation, bloating)

Treatment: Bulk-forming laxatives such as Metamucil can be used to relieve constipation. Increasing fluid intake may relieve the symptoms. A stool softener can be used for relief of constipation. The typical dose is 50 mg; the total dose should not exceed 200 mg/day. Regular exercise and establishing a time of day for defecation decrease constipation. Foods high in bulk such as bran, whole-grain breads and cereal, plus vegetables and fruits should be encouraged. Prune juice and a warm drink at breakfast are helpful for some women. Iron may have to be temporarily eliminated from vitamin and mineral supplementation until constipation is relieved.

Follow-up: As indicated

Sequelae: Straining with bowel movements can contribute to the formation of hemorrhoids.

Prevention/prophylaxis: Adequate fluid intake, high-fiber diet, regular exercise.

Referral: None.

Education: Constipation is common during pregnancy. Laxatives other than bulk-forming laxatives should not be utilized during pregnancy.

DYSPEPSIA

SIGNAL SYMPTOM ▶ burning in the gastric area after eating

| Dyspepsia | ICD-9-CM: 536.8 |

Definition: Dyspepsia is synonymous with indigestion.

Etiology: The pressure of the uterus against the stomach and intestines causes reflux of gastric contents into the esophagus. Increased levels of progesterone contribute to a decrease in gastrointestinal peristalsis and relaxation of the hiatal sphincter.

Occurrence: Common in the third trimester.

Contributing factors: Spicy or fatty foods, large meals.

Signs and symptoms: The woman will report gastric burning, but not chest pain or shortness of breath, upper abdominal pain, diarrhea, or vomiting.

Diagnostic tests: Physical examination including vital signs (CPT code included in general exam code).

Differential diagnosis:

- Cardiac disease
- Gallbladder disease
- Peptic ulcer
- Gastroenteritis

Treatment: Antacids may be taken during pregnancy. Instruct the woman with dyspepsia to follow the package directions for over-the-counter antacids, either calcium-based or aluminum-based. Antacids cannot be taken with tetracycline and should not be taken simultaneously with iron supplementation because they impair iron absorption. The woman should consume small, frequent meals that avoid spicy, fatty, and gas-forming foods. She may need to sleep with her head elevated a few inches to relieve dyspepsia at night.

Follow-up: As indicated to rule out peptic ulcer or gallbladder disease.

Sequelae: None.

Prevention/prophylaxis: Avoid spicy, fatty foods; alcohol; and coffee.

Education: Reassure the woman that dyspepsia resolves with delivery. Sleeping with the head of the bed elevated may relieve dyspepsia. Instruct the woman not to wear restrictive clothing. The pregnant woman should eat small, frequent meals and avoid excessive weight gain.

DYSPNEA

SIGNAL SYMPTOM▶   shortness of breath

| Dyspnea | ICD-9-CM: 786.09 |

Definition: Shortness of breath.

Etiology: An enlarged uterus pressing against the diaphragm prevents full expansion of the lungs and creates dyspnea.

Occurrence: Third trimester prior to descent of the fetal head into the pelvis.

Contributing factors: Women of short stature experience this symptom more than tall women because of the amount of intra-abdominal space. Poor posture, particularly rounding of the shoulders and leaning forward while sitting or standing, contributes to dyspnea.

Signs and symptoms: The woman reports feeling short of breath and perhaps light-headed.

Diagnostic tests: Physical examination including abdominal examination and examination of the heart and lungs (CPT code included in general exam code).

Differential diagnosis:

Cardiac or respiratory disease including upper respiratory infection.

Treatment: Advise the woman to rest, not to wear restrictive clothing, to keep good posture, and to lie in a lateral position while reclining.

Follow-up: As indicated.

Sequelae: None.

Prevention/prophylaxis: Adequate rest, good posture.

Referral: None.

Education: Reassure the pregnant woman that the dyspnea will be relieved when the fetal presenting part descends into the pelvis. Sleeping with her head elevated on a pillow or two may relieve nocturnal dyspnea.

EDEMA

SIGNAL SYMPTOM▶   swelling of the hands and feet

| Edema | ICD-9-CM: 782.3 |

Definition: Edema is swelling caused by accumulation of fluid, most often in dependent areas, primarily during the third trimester.

Etiology: The pressure of the uterus alters venous return to the heart from the legs; consequently, fluid passes into the intracellular spaces. Hormone levels during pregnancy increase capillary permeability, contributing to the edema.

Occurrence: Third trimester.

Contributing factors: None
Signs and symptoms: The woman will report mild edema in her hands and feet that worsens as the day progresses. Edema is decreased in the morning and increases throughout the day, particularly during periods of prolonged sitting or standing.
Diagnostic tests: Physical examination, including vital signs.

Test	Results Indicating Disorder	CPT Code
Urine dipstick for protein	Increased protein	81000
Measurement of urinary output	Decreased urine output	81050

Differential diagnosis:
Generalized edema and facial edema with headache can indicate pregnancy-induced hypertension.
Treatment: Advise the woman with edema related to pregnancy to lie in a lateral recumbent position for resting during the day and sleeping at night. Advise her to decrease prolonged standing or sitting with brief periods of walking. Ask her not to wear constrictive clothing. Have her raise her arms and legs above the level of the heart several times daily to decrease the edema. Her diet should include adequate calories and protein and at least 6–8 glasses of water per day. Salt, sugar, and fats should be consumed in moderation.
Follow-up: As indicated.
Sequelae: None.
Prevention/prophylaxis: None.
Referral: Refer the woman with symptoms of pregnancy-induced hypertension.
Education: Reassure the client that edema during pregnancy is normal and will resolve after delivery. She should avoid sitting or standing for prolonged periods. Instruct the woman not to wear constrictive clothing with the exception of support hose. Advise the woman to take in adequate calories and drink 6–8 glasses of water per day.

EMOTIONAL LABILITY

SIGNAL SYMPTOM▶   feeling "moody"

Emotional lability (excessive)	ICD-9-CM: 301.3

Definition: Emotional lability is commonly called mood swings throughout pregnancy.
Etiology: Hormone levels during pregnancy can create emotional lability. Progesterone has a depressant effect on the nervous system.
Occurrence: Common at any time in the pregnancy or throughout the pregnancy.

Contributing factors: Fatigue, inadequate support system

Signs and symptoms: The pregnant woman may reveal that she has mood swings and cries at times for no apparent reason.

Diagnostic Tests: None.

Differential diagnosis:

- Fatigue related to sleep loss or deprivation
- Fatigue related to iron-deficiency anemia
- Emotional psychiatric disorders (history of mental illness)

Treatment: Increased time for sleep and rest. Social work referral for an inadequate support system. Adequate distribution of calories throughout the day.

Follow-up: As indicated.

Sequelae: None.

Prevention/prophylaxis: Adequate sleep and rest, adequate caloric consumption.

Referral: None.

Education: Explain to the woman that emotional lability is common during pregnancy. Taking "time for herself" is essential, as is adequate rest, sleep, exercise, and diet.

FATIGUE

SIGNAL SYMPTOM ▶ "tired" in spite of adequate rest

Fatigue	ICD-9-CM: 780.79

Definition: Lack of energy or feeling of tiredness, usually during the first trimester of pregnancy.

Etiology: First-trimester fatigue is probably related to the increased physical demands of pregnancy. Fatigue returns in the third trimester, caused by sleep disturbance, decreased exercise, and the physiologic demand of the pregnancy. Fetal movements and urinary frequency may interfere with sleep.

Occurrence: Fatigue is common in the first trimester of pregnancy. Insomnia in the third trimester of pregnancy commonly leads to fatigue.

Contributing Factors: Demanding work schedules and sleep deprivation.

Signs and symptoms: Fatigue despite reported 8 hours or more of sleep per 24-hour period.

Diagnostic tests: Complete blood count to rule out anemia (CPT code: 85025).

Differential diagnosis:

- Anemia with hemoglobin less than 11g/dL
- Depression as measured by history and use of a depression scale.

Treatment: First-trimester fatigue requires adjustment of the woman's schedule to incorporate more sleep. Iron may be prescribed for women with anemia. Amount of oral iron prescribed is dependent upon the blood count results. No sleeping medications should be prescribed for third-trimester insomnia. Describe methods to increase comfort and improve insomnia. Tell patients to avoid exercising in the evening and to avoid caffeine and heavy meals at bedtime. Warm milk may induce sleep.
Follow-up: More frequent prenatal visits may be required for further evaluation of fatigue.
Sequelae: None.
Prevention/prophylaxis: None.
Referral: None.
Education: Explain to the woman that fatigue is expected during the first trimester. Encourage adequate sleep and rest and assist the woman in arranging her schedule to include additional rest. Discuss methods for decreasing insomnia in the third trimester.

HEADACHE

SIGNAL SYMPTOM▶   pain in the forehead

Headache	ICD-9-CM: 784.0

Definition: Headache is the sensation of pain in the forehead; this is apt to occur commonly during the first trimester of pregnancy.
Etiology: Headache during pregnancy is caused by increased circulatory volume, vasodilation caused by high levels of progesterone, and at times low blood sugar.
Occurrence: Headaches are common during pregnancy and especially in the first trimester, particularly in women who have experienced headaches prior to pregnancy.
Contributing factors: History of headache prior to pregnancy, insufficient caloric intake.
Signs and symptoms: Mild headache that is frontal in origin occurring less frequently than daily.
Diagnostic tests: Physical examination including vital signs, ophthalmoscopic examination, and neurologic evaluation (CPT code included in general exam code).
Differential diagnosis: History of headaches must include information on frequency, intensity, and duration, as well as a description of the headache. Knowing what triggers the headache and what relieves it is helpful for evaluation. Pregnancy headache history should not include facial edema; changes in level of consciousness; memory changes; motor, visual, or sensory changes; nausea and vomiting with headache; stiff neck; fever; or eye pain.

Headaches during pregnancy can be related to the pregnancy but can also be related to consumption of alcohol, chemical exposure, food allergies, injury, tension, migraine, sinus infection, or fatigue. One of the symptoms of pregnancy-induced hypertension is headache.

Treatment: Small frequent meals, adequate sleep, relaxation techniques, and acetaminophen 650 mg every 4 hours if needed for relief

Follow-up: Have the client keep a written record of frequency and intensity of headaches. More frequent prenatal visits may be necessary for further evaluation.

Sequelae: None.

Prevention/prophylaxis: Small frequent meals and sufficient rest and sleep.

Referral: Headache related to migraine, pregnancy-induced hypertension, infection, or injury should be referred for evaluation.

Education: Explain to the woman that physiologic changes are producing the headache and that headaches may resolve in the second trimester. Advise her to avoid triggers for the headaches, such as increased stress or certain foods. Frequent small meals may reduce the incidence of headache. Adequate sleep and rest may reduce the incidence of headache.

HEMORRHOIDS

SIGNAL SYMPTOMS▶ pain in the rectal area; bleeding from the rectum

Hemorrhoids (uncomplicated)	ICD-9-CM: 455.6
Complicating pregnancy	ICD-9-CM: 671.8 (+ 5th digit)

Definition: Hemorrhoids are varicosities of the rectum. Hemorrhoids are a common complaint in the third trimester of pregnancy.

Etiology: Hemorrhoids are exacerbated during pregnancy by increased intravascular pressure, constipation, and straining at stool.

Occurrence: Commonly in the third trimester, but may occur at any time during the pregnancy.

Contributing factors: Constipation.

Signs and symptoms: The woman complains of swelling, pain, fullness, or bleeding in the rectal area.

Diagnostic tests:

Test	Results Indicating Disorder	CPT Code
Physical exam including rectal exam	Frank blood	Included in general exam code
Stool for occult blood	Positive	82270
Hemoglobin	Decreased	85018

Differential diagnosis:

- Anal fissures (rectal pain relived by defecation, bleeding, irritation, painful bowel movement)
- Abscessed or thrombosed hemorrhoids. (Thrombosed hemorrhoids look like a clot-containing mass, blue or purple in color, near the anus, and are reported as very painful.)
- Cancerous lesions (positive pathology)
- Condylomata (fleshy warts)

Treatment: Hemorrhoids can be relieved with topical anesthetics such as Preparation H during pregnancy. Encourage the woman to avoid constipation, use sitz baths that are warm or cool, and to use Tucks or similar medicated pads.

Follow-up: As indicated.

Sequelae: None.

Prevention/prophylaxis: Avoid constipation and prolonged standing or sitting.

Referral: Thrombosed hemorrhoids require surgical referral.

Education: Hemorrhoids often resolve after pregnancy. Vaginal delivery exacerbates hemorrhoids, but resolution often occurs during the postpartum period.

MUSCLE CRAMPING IN THE LEGS

SIGNAL SYMPTOM ▶ pain in the calf during the night

Muscle cramping in the legs	ICD-9-CM: 729.82

Definition: Muscle cramping in the legs is the spontaneous contraction of muscles or muscle groups in the legs. It is a common complaint experienced during the second and third trimesters of pregnancy.

Etiology: Cramping occurring in the second and third trimesters is probably related to the pressure of the uterus on the pelvic nerves and blood supply. A calcium imbalance may contribute to the problem.

Occurrence: Cramping occurs most frequently at night and after excessive exercise.

Contributing factors: Inadequate intake or excessive consumption of calcium; excessive exercise.

Signs and symptoms: Cramping in the calf, usually at night, that resolves spontaneously.

Diagnostic tests: Physical examination.

Test	Results Indicating Disorder	CPT Code
Doppler flow studies	Positive for thromboembolic disease	93965

Differential diagnosis:
Thromboembolic disease indicated by positive Homan's sign and/or continuous tenderness in the leg and pain on deep palpation; varicosities should be ruled out.

Treatment: During a cramping episode, pressure against the foot as the woman extends her leg hastens the resolution of the cramping. Excessive or inadequate consumption of calcium should be altered.

Follow-up: As indicated.

Sequelae: None.

Prevention/prophylaxis: Calf-stretching exercises prior to bedtime may be helpful. Adequate calcium intake is necessary for prevention.

Referral: None.

Education: Instruct the woman in calf-stretching exercises.

NAUSEA AND VOMITING

SIGNAL SYMPTOM ▶ nausea with or without vomiting typically, but not limited to, awakening.

Nausea and Vomiting	ICD-9-CM: 787.01

Description: Nausea and vomiting, a common complaint of the first trimester of pregnancy, may or may not be associated with a time of day. Vomiting does not always accompany the nausea.

Etiology: High levels of estrogen and progesterone and the introduction of hCG are probably the cause of nausea and vomiting in the first trimester. Delayed emptying of the stomach is a result of smooth muscle relaxation and hyponatremia. Emotional and dietary factors may also be involved in creating nausea and vomiting.

Occurrence: Over half of all pregnant women in the United States experience these symptoms. The symptoms last until approximately 12–14 weeks of gestation.

Contributing factors: Ingestion of certain foods, the smell of certain foods, preparing food, heat intolerance, and increased workload can contribute to an episode of nausea and vomiting.

Signs and symptoms: Nausea with or without vomiting. Women report nausea and/or vomiting in the first trimester that may or may not be limited to a certain time of day. History of nausea and vomiting should exclude fever, pain, diarrhea, bleeding, or head injury, because these are signs of vomiting unrelated to pregnancy and may require medical evaluation. Vital signs will be normal. Uterine size will be appropriate and fetal heart tones will be audible at 10–12 weeks of gestation. Weight change depends on the severity of the vomiting. If weight loss is greater than 5% of the woman's total weight, hyperemesis gravidarum should be suspected and medical evaluation required.

Diagnostic tests:

Test	Results Indicating Disorder	CPT Code
Urine ketone	Rule out dehydration.	81000
Urine specific gravity	Rule out dehydration.	81000

Differential diagnosis: Differential diagnosis can be performed by history and physical examination, including abdomen examination. Other possible diagnoses are:

- Hyperemesis gravidarum—severe nausea and vomiting with dehydration
- Multiple gestation—more than one fetus diagnosed by ultrasound
- Hydatidiform gestation—abnormal pregnancy diagnosed by ultrasound
- Gastroenteritis—infection in the GI system
- Cholecystitis—infection of gallbladder, radiologic diagnosis
- Inner ear infection—symptoms of ear infection
- Migraine headache—diagnosed by history
- Increased intracranial pressure—related to head injury
- Food poisoning and eating disorder—diagnosed by history

Treatment: Ensure adequate hydration. Intravenous supplementation of fluid may be necessary if the woman is at risk for dehydration. (If the vomiting is severe enough that she cannot retain fluids, she is at risk for dehydration.)

Relaxation techniques may be helpful in relieving nausea. Vitamin B_6 tablets, 50 mg PO, no more than 4 per day, can be helpful in relieving nausea and vomiting. Acupressure applied in the form of wrist bands has been known to be helpful in some women. Eating small, frequent meals and snacks can be effective. Vitamin and mineral supplementation can be discontinued in women with nausea and vomiting until the symptoms have subsided.

Follow-up: More frequent prenatal visits may be required if nausea and vomiting are severe. Hospitalization for hydration is required when dehydration is a risk factor.

Sequelae: If severe and untreated, dehydration can occur, placing both mother and fetus at risk.

Prevention/prophylaxis: Small, frequent meals. Consumption of food such as dry crackers before rising in the morning helps prevent morning nausea and vomiting. Careful selection of diet, including the avoidance of foods that induce nausea, may be helpful. Delegation of food preparation to others has been reported as a method that can decrease nausea in prenatal women.

Referral: Any pregnant woman who cannot retain fluids for a 24-hour period requires referral for medical evaluation.

Education: Explain to the woman that nausea and vomiting during pregnancy are usually confined to the first trimester. The woman must remain hydrated. Remind her to drink fluids.

ROUND LIGAMENT PAIN

Round Ligament Pain	ICD-9-CM: 789.09

Definition: Pregnant women commonly complain of sharp abdominal pain that is relieved spontaneously and is of short duration. The pain is in the area of the round ligament on one side of the abdomen or the other.

Etiology: Growth of the uterus causes the round ligaments to stretch. The round ligaments attach to the top of the uterus, extend anteriorly and inferiorly through the inguinal canal, and attach to the labia majora.

Occurrence: Usually in the second trimester; the woman reports sharp pain on either side or both sides of the uterus.

Contributing Factors: None.

Signs and symptoms: The pain can be intense but is of short duration. The pain may be intensified by quick movements and relieved by resting. There should not be evidence of constipation, contractions, or abdominal pain.

Diagnostic tests: Physical examination including abdominal examination (CPT code included in general exam code).

Differential diagnosis: History should not include contractions, flank or abdominal pain, tender lump or lumps in the groin, or constant pain. Evidence of contractions, cervical dilatation, rebound tenderness, or masses indicates that the pain is not related to round ligaments.

- Preterm labor
- Ectopic pregnancy (first trimester)
- Constipation (bloating, decreased occurrence of defecation—normally 3-5 times per week)
- Gastroenteritis (crampy abdominal pain relieved with vomiting or defecation)
- Appendicitis (abdominal pain in the RLQ that decreases with flexing of right thigh)

Treatment: Rest until the pain subsides. Mild heat to the area of the round ligament may provide relief from aching after the painful episode.

Follow-up: As indicated

Sequelae: None

Prevention/prophylaxis: Avoid sudden movements and move from a lying to a sitting position without placing excessive strain on the abdominal muscles.

Referral: None

Education: Round ligament pain is common during pregnancy. It is frightening to many women because of its intensity. The pain is always of short duration with spontaneous resolution and, at times, with mild aching afterward.

SYNCOPE

SIGNAL SYMPTOM ▶ "dizziness"

Syncope	ICD-9-CM: 780.2

Description: Syncope, reported by the pregnant woman as "dizziness," can occur at any time throughout the pregnancy.

Etiology: Pooling of blood in the lower extremities coupled with expanded blood volume can lead to syncope. Syncope can also be related to nausea and vomiting and low blood sugar.

Occurrence: Syncope can occur at any time during a pregnancy.

Contributing Factors: Prolonged standing, inadequate caloric intake

Signs and symptoms: The woman will report a light-headed feeling or dizziness that lasts for a brief period of time.

Diagnostic tests: Physical examination, including vital signs and otoscopic examination (CPT code included in general exam code)

Test	Results Indicating Disorder	CPT Code
Complete blood count	Hemoglobin, hematocrit decreased	85025
Drug screening	Positive for drug overdose	80100

Differential diagnosis:

- Orthostatic hypotension (decreased BP when moving to the standing position)
- Anemia (low hemoglobin, reduction in RBC mass, decreased hematocrit, fatigue, weakness)
- Hypoglycemia (low blood glucose)
- Toxicity
- Substance abuse (history of drug or alcohol abuse)
- Diseases of the ear

Treatment: Advise the woman to lower her head below her heart if feeling faint. Advise her to change positions gradually, especially from lying to standing. Compression stockings may be helpful.

Follow-up: As indicated.

Sequelae: None.

Prevention/prophylaxis: None.

Referral: None.

Education: A pregnant woman experiencing episodes of syncope must be advised not to drive during episodes of syncope and not to participate in any other activity that may endanger her welfare during an episode of syncope.

URINARY FREQUENCY

SIGNAL SYMPTOM frequent necessity to urinate

| Urinary frequency   ICD-9-CM: 788.41 |

Description: Urinary frequency is a common complaint in the first trimester and last trimester of pregnancy. Differentiation between frequency caused by compression of the bladder and urinary tract infection is essential.

Etiology: During the first trimester the enlargement of the uterus compresses the bladder. During the second trimester, as the uterus moves into the abdomen, this symptom improves. During the third trimester, urinary frequency is related to pressure on the bladder from the distended uterus.

Occurrence: Urinary frequency is a common complaint in both the first and third trimesters.

Contributing factor: Consumption of caffeine.

Signs and symptoms: Increased frequency of urination, sleep disturbance caused by urge to void, involuntary loss of urine.

Diagnostic tests:

Test	Results Indicating Disorder	CPT Code
Urine dipstick	High for protein or glucose or nitrates	81000
Urinalysis	Low specific gravity	81002
Urine culture and sensitivity	Presence of bacteria	87088 and 87181
1 hour post 50-g Glucola serum screening	Positive for gestational diabetes	82950
Nitrazine test, and fern test	Rule out ruptured membranes	87210

Differential diagnosis: History of urinary frequency should not include back pain, fever, hematuria, dysuria, urgency, or pain. Urinalysis and urine culture and sensitivity can be used to rule out urinary tract infection (UTI). The woman reporting urinary frequency should be assessed for polyuria. Polyuria may be a symptom of diabetes, and appropriate screening should be initiated if this is suspected. Nitrazine test and fern test should be performed to rule out ruptured membranes in women who report involuntary loss of fluid.

Treatment: None.

Follow-up: Urine dipstick and examination of the urine with a microscope to rule out UTI at each prenatal visit.

Sequelae: None.

Prevention/prophylaxis: Reduce intake of caffeine.

Referral: None.

Education: Explain to the woman experiencing frequency of urination the anatomic changes responsible for this symptom. Advise her to maintain an adequate fluid intake (6–8 glasses per day). Water intake can decrease prior to retiring for the night, but overall intake must remain at an adequate level. Remind the woman that alcohol and caffeine increase urinary frequency and should be avoided.

UTERINE CRAMPING

SIGNAL SYMPTOM▶ lower abdominal "cramping" similar to menstrual cramping

Uterine cramping	ICD-9-CM: 625.8
Menstrual cramping	ICD-9-CM: 625.3

Description: Uterine cramping is a common complaint in the first and third trimesters of pregnancy.

Etiology: Increased vascular congestion in the pelvis may be the reason for a cramping sensation many women report during the first trimester. In the last trimester of pregnancy, the uterus begins painless, irregular contractions known as Braxton-Hicks contractions. The contractions are thought to be preparation for labor. The cervix does not dilate in response to Braxton-Hicks contractions.

Occurrence: During the first trimester of pregnancy women report a cramping sensation similar to the cramping felt prior to menses. Braxton-Hicks contractions are common during the last weeks of pregnancy. The higher the gravida, the more intense the contractions.

Contributing Factors: None.

Signs and symptoms: Cramping should not be severe, unilateral, abdominal, urinary in origin, or accompanied by bleeding. Physical examination should be within normal limits. There should be no vaginal bleeding, cervical dilatation, adnexal masses, or suprapubic tenderness. With Braxton-Hicks contractions, the woman reports a tightening of the uterus that may or may not be accompanied by a sensation of pelvic pressure. The tightening lasts from a few seconds up to a minute. The contractions are not regular and do not increase in intensity over time. The woman does not report regular contractions, leaking membranes, or symptoms of a UTI. Physical exam will be within normal limits. The pelvic exam will not reveal an increase in cervical dilatation or effacement. Timing of contractions does not reveal a regular pattern. The fetus remains active, and bowel sounds are normal.

Diagnostic tests: Pelvic examination and the monitoring of contractions will rule out active labor and confirm Braxton-Hicks contractions.

Test	Results Indicating Disorder	CPT Code
Serial serum quanti- tative hCG	Evaluate progress of an early pregnancy	84702
Urinalysis Urine culture and sensitivity	Rule out UTI.	81002 87088 and 87181

Differential diagnosis:

- Spontaneous abortion, ectopic pregnancy, and UTI must be ruled out in first-trimester cramping.
- Preterm labor, labor, and UTI must be ruled out in the last trimester.

Treatment: Rest and relaxation and application of mild warmth to the lower abdomen may relieve cramping.

Follow-up: As indicated by the clinical presentation

Sequelae: None.

Prevention/prophylaxis: None.

Referral: None.

Education: Teach the woman the difference between Braxton-Hicks contractions and true labor. Advise her that resting in a lateral position or perhaps walking may relieve the contractions.

VARICOSITIES

SIGNAL SYMPTOMS ▶ aching of the legs, aching of the vulva

Varicosities (ruptured)	ICD-9-CM: 454.9 (+ 5th digit)
In pregnancy	ICD-9-CM: 671.0 (+ 5th digit)

Description: Varicosities are developed during pregnancy, most commonly in the third trimester.

Etiology: Pressure of the gravid uterus causes increased venous stasis. Many women who develop varicosities have a genetic predisposition.

Occurrence: Anytime during the pregnancy, but most commonly during the third trimester.

Contributing factors: Prolonged standing, genetic predisposition.

Signs and symptoms: The woman will report aching and sometimes throbbing in the legs and/or vulva. Twisted and swollen veins are visible, with possible mild swelling below the varicosities.

Diagnostic tests: Physical examination including extremities, testing for Homan's sign, or pain on deep palpation.

Test	Results Indicating Disorder	CPT Code
Doppler flow studies	Rule out venous thrombosis or thrombophlebitis	93965

Differential diagnosis:
Clotting, swelling, redness or tenderness, cyanosis, positive Homan's sign, and/or pain on deep palpation could indicate venous thrombosis or thrombophlebitis.

Treatment: Teach the woman to apply support hose. Instruct her to lie flat and raise her legs to drain the veins. While her legs are elevated, roll on the stockings or pantyhose. She should apply the stockings upon arising in the morning and not remove them until bedtime. She should not cross her legs, wear tight knee-high stockings, or high-heel shoes. She should elevate her legs above the level of the heart at least twice daily (a recliner is perfect for this) and avoid prolonged periods of sitting or standing. Sanitary napkins applied snugly to the vulva may help relieve vulvar varicosities.

Follow-up: As indicated.

Sequelae: None.

Prevention/prophylaxis: Support hose during pregnancy, rest periods during episodes of prolonged sitting or standing.

Referral: Thrombophlebitis and deep vein thrombosis require referral.

Education: Teach the woman how to apply support stockings. Advise her not to gain excessive weight during the pregnancy.

MANAGEMENT OF THE COMPLICATIONS OF PREGNANCY

DIABETES IN PREGNANCY

SIGNAL SYMPTOMS none

| Diabetes in pregnancy | ICD-9-CM: 648.80 |

Description: Pregnant women with diabetes can be classified into three groups. The first is gestational diabetes, with women developing diabetes for the first time while pregnant. The second is preconceptual diabetes without diabetic sequelae, both insulin- and non–insulin-dependent. The third is preconceptual diabetes with significant diabetic sequelae.

Etiology: Carbohydrate intolerance of varying severity resulting from pre-existing disease or as a consequence of changes in maternal metabolism related to pregnancy.

Occurrence: Gestational diabetes has an incidence of 2%–13% for all pregnant women.

Age: Not significant.

Ethnicity: Not significant.

Contributing Factors: Family history of diabetes, obesity, previous delivery of an infant weighing less than 4000 g.

Signs and symptoms: Gestational diabetes is usually without symptoms; it has been demonstrated that over one half of all women diagnosed have no significant risk factors and are under 30 years of age.

Diagnostic tests: All pregnant women should be screened for gestational diabetes at 24–28 weeks of gestation. Screening for gestational diabetes is a serum glucose measurement 1 hour post 50-g Glucola ingestion drawn at any time of the day (see also Figure 12- 2).

Test	Results Indicating Disorder	CPT Code
Serum glucose level 1 hour post 50-g Glucola ingestion drawn at any time of the day. The patient need not be fasting.	Greater than 140 mg mandates a 3-hour glucose tolerance test (GTT).	82951 and 82952 for each additional test above 3
Gestational diabetes is diagnosed when two or more values meet or exceed the following:	Fasting $>$ 105 1 hour $>$ 190 2 hours $>$ 165 3 hours $>$ 145	

Differential diagnosis: Inaccurate laboratory diagnosis.

Treatment: Women with pre-existing diabetes, prior to conception, may be insulin-dependent or non–insulin-dependent. All pregnant women

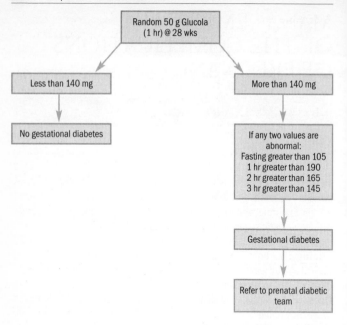

Figure 12–2. Diagnosis of gestational diabetes.

with diabetes will require insulin during the pregnancy. Oral hypoglycemics are not utilized during pregnancy. The desired outcome of diabetes and pregnancy is a healthy mother and a healthy baby. The route to that outcome is the maintenance of a maternal environment that is euglycemic throughout the pregnancy. This is maintained with proper diet, insulin therapy, and home glucose monitoring. Antepartum fetal surveillance is an important tool used throughout the pregnancy. Prenatal care for diabetic women is provided by a team consisting of perinatologist, endocrinologist, obstetrician, neonatologist, nutritional therapist, and nurse. An individualized plan of care is designed and carried out by the team.

Follow-up: Care as necessary to achieve diabetic control.

Sequelae: Polyhydramnios, pregnancy-induced hypertension, ketoacidosis, dystocia, congenital anomalies, macrosomia, and urinary tract infection.

Prevention/prophylaxis: Appropriate prenatal screening and referral

Referral: Diabetes and pregnancy require referral to a team of healthcare providers that includes a perinatologist and an endocrinologist. Pregnancy for the woman with diabetes is substantially risky for both mother and fetus, and requires very close and specialized medical and nursing care.

Education: Importance of prenatal care including screening for diabetes. Importance of maternal cooperation and participation in developing a health-care plan that achieves diabetic control

ECTOPIC PREGNANCY

SIGNAL SYMPTOMS▶   none; abdominal pain

Ectopic Pregnancy	ICD-9-CM: 633.90
Affecting fetus	ICD-9-CM: 761.4
Tubal	ICD-9-CM: 633.10

Definition: Implantation of a fertilized ovum in a site other than the endometrium of the uterus.

Occurrence: Many early ectopic pregnancies are reabsorbed and undiagnosed. Approximately 1 in 44 pregnancies is ectopic.

Age: Childbearing age.

Ethnicity: Not significant.

Contributing factors: Risk determinants for ectopic pregnancy include a history of salpingitis, previous tubal surgery, advanced maternal age, postcoital estrogen contraceptives, progesterone-containing intrauterine devices, ovarian hyperstimulation, in vitro fertilization, and previous ectopic pregnancy.

Signs and symptoms: Signs and symptoms of pregnancy, plus one-sided lower abdominal pain with possible referred shoulder pain. Ectopic pregnancy can occur without any symptoms.

Diagnostic tests: Laboratory and ultrasonographic testing are the cornerstones of diagnosing ectopic pregnancy.

Test	Results Indicating Disorder	CPT Code
hCG	Slower rise in levels of beta hCG than is seen in normal pregnancies	84702
Ultrasound	No visible yolk sac at 5 weeks seen or adnexal mass present	76801
Serum progesterone	Commonly depressed in women with abnormal gestations	84144

The measurement of hCG is essential to the diagnosis of pregnancy. Measurements of quantitative beta hCG in a serial fashion have been shown to be of diagnostic value for ectopic pregnancy. Levels of serum hCG are known to rise exponentially in early gestation. hCG levels normally increase by at least 66% every 2 days and more than double every 3 days. Pregnancies that deviate from this pattern are typically abnormal. Beyond 6 weeks of pregnancy, the normal rate of increase slows and may take more than 1 week to double. Ectopic pregnancies generally demonstrate a slower rise in levels of beta hCG than is seen in normal pregnancies.

Ultrasound must be combined with serial hCG to diagnose ectopic pregnancy. Using a vaginal probe, visualization of the gestational sac becomes possible at the time of missed menses. The diameter of the sac normally continues to increase daily and by 40 days from last menstrual period approximates 10 mm. A yolk sac normally becomes visible at 5 weeks of pregnancy within the developing gestational sac, confirming the presence of embryonic tissue within the uterine cavity. Deviations from these patterns coupled with adnexal mass and abnormal serum beta hCG level confirm the diagnosis of ectopic pregnancy.

Measurement of serum progesterone is an additional method of evaluation of early pregnancy. Progesterone measurements are commonly depressed in women with abnormal gestations. Measurement of serum progesterone may complement serial hCG and ultrasound measurements (see Figure 12–3).

Differential diagnosis:

- Ruptured ovarian cyst (mid-cycle pain, sharp pain, tenderness)
- PID (lower abdominal tenderness, cervical motion tenderness, and adnexal tenderness are the hallmark symptoms)
- Normal pregnancy
- Irritable bowel syndrome (recurrent, intermittent crampy abdominal pain, alternating constipation and diarrhea, gas, bloating)
- Appendicitis (RLQ abdominal pain that decreases with flexing of right thigh)

Treatment: Improved detection of ectopic pregnancy allows for greater treatment options. For symptomatic patients in need of acute care, serial examination is not appropriate. In an emergency, rapid urine pregnancy test followed by ultrasound will establish the diagnosis. Laparoscopy is definitive for diagnosis and may be the route for treatment of choice. The choice of surgical technique is determined by condition of the tube, location of the gestation, and size of the gestation. Laparoscopy or laparotomy, linear salpingostomy, segmental resection, or salpingectomy is performed. Linear salpingostomy is the procedure of choice for the treatment of ectopic pregnancy that is not ruptured. Medical therapy, if appropriate, involves the use of methotrexate.

Follow-up: Dependent upon treatment, Rh immunoglobulin to all Rh-negative women.

Sequelae: Ruptured ectopic pregnancy. Subsequent conception rate after linear salpingostomy is 60%, and recurrent ectopic rate is about 13%.

Prevention/prophylaxis: Avoid contributing factors when possible.

Referral: Ectopic pregnancy requires physician referral for medical or surgical intervention.

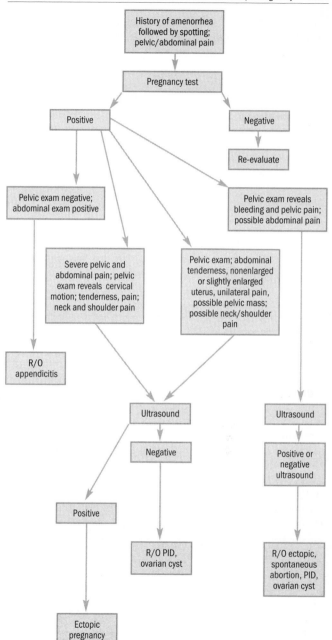

Figure 12–3. Ectopic pregnancy.

Education: Importance of early initiation of prenatal care. Importance of contact with health-care providers in any episode of abdominal pain in early pregnancy

PLACENTAL ABRUPTION

SIGNAL SYMPTOM▶   vaginal bleeding

Placental abruption	ICD-9-CM: 641.2 (+ 5th digit)

Definition: Placental abruption is defined as premature separation of the normally implanted placenta prior to the delivery of the fetus. The degree of separation may be partial or complete. It is also known as *abruptio placentae*.

Etiology: Cause is unknown, but there is an association with hypertension.

Occurrence: Third-trimester bleeding occurs in approximately 4% of pregnancies. Of instances of third-trimester bleeding, 30% are the result of abruptio placentae.

Age: More likely to occur in women older than age 35.

Ethnicity: Not significant.

Contributing factors: Multiparity, pregnancy-induced hypertension, use of cocaine, and trauma.

Signs and symptoms: Symptoms can range from minimal vaginal bleeding to severe hemorrhage. Cause is unknown, but there is an association with hypertension. The typical history is that of an acute onset of vaginal bleeding associated with abdominal pain. The degree of bleeding varies. Uterine tenderness is common. Uterine irritability or preterm labor may be evident. Bleeding from abruption can be concealed. This occurs when the edges of the placenta remain attached to the uterine wall so that the bleeding is contained within the retroplacental space and therefore no vaginal bleeding is observed. Diagnosis is made by ultrasound (see Figure 12–4).

Diagnostic tests: Physical examination reveals vaginal bleeding. Ultrasound confirms placental abruption. Vaginal exam is delayed until placenta previa is ruled out.

Test	Results Indicating Disorder	CPT Code
Ultrasound	Confirms separation of the placenta	76801 (less than 14 weeks) 76805 (greater than or equal to 14 weeks) 76816 (limited– position, placenta, heart rate)

Differential diagnosis:

- Placenta previa (painless vaginal bleeding in the third trimester; diagnosis made by ultrasound)

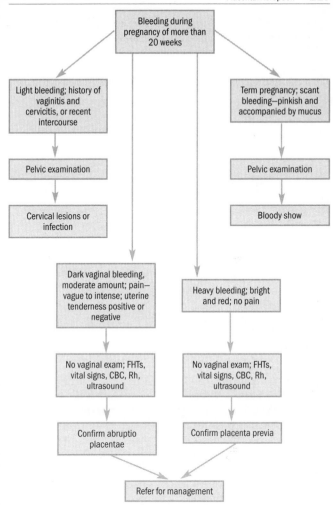

Figure 12–4. Bleeding during pregnancy of more than 20 weeks.

- Hematoma (history of trauma)
- Ruptured appendix (high fever, increased WBC with left shift, tenderness over the site of the appendix, severe pain)
- Ruptured ovarian cyst (mid-cycle pain, sharp pain, tenderness)

Treatment: Once the diagnosis of abruption has been made, management will be determined by the severity of the abruption. The majority of fetuses are delivered, with the severity of the situation determining the route of delivery.

Follow-up: Dependent upon treatment.

Sequelae: The most common complication of placental abruption is maternal hemorrhage. The blood loss can be significant. There is a risk for disseminated intravascular coagulation (DIC). Abruption is the most common cause of DIC in pregnancy.

Prevention/prophylaxis: Avoidance or appropriate treatment of contributing factors.

Referral: Physician referral is necessary.

Education: Importance of reporting episode of vaginal bleeding during pregnancy.

PLACENTA PREVIA

SIGNAL SYMPTOM ▶ vaginal bleeding

| Placenta previa | ICD-9-CM: 641.1 (+ 5th digit) |

Definition: Placenta previa is defined as the implantation of the placenta over the cervical os. Placenta previa is complete if the placenta totally covers the os and partial if only a portion of the os is covered. "Marginal" is the term used to describe a placenta that extends to the os but does not cover it. If the placental site is in the lower uterine segment but not touching the cervix, the diagnostic term used is "low-lying placenta."

Etiology: Placental implantation in the lower uterine segment.

Occurrence: Once in 200 pregnancies.

Age: Childbearing.

Ethnicity: Not significant.

Contributing factors: Multiparity, uterine surgical scars.

Signs and Symptoms: The typical symptom of placenta previa is painless vaginal bleeding in the third trimester (see Figure 12–4).

Diagnostic tests: Diagnosis is made by ultrasound. Because of the widespread use of ultrasound prenatally, diagnosis of placenta previa in asymptomatic women is common. The diagnosis of placenta previa should be reserved for patients beyond 24 weeks of gestation. Growth of the lower uterine segment results in the appearance of the placenta that is located close to the os "migrating" away from the cervix. If ultrasound performed earlier than 24 weeks shows placenta previa, sonograms should be repeated to validate "migration." Vaginal examination is delayed until ultrasound rules out placenta previa.

Test	Results Indicating Disorder	CPT Code
Ultrasound	See explanation above	76801 (less than 14 weeks) 76805 (greater than or equal to 14 weeks) 76816 (limited—position, placenta, heart rate)

Differential diagnosis:

- Abruptio placentae (vaginal bleeding to severe hemorrhage, confirmed by ultrasound)
- Other causes and sources of bleeding, such as rectum, bladder, or genital infection or laceration

Treatment: Management of placenta previa is based upon maternal and fetal stability and gestational age. Route of delivery is determined by the extent of the disorder and the maternal and fetal condition.
Follow-up: Serial ultrasounds.
Sequelae: None.
Prevention/prophylaxis: None.
Referral: Physician consultation is required.
Education: Stress the importance of reporting vaginal bleeding during pregnancy to a health-care provider.

PREGNANCY-INDUCED HYPERTENSION

SIGNAL SYMPTOMS none; headache, visual disturbances

Pregnancy-induced hypertension ICD-9-CM: 405.9

Description: Hypertension during pregnancy is well-recognized as a significant risk for both mother and fetus. Hypertension is the number one cause of maternal death. Perinatal morbidity and mortality are associated with premature delivery, intrauterine growth retardation, and placental abruption related to hypertension.

Pregnancy-induced hypertension (PIH) develops as a consequence of pregnancy, occurs after 20 weeks of gestation, and regresses following delivery. Chronic hypertension is diagnosed prior to pregnancy or is evident prior to 20 weeks of gestation. Chronic hypertension can be superimposed by PIH.

PIH affects the cardiovascular system as well as the coagulation system, central nervous system, and the hepatic and renal systems.
Etiology: Unknown. Significant family history increases the risk of PIH.
Occurrence: The incidence of PIH ranges from 5%–10%, with a significant increase in primigravidas, multiple gestations, diabetic pregnancies, and in women with pre-existing hypertension of any origin, or renal disease.
Age: Adolescents and women over 35 years are at greater risk of PIH.
Ethnicity: Incidence of PIH in all pregnancies is 6%–8%. Incidence of PIH among pregnant African-American women is 15%–20%.
Contributing factors: Primigravida, diabetes, and multiple gestations.
Signs and symptoms: Blood pressure (BP) elevated above 140/90 mmHg on at least two occurrences; proteinuria over 300 mg in a 24-hour

collection; and edema. The woman may report headache and/or visual disturbances (see Table 12–1).

Diagnostic tests: There are no specific tests to distinguish chronic hypertension from PIH; therefore, the diagnosis is based on history and physical examination. The diagnostic criteria for PIH are hypertension (BP more than 140/90 or elevation of systolic more than 30 mmHg and diastolic more than 15 mmHg) documented at least twice; proteinuria with a random specimen $1+$ or greater or more than 300 mg in 24-hour collection; and nondependent edema, especially of the hands or face.

PIH is classified as either mild or severe. It is diagnosed as severe if any of the following are present: BP greater than 160/110, proteinuria greater than 5 g/24 hours, oliguria less than 20–30 mL/hour, significant visual symptoms or headache, HELLP syndrome (*h*emolysis, *e*levated *l*iver enzymes, *l*ow *p*latelets), eclampsia, or pulmonary edema.

Test	Results Indicating Disorder	CPT Code
24-hour urine	Proteinuria < 5 g/24 hrs or <300 mg; oliguria >20-30 ml/hr	81050
Liver enzymes	Elevated	84460 and 84450
Platelets	Low	85576
Sputum sample	Hemolysis	89350
Chest X-ray posteroanterior and lateral	Pulmonary edema	71020
Toxoplasma antibody	Elevated with physical signs of: hypertension, nonpitting edema, eclampsia, visual symptoms, headache	86777

Differential diagnosis:

Essential or chronic hypertension or HELLP syndrome.

Treatment: Management decisions for PIH include consideration of the severity of the disease and maternal and fetal well-being. Definitive treatment of PIH is delivery. Decision to deliver must consider the risks to the mother of prolonging the pregnancy versus risks to the fetus at delivery. Mild PIH is usually managed with frequent assessment and evaluation of mother and fetus until delivery is determined to be a reasonably safe

Table 12–1 Classification of Hypertensive Disorders Complicating Pregnancy

- Pregnancy-induced hypertension:
  Hypertension develops during pregnancy and resolves postpartum.
  1. Hypertension (without proteinuria and edema)
  2. Hypertension (with proteinuria and edema)
     a. Mild
     b. Severe
  3. Hypertension, proteinuria, edema, convulsions
- Pregnancy-aggravated hypertension
  Underlying hypertension aggravated by pregnancy
- Coincidental hypertension
- Chronic hypertension that precedes pregnancy and persists postpartum

option. Severe PIH is a difficult management dilemma. Treatment options must be weighed against benefit. The route of delivery is dependent upon the maternal and fetal condition.

Follow-up: Dependent upon severity of symptoms.

Sequelae: None after delivery.

Prevention/prophylaxis: Unknown.

Referral: Referral to a physician is necessary.

Education: Stress the importance of maintaining a therapeutic plan of care.

PREMATURE RUPTURE OF MEMBRANES

SIGNAL SYMPTOM▶ fluid from the vagina

Premature rupture of membranes	ICD-9-CM: 658.1 (+ 5th digit)

Definition: Amniotic and chorionic membranes rupture prior to term pregnancy.

Etiology: The etiology of premature rupture of membranes (PROM) is multifactorial. Factors associated with PROM are cervical incompetence, multiple pregnancy, polyhydramnios, genetic conditions, and exogenous effects on the properties of the membranes.

Occurrence: The incidence of PROM for all pregnancies is 3%–18%.

Age: Less than 17 years or greater than 35 years of age.

Ethnicity: There is increased incidence in African-American women.

Contributing factors: Chorioamnionitis, endometritis, incomplete cervix, and multiple pregnancy.

Signs and symptoms: Gush of fluid from the vagina or slow fluid "leak" from the vagina.

Diagnostic tests: Rupture of membranes is diagnosed with history of fluid escaping from the vagina and testing that includes pooling of amniotic fluid, Nitrazine testing, or staining of fetal cells. Initial examination should be performed with a sterile speculum. An amniotic fluid sample is obtained from the posterior vaginal vault. Culture for group B streptococci should also be obtained.

Test	Results Indicating Disorder	CPT Code
Nitrazine testing or staining of fetal cells	Positive for amniotic fluid	87210
Culture for group B streptococci	Negative	82802

Differential diagnosis:

Leakage of urine (evaluation of fluid).

Treatment: The principle guiding the management of patients with PROM involves attempts to prolong the pregnancy until fetal lung maturity is attained.

Follow-up: Dependent upon medical management.
Sequelae: Preterm birth.
Prevention/prophylaxis: Treatment of infection.
Referral: Physician referral is required.
Education: Teach the patient the signs and symptoms of preterm labor.

PRETERM LABOR AND DELIVERY

SIGNAL SYMPTOM▶ uterine contractions

Preterm labor and delivery	ICD-9-CM: 6.44.2 (+ 5th digit)

Definition: Preterm delivery is defined as delivery at less than 37 weeks of gestation, and is a major cause of neonatal morbidity and mortality.
Etiology: In the United States, 75% of the neonatal deaths result from premature delivery. Approximately one third of premature delivery is a result of maternal or fetal complications such as hypertension, abruption, or multiple pregnancy. One third is a result of premature rupture of membranes, and one third is from unknown causes. Maternal infections outside of the uterus are associated with premature labor, with a special emphasis on infection of the urinary tract. Anatomic variations of the uterus account for a small percentage of premature labor.
Occurrence: 9%–10% of all pregnancies.
Age: Increased risk for women under age 17 or over 34.
Ethnicity: More common in African-American women.
Contributing factors: Risk factors associated with premature labor are multiple gestation, diethylstilbestrol (DES) exposure, uterine anomaly, cervical dilatation, previous preterm labor, history of cone biopsy, history of second-trimester abortion, and uterine irritability. Scoring systems have been published and are available for use. Congenital malformations, particularly those associated with oligohydramnios, can result in premature labor. The high frequency of small-for-gestational-age infants among preterm deliveries supports the association of placental insufficiency with preterm labor. Genital tract infection leading to intra-amniotic infection has been proposed as a cause of preterm labor (see Table 12-2).
Signs and symptoms: Uterine contractions and cervical change.
Diagnostic tests: Physical examination.

Test	Results Indicating Disorder	CPT Code
Electronic monitoring	Positive for regular contractions	59020
Ultrasound	Low amniotic fluid; positive for cervical dilation	76805

Differential diagnosis:
- False labor (no progression of labor)
- Urinary tract infection (positive culture)

Table 12–2 Risk Factors for Premature Labor

Type of Risk	Risk Factor
Demographic Risks	• Age under 17 or over 34 • Low socioeconomic status • Unmarried • African-American race • Low educational level
Medical Risks	• Parity of 1 or more than 4 • Genitourinary anomalies/surgery • Previous low birth weight, preterm labor • Multiple spontaneous abortions • Low weight for height
Risks in Current Pregnancy	• Multiple gestation • Hypertension • First- or second-trimester bleeding • Spontaneous rupture of membranes • Anemia or hemoglobinopathy • Fetal anomalies • Hyperemesis gravidarum • Short interpregnancy interval • Oligohydramnios • Isoimmunization • Incompetent cervix
Environmental Risks	• Smoking • Alcohol or substance abuse • High altitude • Poor nutritional status • Exposure to toxic compounds

Adapted from Youngkin, E, and Davis, M, Women's Health: A Primary Care Clinical Guide. Norwalk, CT: Appleton & Lange, 1994.

Treatment: A woman determined to be at risk for premature labor by use of a scoring system, cervical change, or increased uterine activity must be followed with frequent pelvic exams, have strenuous physical activity limited, and have her work environment altered. Vaginal infection must be identified and treated. Abstinence from sexual intercourse is recommended.

Home uterine activity monitoring is one of the tools available to help the woman identify preterm labor. Telephone transmission of external monitoring for labor awareness is very useful for evaluation. Prophylactic tocolytics may be used. Tocolytic therapy is usually restricted to between 24 and 34 weeks of gestation. Evaluation of fetal maturity is a critical part of the management of preterm labor. The use of steroids to enhance pulmonary maturity has been studied and shows beneficial effect.

Survival rates of preterm infants born in tertiary-care centers are higher than survival rates of those transferred to centers after delivery. Transport to a tertiary-care facility prior to delivery should be initiated when this can be accomplished safely. Method of delivery will be determined by fetal weight, presentation, and establishment of labor.

Follow-up: Dependent upon management.

Sequelae: None after delivery.
Prevention/prophylaxis: Treatment of infection during pregnancy.
Referral: Physician referral is required.
Education: Stress the importance of prenatal care.

SPONTANEOUS ABORTION

SIGNAL SYMPTOMS▶ vaginal bleeding, uterine cramping

Spontaneous abortion	ICD-9-CM: 637.9 (+ 5th digit)

Definition: Termination of pregnancy before fetal viability is the definition of abortion.
Etiology: Unknown, with genetic abnormalities the most common suspected etiology.
Occurrence: The incidence of spontaneous abortion is approximately 10%. The actual number is difficult to ascertain because many spontaneous abortions are not diagnosed. More than 80% of abortions occur in the first 12 weeks of pregnancy.
Age: Childbearing.
Ethnicity: Not significant.
Contributing factors: Chromosomal anomalies account for the majority of these terminations, with abnormal development of the zygote, embryo, or early fetus noted. Maternal factors associated with spontaneous abortion include chronic infection, hyperthyroidism, diabetes, progesterone insufficiency, drug use, environmental toxins, autoimmune mechanisms, or uterine defects.
Signs and symptoms: Hemorrhage and necrotic changes in the tissues usually accompany spontaneous abortion. There may be no visible fetus in the sac on ultrasound examination, leading to diagnosis of a blighted ovum. Spontaneous abortion at times involves passing of all of the products of conception with no interference from a provider. Complete abortion can be verified with serial decreasing beta hCG titers. If any products of conception are retained as indicated by pelvic examination and beta hCG titers, dilatation and evacuation (D&E) must be performed.

"Threatened abortion" is the term used when vaginal bleeding occurs during the first half of pregnancy. Bleeding can range from slight to heavy. In inevitable abortion, there is rupture of membranes and cervical dilatation. Under these conditions abortion is almost certain. "Missed abortion" is the term used to indicate that products of conception are not viable; however, bleeding and contractions do not follow. Careful palpation and measurement of the uterus at prenatal examinations will reveal no growth of the uterus, and fetal heart tones will be absent. Retained nonviable products of conception, particularly those in the second trimester, can lead to coagulation defects and should be terminated (see Figure 12-5).

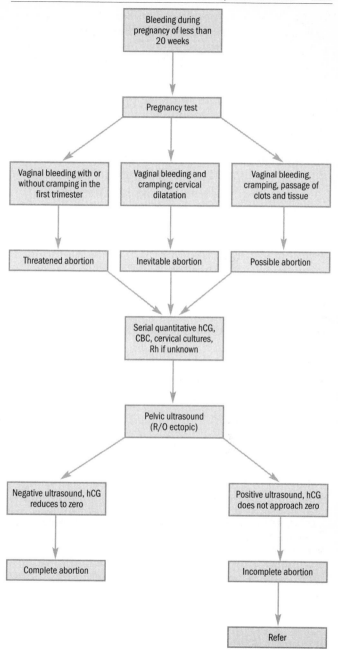

Figure 12–5. Bleeding during pregnancy of less than 20 weeks.

Diagnostic tests: Complete abortion can be verified with serial decreasing beta hCG titers. Threatened abortion requires ultrasound for confirmation of fetal viability and pelvic examination to determine cervical dilatation. In many cases a series of ultrasounds is required to monitor fetal growth and viability.

Test	Results Indicating Disorder	CPT Code
Serial beta hCG titers	Decreasing	84703 × 3
Ultrasound	Cervical dilatation	76805

Differential diagnosis:

- Ectopic pregnancy (Positive signs of pregnancy with one-sided lower abdominal pain, serial beta hCG in series can be helpful in the diagnosis.)
- Infection (positive culture)
- Malignancy (positive pathology report)

Treatment: Serial hCG until resolution, D&E, or induction of labor.

Follow-up: According to treatment.

Sequelae: Infection and bleeding if unresolved.

Prevention/prophylaxis: None.

Referral: Consultation with a physician for management plan is recommended.

Education: Teach the patient to notify the health provider if bleeding during pregnancy occurs.

REFERENCES

ACOG News Release, November 29, 2002.

Alexander, G, and Kotelchuck, M: Assessing the role of the effectiveness of prental care: history, challenges, and directions for future research. Public Health Reports, 116(4), Jul/Aug 2001.

Anderson, C: Battered and pregnant. AWHONN Lifelines, 6(2), April/May 2002.

Bates, B: A Guide to Physical Examination and History Taking. Lippincott, Philadelphia, 1991.

Frey, K: Preconception care by the nonobstetrical provider, Mayo Clinic Proceedings 77(5):469, 2002.

Gant, N, and Cunningham, F: Basic Gynecology and Obstetrics. Appleton & Lange, Norwalk, CT, 1993.

James, D: Maternal screening and treatment for group B streptococcus. JOGNN 30(6), Nov/Dec 2001.

Jones, S: Genetic based and assisted reproductive technology of the 21st century. JOGNN 28(6), Supp 1, 1999.

Klerman L, et al: A randomized trial of augmented prenatal care for multiple-risk Medicaid-eligible African-American women. Amer J Public Health 91(1):105, 2001.

McCormick G, Thyer B, Panton T, Meyers L: The association between appointment-keeping and birth outcome in the prenatal care program for high risk women. J Family Social Work 4(1), 2000.

Morrison, B: The nurse-midwifery process of prenatal care. University of Illinois at Chicago, 2000.

Olds, S, London, M, and Ladewig, P: Maternal and Newborn Nursing. Addison Wesley, Menlo Park, CA, 1996.

Todd S, LesSala, K, Neil-Urban, S: An integrated approach to prental smoking cessation interventions. MCN 26(4), Jul-Aug 2001.

Twizer, I et al: Lack of prenatal care in a traditional society: is it an obstetric hazard? J Reprod Med 46(7), 2001.

Warriner, S: Women's views on being weighed during pregnancy. Brit J Midwifery 8(10), 2000.

Williamson, R: Prevention of birth defects: folic acid. Biological Research for Nursing 3(1), 2001.

Youngkin, E, and Davis, M: Women's Health. Appleton & Lange, Norwalk, CT, 1994.

Chapter 13

POSTPARTUM CARE

PHYSIOLOGY AND NURSING CARE AFTER DELIVERY

Uterus

Immediately after delivery the uterus is approximately at the level of the umbilicus, and remains there for approximately 2 days, after which it begins a gradual descent into the pelvis. Oxytocin causes the myometrium, the thick muscular walls of the uterus, to contract, thereby compressing exposed placental blood vessels and slowing the uterine bleeding. Uterine bleeding in the postpartum woman is controlled by contraction of the uterus; therefore, careful assessment of the fundus of the uterus immediately following delivery is important. The fundus of the uterus should be palpated for contraction every 15 minutes for the first hour after delivery, every 30 minutes for the next hour, hourly for the next 2 hours, and every 8 hours until discharge to home. The consistency of uterine contraction should be noted, as should the placement of the fundus. (A full bladder can interfere with the placement and contraction of the uterus.) A uterus felt to be "boggy" should be massaged to stimulate contraction. Many factors can interfere with the contraction of the uterus immediately after delivery. These factors are anesthesia, manipulation at birth, multiparity, full bladder, retained placenta, and infection. If the postpartum woman has any of these risk factors, her fundus must be evaluated very frequently immediately after delivery.

If the woman has delivered by cesarean section, anesthesia permits uterine palpation in the immediate postpartum period. After the effects of anesthesia have ended, palpation of the uterus is performed gently and with guidance from the woman. Lifting of the head tightens abdominal muscles, making palpation even more difficult. Ask the woman to keep her head down during the examination.

Lochia

The lochia in the early postpartum phase, approximately 3 days, is rubra containing blood and deciduous tissue. Exfoliation or sloughing is in process after delivery. In approximately 3 weeks, new endometrium will form. In approximately 6 weeks, the placental site is healed. Healing occurs without scarring. In the immediate postpartum period, the amount of lochia is used as an additional assessment of uterine contraction. Lochia immediately following delivery is heavy, meaning that it would saturate a pad within an hour. It also increases in flow upon arising, with breastfeeding, and with exertion. Clots in lochia serosa may be present but are small in size. Numerous clots, foul smell, and excessive bleeding require further assessment.

Lochia becomes lochia serosa after the first 3 days following delivery. This lochia contains primarily serous fluid, deciduous tissue, leukocytes, and erythrocytes. Its color is pink or brown with a serosanguineous consistency. It should not have a foul odor and should not saturate pads.

Lochia alba appears at approximately day 10 after delivery and consists primarily of leukocytes. It should not saturate pads nor return to red or pink discharge. Lochia alba persists for approximately 2–3 weeks.

Vital Signs

Vital signs should remain stable during the postpartum period. Vital signs are taken simultaneously with assessment of the uterus and lochia. Blood pressure should not alter during the postpartum period; however, slight bradycardia may be present for the first 6–8 days after delivery. Postpartum women are susceptible to orthostatic hypotension because their cardiovascular system adjusts to the nonpregnant state. Temperature elevation up to 100.4° F can be related to dehydration in the first 24 hours after delivery. Persistent or recurrent fever at or above this level could indicate infection.

Vagina and Perineum

The vagina and perineum are stretched and edematous immediately after vaginal delivery. Bruising may or may not be present. Extensive edema or hematoma requires further evaluation. Ice packs to the perineum in the early postpartum period help to relieve perineal discomfort and decrease edema.

The bladder is edematous and hypotonic following vaginal delivery. The woman experiences decreased sensation and may not recognize the urge to void. The bladder should be palpated for distention frequently during the first postpartum day. If the woman's bladder is distended and she cannot void, pouring warm water over the perineum may be helpful. Catheterization is performed only if necessary. The postpartum woman is susceptible to urinary tract infection, and catheterization increases this risk.

Breasts

Breast engorgement occurs at approximately 48–72 hours following delivery. After delivery, the inhibiting effects of estrogen and progesterone decrease, allowing the luteinizing hormone to initiate lactation. Infant sucking stimulates oxytocin production, allowing the milk to "let down." The breasts are usually soft during the first 2 days after delivery and become substantially larger and firmer on postpartum day 3. Congestion known as engorgement is caused by hormonal change that produces venous stasis and seeping of fluid. When a regular breastfeeding pattern is established, the breasts soften and become more comfortable. Nursing mothers can develop soreness and even cracking and bleeding of the nipples. Engorgement makes "latching on" by the infant more difficult, and can result in sore nipples. Breasts should be checked daily while caring for postpartum women. Snug brassieres can help to relieve engorgement. Sore nipples can be relieved with topical medication.

Medication to relieve engorgement is not recommended currently for postpartum women. Women who do not choose to breastfeed should be instructed to relieve engorgement with a tight-fitting bra and no stimulation to the breasts.

In summary, postpartum assessment includes evaluation of vital signs, breasts, uterus, lochia, perineum, incision (if present), and legs (for thrombophlebitis). Postpartum assessment should be performed immediately after delivery, then at scheduled intervals over the next few days and weeks until 6 weeks post-delivery. Immediate assessment occurs in the hospital or birthing suite. Follow-up assessments can occur in outpatient settings or in the woman's home.

POSTPARTUM CARE

Shortened hospital stays are requiring changes in the delivery of postpartum care. In the Canadian system, which is publicly funded, postpartum care is provided by public health nurses in the woman's home (Gypton, 1995). Instructions about care of the perineum and breasts, the possibility of postpartum depression, resumption of sexual intercourse and contraception, diet, and exercise should begin after delivery in the hospital or birthing center and continue at intervals throughout the postpartum period. Frequency of visits is dependent upon nursing assessment after delivery (see Table 13–1).

Health-related problems can occur in the postpartum period. Mastitis, uterine infection, incontinence, and thyroiditis can occur in the postpartum period. In a review of all postpartum deaths in the developing countries and the United States, 60% of maternal deaths occurred in the postpartum period. 45% of those deaths occurred within one day of delivery. 65% occurred within one week, and 80% occurred within 2

Table 13-1 Postpartum Assessment

Area Assessed	Findings, Day 1	Findings, Days 2-3
Vital Signs		
Temperature	Elevated (100.4° F)	Normal
Pulse rate	40-70 beats per minute	Bradycardia or normal
Blood pressure	Normal	Normal
Involution		
Uterus	Fundus at umbilicus	1-2 cm below umbilicus
Lochia	Rubra	Rubra to serosa
Abdomen		
	Soft	Soft
Perineum		
	Edematous	Less edema
Breasts		
Consistency	Soft, colostrum	Firm, large, warm
Nipples	Intact	May be reddened, sore
Lactation	Colostrum	Milk
Legs		
	Pretibial, pedal edema	Edema minimal
Elimination		
Voiding	Up to 3000 mL	Decreasing amount
Defecation	None	Bowels move
Discomfort		
	Perineum aching, hemorrhoid pain, generalized aching	Less perineal pain, less hemorrhoid pain
Energy Level	Fatigued	Tired
Appetite	Often thirsty	Very hungry
Emotional State	Euphoric, excited	Happy, concerned

weeks (Li et al, 1996). Horon et al. (2001) reviewed all pregnancy-associated deaths in Maryland from 1993 to 1998 via death certificates. Of the 247 pregnancy-associated deaths, homicide was the leading cause of death during pregnancy and within one year after pregnancy. In a study of teen victims of domestic violence (Mortensen et al., 2002), the highest prevalence for interpersonal violence was at three months postpartum. 75% of the victims reported violence in the two-year period after delivery, and the majority of the victims did not experience violence prior to the delivery.

Prevention of postpartum deaths requires primary prevention, early detection, and treatment. Excellent postpartum care is the method by which these goals are accomplished.

Follow-up visits should be scheduled at more frequent intervals for women who deliver by cesarean section. Follow-up assessment should include, as a minimum, the following components: physical exam, laboratory testing, assessment of family adjustment, and contraceptive counseling.

Postpartum Evaluation at Four to Six Weeks

By 4–6 weeks after delivery, the uterus has returned to its nonpregnant state; the lochia is lochia alba, which contains primarily leukocytes, and is scant, and the vagina and perineum are regaining tone. Physical examination includes general health assessment. Vital signs are taken. Extremities are assessed for varicosities. Abdominal exam includes inspection for striae, diastasis, hernias, masses, tenderness, and lymph nodes. If cesarean section was the method of delivery, healing of the incision should be assessed.

Breast examination should be performed. The lactating breast will be full without redness or masses. The nonlactating breast should be soft, without masses or lymphadenopathy. Milk may discharge from a nonlactating breast for up to 3 months after delivery.

External genitalia should be without edema or lesions and the episiotomy, if present, should be well healed. The vagina should have rugae. The cervical os should be closed. The uterus should be 4–6 weeks' size and nontender. The rectum should be free of hemorrhoids and have good sphincter control. Pelvic musculature is evaluated for return to the nonpregnant state. Kegel exercises are suggested to women with relaxed musculature. Schedule a follow-up visit after several weeks of Kegel exercises to re-evaluate strength of pelvic musculature, particularly in the presence of cystocele or rectocele.

Antepartum and postpartum hemoglobin levels should be compared to determine the necessity for continued iron therapy and further testing. Rubella vaccination should be given after delivery to nonimmunized women. Date of next Pap smear should be planned. Glucose tolerance testing for women who were diagnosed with gestational diabetes should be requested.

Postpartum assessment of mental status and family adjustment postdelivery is an important part of postpartum care. Family adjustment includes discussion and counseling surrounding the issues of integration of the baby into the family structure, rest and sleep habits, appetite and diet, activity level, exercise program, plans for return to employment, coping ability in caring for the baby, and any problems with the baby.

Horowitz and Damato (1999) reported categories of maternal stressors. In their research, areas of stress identified by postpartum women were: work/school, sleep/rest, adjustment/own needs, health/body image, organization of life, child care, day care, housework, future challenges, finances, housing, time, partner, and family. Areas of satisfaction identified by the same postpartum women were: participating in relationships, sharing a future, being proud to be a mother, enjoying a healthy baby, and caring for a child.

Martell (2001) conducted an interview study and reported that postpartum women are "heading toward the new normal." Factors in this process according to postpartum women interviewed are appreciating the body, settling in, and becoming a family.

Resumption of sexual intercourse must be discussed with postpartum women, along with use of contraceptives. Lactation suppresses ovulation, but there is difficulty with determining when ovulation will return. Contraception must be utilized for women who do not desire conception during lactation. Lactation creates a vaginal dryness that must be countered with lubrication during intercourse. Temporary methods of birth control discussed with postpartum women include barrier methods, hormonal methods, and use of spermicidal agents. Oral contraceptives and progestin-only contraceptives can be utilized by lactating women, but a decrease in milk production is possible. This possibility must be discussed with women who desire the use of hormonal contraceptives.

MANAGEMENT OF POSTPARTUM COMPLICATIONS

PERINATAL LOSS

SIGNAL SYMPTOMS ▶ bleeding, no fetal heart tones, spontaneous abortion

Perinatal Loss	ICD-9-CM: 637.9 (+ 5th digit)

Definition: Loss of a pregnancy.

Etiology: Early pregnancy loss is related at least 50%–60% of the time to a karyotypic abnormality. As gestation progresses, the proportion of losses arising from genetic factors decreases and those arising from maternal or environmental factors increase. In the third trimester only 5% of stillborns have chromosomal aberrations. When there is a stillborn infant without any obvious cause, a genetic etiology should be sought.

Occurrence: 10%–20% of all pregnancies.

Age: Childbearing.

Ethnicity: Not significant.

Contributing Factors: Maternal infection, anatomic abnormalities of the uterus, maternal chronic disease.

Signs and symptoms: Delivery of products of conception or a nonviable infant.

Diagnostic tests:

Test	Results Indicating Disorder	CPT Code
Serial beta human chorionic gonadotropin (BHCG) levels in the first trimester	Decreasing	84702 × 3
After second or third-trimester delivery, a thorough examination of the fetal remains	Appear to be abnormalities present. Photographs should be taken.	Included in physical exam code
Autopsy	Aid in diagnosis	88020
Karyotype	Abnormalities	85130

Differential diagnosis: Ectopic pregnancy (positive signs of pregnancy with one-sided lower abdominal pain; serial beta hCG in series can be helpful in the diagnosis)

Treatment: Bed rest, first trimester: dilation and evacuation (D&E) if BHCG levels do not fall to zero. Second- and third-trimester loss may require cervical ripening and induction of labor.

When a prenatal diagnosis of a lethal anomaly has been established, some women choose to continue their pregnancy. An article on perinatal hospice care appeared in the American Journal of Obstetrics and Gynecology in September, 2002. The authors encourage the application of hospice concepts, both structured and compassionate, to perinatal loss.

Follow-up: Follow-up depends on treatment strategy. Helping a woman cope with the loss of a pregnancy is both rewarding and challenging. Circumstances surrounding the loss can carry ramifications that last a lifetime. Assisting a woman to cope with her loss with comfort and dignity is important in both the immediate aftermath of the loss and in the long-term adjustment. Perinatal grief management is important and necessary.

Sequelae: Retained fetal loss increases the risk of an infection and bleeding. The loss of a family member can bring about reminders of what may have been long after the initial pain has subsided.

Prevention/prophylaxis: None.

Referral: Physician referral is required.

Education: Signs and symptoms of infection should be reviewed with the woman.

POSTPARTUM DEPRESSION

SIGNAL SYMPTOMS sadness, frequent crying, insomnia

Postpartum depression	ICD-9-CM: 648.4 (+ 5th digit)

Definition: Depression after delivery of an infant.

Etiology: Mood disorder with postpartum onset.

Occurrence: Postpartum depression develops in approximately 10% of all postpartum women. The greatest risk occurs at approximately 4 weeks after delivery.

Age: Childbearing.

Ethnicity: Not significant.

Contributing factors: Risks for postpartum depression include primiparity, history of postpartum depression, lack of social support, and lack of stable relationships.

Signs and symptoms: Symptoms of postpartum depression are the same as those of any major depression: sadness, frequent crying, insomnia, appetite change, difficulty concentrating, feelings of worthlessness, feelings of inadequacy, lack of concern about personal appearance, persistent anxiety, and irritability toward others.

Diagnostic tests: Patient history of depression. Depression inventory testing.

Differential diagnosis: The new mother may experience some degree of baby "blues" a few days after delivery. This is the result of many factors, some of which are emotional letdown following delivery, physical discomfort of the immediate postpartum period, fatigue, and anxiety.

Mild and transient "postpartum blues" are treated with anticipatory guidance and counseling. If the blues are mild and self-limiting, there is minimal concern. Depression, which is not a normal accompaniment of childbearing, requires investigation. There is no evidence that pregnancy itself causes depression, but it may precipitate underlying disease. Postpartum depression must be identified and treated.

Treatment: Hospitalization, medication, psychotherapy.

Follow-up: As per treatment protocol.

Sequelae: Dependent on severity.

Prevention/prophylaxis: None.

Referral: Psychiatric referral.

Education: It is important to report feelings of sadness following delivery to a health-care provider.

POSTPARTUM HEMORRHAGE

SIGNAL SYMPTOM▶ significant blood loss within 24 hours of delivery

Postpartum hemorrhage (after delivery)	ICD-9-CM: 666
24 hours after delivery	ICD-9-CM: 666.2 (+ 5th digit)
Retained placenta	ICD-9-CM: 666.0 (+ 5th digit)
Third stage	ICD-9-CM: 666.0 (+ 5th digit)

Definition: Postpartum hemorrhage has been defined as blood loss of more than 500 mL during the first 24 hours after delivery. This definition is difficult to use since blood loss is estimated at delivery with the estimate often one half of the actual loss.

Etiology: The two most important causes of immediate postpartum hemorrhage are uterine atony and laceration of the cervix and vagina. The overdistended uterus is likely to be hypotonic after delivery. Thus the woman with a large fetus, twins, or polyhydramnios is prone to postpartum hemorrhage. Labor initiated or augmented with pitocin is more likely to be followed with atony and hemorrhage. Postpartum hemorrhage can also be related to retained placental tissue interfering with uterine contraction. Trauma can lead to postpartum hemorrhage. Examples of trauma can be related to delivery of large infants, midforceps deliveries, and forceps rotations.

Occurrence: Of women delivering vaginally, 5% lose more than 1000 mL of blood. Postpartum hemorrhage is the cause of one quarter of the deaths from obstetric hemorrhage.

Age: Childbearing.

Ethnicity: Not significant.

Contributing factors: Delivery of large infant, forceps delivery, multiple gestation, and polyhydramnios. Rarely, postpartum bleeding is related to a coagulation disorder. In women with obstetrical and/or medical complications of pregnancy, disseminated intravascular coagulation (DIC) can occur, resulting in acceleration of the coagulation system and activation of the fibrinolytic system.

Signs and symptoms: Heavy vaginal bleeding after delivery.

Diagnostic tests:

Test	Results Indicating Disorder	CPT Code
Ultrasound	Retained placental fragments	76856

Differential diagnosis: Vulvar hematoma may cause excruciating pain and is diagnosed with the sudden appearance of a tense and sensitive mass covered by discolored skin or mucous membrane.

Treatment: The cause of the hemorrhage must be determined prior to initiation of treatment. Atony of the uterus should be considered first. If the uterus is "boggy," massage is appropriate, and at times oxytocin must be administered. The role of lacerations in postpartum bleeding must be ascertained. Any lacerations creating excessive bleeding must be repaired. Vulvar hematoma is treated with prompt incision and evacuation of blood with ligation of the bleeding points.

Follow-up: According to therapy.

Sequelae: Anemia.

Prevention/prophylaxis: Treat causative factor or factors.

Referral: Consultation with a physician is required.

Education: Postpartum women should be taught the normal phases of involution, including type and amount of vaginal discharge.

POSTPARTUM INFECTION

SIGNAL SYMPTOMS ▶ fever, chills, abdominal pain, incisional pain or breast pain

Postpartum Infection (major)	ICD-9-CM: 670 (+ 4th digit)
Minor	ICD-9-CM: 646.6 (+ 5th digit)

Definition: Infection following delivery can occur in the pelvis, breast, or urinary tract. The likelihood of pelvic infection is related to the length of time the membranes were ruptured prior to delivery, the number of examinations the woman had during labor, the amount of manipulation at the time of vaginal delivery, the size and number of incisions and lacerations, and operative method of delivery.

Etiology: Organisms that invade the placental site, incision, and lacerations are typically those that normally colonize the cervix, vagina, and perineum. Most of the organisms are of low virulence and seldom cause infection in healthy tissues. The most common causative agents of postpartum infection are anaerobic streptococci, clostridia, β-hemolytic streptococci, *Escherichia coli,* and *Klebsiella.* Infection of episiotomy and repaired lacerations is unusual considering the degree of bacterial contamination to which the site is exposed.

Occurrence: Unknown.

Age: Childbearing.

Ethnicity: Not significant.

Contributing factors: Size and number of incisions or lacerations if related to infection. Uterine infection is more common following cesarean delivery, particularly if the cesarean followed long labor with multiple pelvic examinations. Length of time that membranes are ruptured is related to infection.

Signs and symptoms: Postpartum uterine infection involves the decidua, myometrium, and parametrial tissues. Symptoms are fever, chills, and abdominal pain. There is bilateral tenderness elicited on bimanual examination, and the lochia has a foul odor.

If infection of an incision occurs, wound edges become red and swollen and sutures may tear through edematous tissue, causing wound gaping. Drainage may be serous or frankly purulent. Complete breakdown of the repair site may occur.

Pain and dysuria are symptoms of episiotomy infection or urinary tract infection (UTI) (see Figure 13–1).

Symptoms of mastitis rarely occur prior to the first week after delivery, and as a rule do not occur until the third or fourth week of lactation. Engorgement precedes inflammation. Rise in temperature occurs early in the infection process. The breast becomes reddened, hard, and painful. The most common organism is *Staphylococcus aureus,* the source of which is the infant's mouth and throat.

Diagnostic tests:

Test	Results Indicating Disorder	CPT Code
Culture and sensitivity of urine or wound	Positive culture	87088 (urine culture) 87070 (wound culture) 87181 (sensitivity)
Pelvic and breast examination	Masses or pus or inflammation seen or palpated	Included in general physical

Differential diagnosis:

- Suture irritation (redness, soreness)
- Bladder infection (confirmed by lab studies)

Treatment: Treatment of postpartum infection consists of establishing drainage and administering broad-spectrum antibiotics by oral route or, in the event of severe infection, by intravenous route. Symptoms of endometrial infection rarely occur prior to 5 days after delivery. Antibiotics are used to treat endometrial infection.

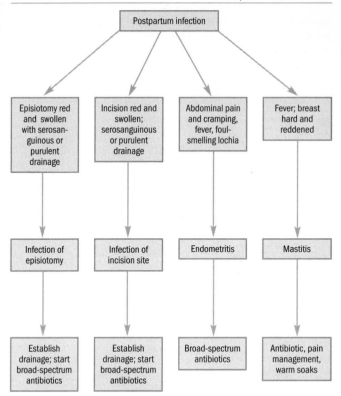

Figure 13-1. Diagnosis of postpartum infection.

 Clinical Pearl: Wound infection is treated with cleansing the wound followed by antibiotics.

Culturing the wound prior to cleansing is recommended.

Urinary tract infection can occur after delivery. Manipulation and use of catheters contribute to this infection. Women experience pain with urination and frequency of urination. Treatment is with broad-spectrum antibiotics after urinary culture and sensitivity to identify the organism involved.

For mastitis, treatment involves antibiotics, acetaminophen for pain and fever, warm soaks on the affected breast, and frequent nursing on the infected breast.

Follow-up: Repeat culture and sensitivity following resolution of infection.

Sequelae: None after therapy.

Prevention/prophylaxis: Appropriate management of labor and delivery.

Referral: For unresolved infection, physician referral is required.

Education: Stress to the postpartum woman the importance of reporting fever and pain postpartum.

SUBINVOLUTION OF THE UTERUS

SIGNAL SYMPTOM excessive bleeding 1–2 weeks following delivery

Subinvolution of the uterus	ICD-9-CM: 621.1
Postpartum	ICD-9-CM: 674.8 (+5th digit)

Definition: "Subinvolution of the uterus" is the term utilized when excessive vaginal bleeding occurs in the nonimmediate postpartum period.

Etiology: Prolongation of the involution process.

Occurrence: Unknown.

Age: Childbearing.

Ethnicity: Not significant.

Contributing factors: Subinvolution accompanied by pain and fever indicates a relationship with endometritis. Multiparity and cesarean delivery may contribute to subinvolution.

Signs and symptoms: The woman experiences excessive vaginal bleeding with or without fever and pain 1–2 weeks after delivery. The bleeding can be related to retained placental fragments or abnormal involution at the placental site. A subinvoluted uterus will feel "boggy" and tender.

Diagnostic tests:

Test	Results Indicating Disorder	CPT Code
Complete blood count (CBC)	Signs of inflammation	85025
Cervical culture	Negative	87070
Serum human chorionic gonadotropin (hCG)	Higher than expected for postpartum	84702
Pelvic ultrasound	Endometritis, placental remains	76856

Differential diagnosis:

- Infection of the endometrium (fever, chills, positive culture)
- Cystitis (positive culture)
- Retained placental fragments (pelvic ultrasound)

Treatment: The treatment for subinvolution depends on the cause.

Follow-up: Outpatient visits are necessary to ensure resolution.

Sequelae: None.

Prevention/prophylaxis: None.

Referral: If resolution does not occur in a timely fashion, refer to an obstetric and gynecologic physician.

Education: Stress the importance of reporting excessive vaginal bleeding during postpartum period.

THROMBOPHLEBITIS

SIGNAL SYMPTOMS fever, pain and swelling in leg; positive Homan's sign

Thrombophlebitis (superficial)	ICD-9-CM: 671.2 (+ 5th digit)
Deep	ICD-9-CM: 671.3 (+ 5th digit)

Definition: Thrombophlebitis is an infection of the lining of a vessel in which a clot attaches to a vessel wall. Thrombophlebitis may affect the veins in the leg or pelvis after delivery. Thrombophlebitis can be superficial or deep. If superficial, only the surface venous system is involved. If deep, changes take place in the deep veins of the calf, thighs, or pelvis. With deep venous involvement, there is a risk of pulmonary embolism.

Etiology: Thrombophlebitis occurs after delivery and is related to the increased clotting factors during this period.

Occurrence: The incidence is less than 1% of postpartum women, with onset usually between the tenth and twentieth postpartum day.

Age: Thrombophlebitis occurs more frequently with increased maternal age.

Ethnicity: Not significant.

Contributing factors: History contributing to deep vein thrombosis (DVT) includes obesity, operative delivery, long labor, post-delivery infection, past history of DVT, and varicosities.

Signs and symptoms: DVT symptoms include positive Homan's sign, elevated temperature, pain in the leg, swelling and tenderness of the leg, and/or groin pain.

Diagnostic tests:

Test	Results Indicating Disorder	CPT Code
Doppler flow studies	Positive for obstruction/thrombi	93970
CT or MRI scanning of the pelvis	Positive for obstruction/thrombi	72193 (CT) with contrast 72196 (MRI) with contrast

Differential diagnosis: Edema of the leg or leg pain unrelated to thrombophlebitis.

Treatment: Superficial thrombophlebitis is treated with application of continuous moist heat to the extremity and elevation of the extremity. DVT is treated with anticoagulant therapy, bed rest, elevation of the extremity, and analgesia.

Follow-up: As per treatment regimen.

Sequelae: Risk of reoccurrence following delivery or surgery. DVT can precede pulmonary embolism. The incidence is 1 in 5000 deliveries.

Prevention/prophylaxis: Early ambulation after delivery reduces the incidence of thrombophlebitis.

Referral: For diagnostic testing. Refer to a physician if Doppler study is positive.

Education: Stress the importance of reporting signs and symptoms of thrombophlebitis to a health-care provider.

REFERENCES

Chalmers, B, et al: WHO principles of perinatal care: the essential antenatal, perinatal, and postpartum care course. Birth 28(3), 2001.

Gant, N, and Cunningham, F: Basic Gynecology and Obstetrics. Appleton & Lange, Norwalk, CT, 1993.

Gypton, A, and McKay, M: The Canadian perspective on postpartum home care. JOGNN 24(2), Feb 1995.

Harrykissoon, S, et al: Prevalence and patterns of intimate partner violence among adolescent mothers during the postpartum period. Arch Pediatr Adolesc Med 156, 2002.

Hiller, J, et al: Education for contraceptive use of women after childbirth. Cochrane Database of Systematic Reviews (3):1863, 2002.

Hoeldtke, N, and Calhoun, B: Perinatal hospice. Amer J Obstet Gynecol 185(3), Sept 2002.

Horon, I, et al: Enhanced surveillance for pregnancy-associated mortality: Maryland 1993–1998. JAMA 285, 2001.

Horowitz, J, and Damato, E: Mother's perceptions of postpartum stress and satisfaction. JOGNN 28(6), 1999.

Li, X, et al: The postpartum period: the key to maternal mortality. International J Gynaecol Obstet 54(1), 1996.

Martell, K: Heading toward the new normal: A contemporary postpartum experience. JOGNN 30(5), 2001.

Mortensen, P: Pregnant adolescents. MCN 28(1): 2002.

Quistad, C: How to smooth Mom's postpartum path. RN 40, April 1994.

Stover, A, and Marnejon, J: Postpartum care. American Family Physician 52(5), 1995.

Youngkin, E, and Davis, M: Women's Health. Appleton & Lange, Norwalk, CT, 1994.

Chapter 14

MENOPAUSE

MENOPAUSE

SIGNAL SYMPTOMS ▶ irregular bleeding, hot flashes

Menopause	ICD-9-CM: 627.2
Surgical menopause	ICD-9-CM: 627.4
Premature menopause	ICD-9-CM: 256.31
Premature postsurgical menopause	ICD-9-CM: 256.2

Description: Menopause, which is marked by estrogen deficiency, is not a disease of the endocrine system; rather, it is a transition and an indicator of continuing maturity. The term menopause refers to the cessation of menses, usually defined retrospectively after 12 months of amenorrhea. Menopause marks the end of reproductive years for women.

More than 30 million U.S. women are now at or beyond menopause. At least 6 million women will reach this stage of life in the next decade. A woman at the age of 50, the average age for menopause in the United States, has a life expectancy of approximately 30 more years. Menopause is, therefore, a transition to approximately 30 postreproductive years. Reproductive capability ceases with menopause, but women's sexuality does not change. Women can remain sexually active throughout their lifetime. Presence of a partner has been shown to be the most important indicator for sexual activity in postmenopausal women.

Perimenopause is a term used to define the period of time surrounding the menopause. Perimenopause begins with changes that indicate a transition is occurring, and ends after the cessation of menses and perimenopausal symptoms.

Mid-life is a term used to define the perimenopausal and early menopausal years.

Natural menopause refers to menopause occurring without medical intervention. **Surgical menopause** refers to menopause occurring as a result of the surgical removal of the ovaries.

Etiology: A decrease in estradiol and progesterone levels produces perimenopausal symptoms. Most notable among those symptoms are hot flashes or flushes, sleep disturbance, genitourinary complaints, skin changes, changes in muscle strength, and changes in memory. It is a complex interaction of factors involving hormonal changes, vasomotor phenomena, neurotransmitters, and psychological factors. Perimenopausal women are more likely to report symptoms of headaches, back pain, stiff joints, and tiredness than are postmenopausal women. Postmenopausal women reported more hot flushes and night sweats.

Occurrence: The average American woman now lives one third of her life after menopause. Women do not report depression related to loss of reproductive function. They do report concern about the symptoms related to menopause. Loss of reproductive function is reported to be a "relief" to many women.

The most frequently reported symptom of perimenopause is hot flashes. 70% of women experience hot flushes (Rymer, 2000). This symptom brings perimenopausal women to health-care providers most often. Hot flashes are experienced by approximately 75% of women around the time of menopause. This symptom is often the first indicator of transition.

Age: The median age for menopause in the United States is 50–51 years.

Contributing factors: The variability of women's symptoms indicates that pure biology is not the only explanation. Other factors that may influence symptoms are heredity, diet, weight, exercise patterns, and stress levels.

Ethnicity: The impact of menopause on women's health and overall well-being is currently being studied. Of note is a lack of research on non-Caucasian women and health and menopause. What is known to date is that any woman with an early natural menopause has a stronger risk for vasomotor symptoms (hot flashes and night sweats), more sexual difficulties, and more trouble sleeping. All types of symptoms are more common in women who have had a hysterectomy or are users of hormone replacement therapy (Kuh et al., 1997).

Signs and symptoms:

Irregular Bleeding: Menstrual cycles become irregular prior to menopause. Irregularity is usually related to anovulatory cycles. Bleeding may become infrequent, prolonged, heavy, or intermenstrual.

Hot Flashes:

- Hot flashes can occur for 30 seconds or for several minutes at intervals lasting for months or years. They can occur at any time of the day or night.

- Hot flashes are sudden, transient feelings of warmth accompanied by flushing and sweating. Women will feel a need to remove their coats or sweaters or to kick off their blankets. Estrogen withdrawal is related to hot flashes, but exactly how is poorly understood. Estrogen replacement can relieve hot flashes, but low estrogen levels are not sufficient to produce hot flashes. (Prepubertal girls with low estrogen levels do not experience hot flashes. Women with hypothalamic amenorrhea do not experience hot flashes.) However, in perimenopausal women, the lower the estrogen level, the more likely the symptom.

- Episodes usually diminish in frequency and severity over time.
- Hot flashes increase in warm weather; confined spaces; and after consumption of caffeine, alcohol, or spicy foods.
- Women who experience surgical menopause tend to have more hot flashes than women who experience natural menopause.
- After menopause, the prevalence of hot flashes is highest in the first 2 years.

Urogenital Changes/ Stress Incontinence: Decrease in estrogen causes tissue changes. The tissues of the vagina, urethra, vulva, and trigone of the bladder contain large numbers of estrogen receptors. These tissues atrophy when estrogen is reduced. The vulva loses subcutaneous fat and the epidermis and vaginal epithelium becomes thinner. Vaginal glycogen level decreases, leading to a less acidic vagina. (A less acidic environment increases susceptibility to infection.) General lubrication and lubrication accompanying sexual arousal also decreases (see Figure 14–1). Stress incontinence may be related to perimenopausal changes.

Diagnostic tests:

Test	Results Indicating Disorder	CPT Code
Pap smear	Rule out for carcinoma	88142
Endometrial sampling	Rule out for carcinoma	58100
Pelvic exam	Vulva with decreased subcutaneous fat; epidermis and vaginal epithelium thin; rule out carcinoma	Included in physical exam code
Estrogen level	Decreased	82672 (total); 82671 (fractionated)
pH of vagina	Less acidic	83986
FSH level	Increased	83001
LH level	Increased	83002
Serum pregnancy test	Negative	84702
Wet prep	Atrophic basal cells; no other causes of vaginitis	87210
Mammogram	Rule out carcinoma	76091 bilateral 76090 unilateral

Differential diagnosis:

- Pregnancy and other causes of missed menstrual periods; other irregularities or abnormalities of menstruation; or both
- Anxiety and other physiologic states occurring in the absence of menopause

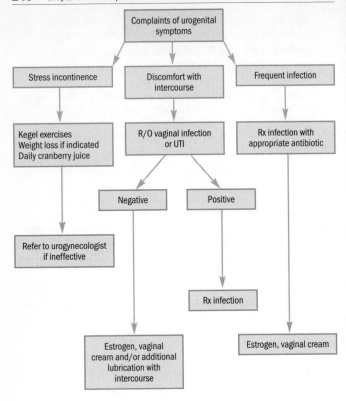

Figure 14–1. Urogenital changes, perimenopausal and postmenopausal.

- Alternative explanations for any nonspecific symptoms of menopause, such as headaches, fatigue, stress, and tension
- Cancer

Treatment:

Therapies for irregular bleeding include reassurance, hormonal treatment, or endometrial ablation (see Figure 14–2).

Treatment for hot flashes includes reassurance, hormone replacement therapy, "alternative therapies" such as black cohosh, and weight loss in overweight women.

Topical or systemic estrogen decreases these symptoms. Sexually active women have less vaginal atrophy than women who are not sexually active.

Regular consumption of cranberry juice (300mL daily) reduces the risk of bladder infection. To reduce stress incontinence, the urethral

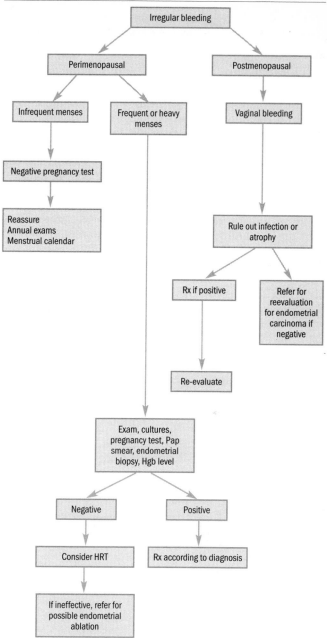

Figure 14–2. Irregular bleeding.

sphincter can be strengthened with Kegel exercises (see Appendix, Chapter 12). Stress incontinence is not affected by estrogen levels.

Hormone Replacement Therapy

Rationale: The rationale for HRT is that hormone shifts cause menopausal symptoms. Women with perimenopausal symptoms interfering with their daily lives should consider HRT. In May 2002, the Women's Health Initiative (WHI) clinical trial found that a combination of estrogen and progesterone prescribed to postmenopausal women increases the risk of invasive breast cancer, heart disease, stroke, and pulmonary embolism. Combination hormone therapy reduces bone fractures and colon cancer, but not enough to outweigh the other risks. Also, in May of 2002, an epidemiologic study was published suggesting that estrogen replacement therapy, when used alone for 10 years or more, increases the risk of ovarian cancer. The WHI study calls into question the *long term* use of HRT in healthy women (Women's Health Initiative, May, 2002). Use of estrogen to reduce the incidence of Alzheimer's disease has had disappointing results (Knopman, 2002). The benefit of the temporary use of estrogen in controlling disruptive symptoms of menopause is currently being challenged.

Contraindications: Contraindications for HRT are stroke, breast cancer, liver disease, pancreatic disease, history of thrombophlebitis, recent myocardial infarction, endometrial adenocarcinoma, estrogen-dependent tumors, and undiagnosed vaginal bleeding (see Table 14–1).

Forms of administration:

HRT can be supplied in oral form, patches applied to the skin, and in cream form.

- Oral administration is usually estrogen 0.625 mg daily with 2.5 mg progesterone daily. Progesterone is necessary to protect the uterus. It is not necessary to prescribe progesterone following hysterectomy.
- Skin patches are applied once or twice per week on a dry, hairless area of the body, but not on the breast. Patches are a lower dose of estrogen than oral administration, 0.05 mg most commonly, and the estrogen is absorbed directly. Estrogen skin patches are given with oral progesterone when the uterus is present.

Table 14–1 Contraindications to Estrogen Therapy

Absolute	Relative
Unexplained vaginal bleeding	Seizure disorders
Acute liver damage	High levels of triglycerides
Recent vascular thrombosis	High levels of lipids
Carcinoma of the breast	Migraine headaches
Carcinoma of the endometrium	Atraumatic thrombophlebitis
	Current gallbladder disease

- Cream containing estrogen 0.3 mg is used for vaginal effect only; 2 g daily for 1–2 weeks intravaginally, followed by 2 g once or twice weekly for maintenance is the recommendation.
- Prolonged estrogen therapy unopposed by progestin causes hyperplasia of the endometrium and a four- to six-fold increase in endometrial cancer. Regular addition of a progestin negates the risk and provides protection.

Considerations for HRT therapy:

- HRT alleviates vasomotor and urogenital discomfort. This finding is well established.
- HRT or alendronate (Fosamax) are utilized to treat osteoporosis and decrease the fracture risk.
- HRT has a favorable impact on the risk of colon cancer.

The right medication for the correct period of time is the issue for women who choose HRT. History and symptoms will dictate what drug or combination of drugs and in what form. The most commonly prescribed regimens provide a baseline from which to begin therapy. Side effects and decrease in symptoms guide the modification of dose and route of administration.

Follow-up: For patients with menopausal symptoms, a yearly physical with Pap smears and pelvic exam is sufficient. For those on hormone replacement therapy, blood pressure checks should be done every six months for first year, and annual Pap smears. For both types of patients, frequent follow-up is needed to counsel the patient and deal with psychological and other aspects of menopausal syndrome.

Sequelae:

- Change in Physical Strength at Menopause: Decrease in grip strength has been noted in postmenopausal women. Women report less physical strength following menopause.
- Memory Problems and Difficulty Concentrating: Cerebral perfusion declines with age. Women have higher blood flow values than men until menopause occurs. The connections between menopause and memory are being studied. Results from recent controlled trials have not consistently shown a beneficial effect of estrogen therapy on cognitive function of women.
- Sleep Changes: Night "sweats," psychological distress, and sleep apnea can create sleeping problems in perimenopausal and postmenopausal women. Hot flashes, often called night sweats, can disrupt sleep. Apnea caused by blockage of the air passage during sleep causes arousal in order to breathe. Apnea is associated with upper-body obesity in women. Symptoms of apnea are daytime sleepiness, persistent tired feelings, and loud snoring at night with gasps.
- Visual Changes: Decreased ability to accommodate to close items is common in women over 40 years. Presbyopia, difficulty seeing things close up, is a common diagnosis.

- Cataracts are protein deposits in the lenses of the eyes. Early cataract signs are blurred vision and night vision problems. Cataracts require diagnosis and surgical treatment.
- Glaucoma is an increase in pressure within the eye. This pressure can damage the optic nerve.

Prevention/prophylaxis:

Risk assessment: The leading causes of death for women aged 45–54 in order of incidence are malignancy, heart disease, cerebrovascular disease, accidents, liver disease, suicide, chronic obstructive pulmonary disease (COPD), diabetes, pneumonia, and homicide. For women aged 55–64, the causes of death in order of incidence are malignancy, heart disease, COPD, pneumonia, diabetes, liver disease, accidents, suicide, and homicide. Women with a natural menopause at age 40–44 years experience an increased risk for cancer-related mortality. No age-related increased mortality rate is seen among women who experience surgical menopause.

Refer to Chapter 1 for discussion of screening for malignancy in these age groups. Secondary prevention strategies for malignancy include breast examination and mammography. Regular Pap smears and pelvic examinations are part of the screening process for malignancy.

Screening for cancer includes accurate taking of both personal and family history. Tamoxifen has been found to be a useful drug for women who are a significant risk for breast cancer (see Chapter 1). Referral for tamoxifen treatment should be considered for all high-risk perimenopausal women.

Perimenopausal and postmenopausal women should be encouraged to have regular screening for breast cancer, but should also be warned concerning the risk of false positives. A research article in the *New England Journal of Medicine* (Elmore et al, 1998) revealed that in each woman the cumulative risk of a false-positive breast cancer screening after 10 screenings was 49.1% for mammograms and 22.3% for breast examination.

Cardiovascular disease in women is related to obesity, plasma lipid levels, hypertension, diabetes, cigarette smoking, sedentary lifestyle, and lack of estrogen. Improvement in any of these factors improves cardiovascular status. Blood pressure screening should be performed at every health-care encounter. The following Education section contains a discussion about health promotion related to reducing the risk of cardiovascular disease in women.

Referral:

- Any patient with a history of contraindications for hormone replacement therapy (see below).
- Any patient who develops genital bleeding while on hormone replacement therapy, other than those women who have predictable progesterone withdrawal bleeding.

- Any patient with severe complications.
- Any patient with abnormal findings on diagnostics, such as cancer.

Education:

Health Promotion

Cardiovascular: A significant health risk facing perimenopausal and menopausal women is cardiovascular disease. The risk for heart disease begins to rise at age 45. The Framingham Study reported that the risk for cardiovascular disease for women triples after menopause and premature menopause increases the risk. Modifiable risk factors for cardiovascular disease are lack of exercise, poor diet, smoking, and estrogen levels.

Exercise: A regular exercise routine is recommended for all perimenopausal and postmenopausal women to overcome the natural tendency for decreased strength. More active and physically fit women experience less cardiovascular disease. When active people do develop cardiovascular disease, it occurs later in life and is less severe. Fitness can also prevent bone mineral loss. Exercise decreases the risk for falls and can increase flexibility. Exercise helps prevent depression and anxiety. Perimenopausal and menopausal women who exercise have fewer hot flashes, less symptoms of depression, improved memory, and less difficulty sleeping. They also have fewer digestive complaints. The Centers for Disease Control tell us that American women are sedentary and that activity level decreases at mid-life. Thus, increasing physical activity for women is an objective for all women's health nurse practitioners.

Women's leisure time is often filled with the priorities of others, making time for exercise difficult to find. Finding a mode of activity suitable for each woman is a challenge for practitioners. Women in mid-life who are successful in exercising regularly often choose activities that can be done in and around their homes, using time as it becomes free. Examples of these activities are walking, exercising with videos, and riding a stationary bicycle. Exercising for 20–30 minutes three to four times per week is the current recommendation (see Chapter 1). Suggest to women that they explore exercise activities that are reasonable for them to pursue within their current lifestyle, and suggest that the exercise activity be something that they enjoy.

Nutrition

- Limiting fat intake, particularly after the effective protection of estrogen is removed at menopause, is an important dietary goal. The nutritional goal for menopausal women is 15% protein, 55% carbohydrates, and 30% or less fat.
- Daily calorie requirements for maintenance decrease at menopause. Weight will increase after menopause unless there is increased activity or decreased intake of calories. The recommended daily allowance (RDA) for women over 50 is 80%–85% of the 2200 calories recommended for young adults.

- Calcium intake of 800 mg/day is sufficient for active women under 50. After 50, calcium intake should be increased to 1200–1500 mg/day. Postmenopausal women not on HRT should consider 1500 mg/day of calcium intake.
- The need for iron decreases to 10 mg/day from 15 mg after menopause.
- A diet high in complex carbohydrates (high fiber) may reduce the incidence of colon cancer and may avoid constipation that is common in women in mid-life.
- Eight to ten 8-oz glasses of water daily is recommended.
- Weight reduction should be encouraged in overweight perimenopausal and menopausal women. Obesity is associated with cardiovascular disease.

Smoking Cessation: Smoking is associated with lung cancer, coronary artery disease, cerebrovascular disease, cervical cancer, hypertension, and respiratory disease. Women in mid-life who smoke are more likely to be heavy smokers and less likely to quit than younger women. Quitting smoking for 10 years reduces the risk of lung cancer by 30%–50%, according to the Centers for Disease Control and Prevention. Women who quit smoking reduce their risk for cardiovascular disease by 24% within 2 years of stopping.

Women report that they smoke to reduce their weight and to reduce stress. Advise mid-life women to stop smoking and address these two concerns. Other avenues for stress reduction and maintenance of weight should be explored. Address a woman's concerns and barriers to stopping. Help her decide on a quit date. Provide her with reassurance. Nicotine gum and patches may be helpful both with stopping smoking and with preventing weight gain. Antidepressants have demonstrated efficacy in aiding smoking cessation.

Stress Management: Sleep disruption can be reduced by treating hot flashes. Stress management may decrease sleep disruption. Any indicator of sleep apnea requires referral for evaluation and treatment.

Visual Adjustments: For women who have never worn glasses and who now have symptoms of presbyopia, drugstore nonprescription glasses may be all that are necessary. If these are not effective, prescriptive lenses are necessary. Decreased exposure to the sun decreases the likelihood of cataract formation. Daily consumption of vitamin C also decreases the likelihood of cataract formation. Glaucoma can be controlled if diagnosed early. The pressure within each eye should be checked at all eye examinations.

OSTEOPOROSIS

SIGNAL SYMPTOM▶   fractures of hip or spine; most cases, however, are asymptomatic

| Osteoporosis (generalized) | ICD-9-CM: 733.00 |
| Postmenopausal osteoporosis | ICD-9-CM: 733.01 |

Description: A heterogeneous group of diseases resulting in a reduction in bone mass per unit volume to a level below the level required for adequate mechanical support. The ratio of mineral to matrix material remains normal. This reduction may ultimately lead to fractures, most frequently in the hip, spine, and wrist.

Etiology: Multiple known causes for osteoporosis include corticosteroid therapy, chronic heparin therapy, prolonged immobilization, thyrotoxicosis, Cushing's disease, malabsorbtion, renal tubular acidosis, and multiple myeloma. Most cases are of unclear etiology. After menopause women undergo a rapid phase of calcium loss from bone that continues for approximately 5–7 years, followed by a slower annual calcium loss. Estrogen replacement delays the rapid phase of calcium loss; after hormonal replacement is stopped the rapid phase will begin.

Occurence: 20 million women currently have osteoporosis. According to the National Osteoporosis Foundation, the overall cost of acute and long-term care associated with osteoporosis exceeds $10 billion annually. (Health-care costs are related primarily to the morbidity and mortality associated with fractures [Hulley, 1998].)

Age: Loss of bone mineral density begins in women around the age of 30. The rate increases after age 40, and escalates further after menopause.

Ethnicity: African-American women have denser bones than Caucasian women.

Contributing factors: Bone loss is influenced by age, female sex, menopausal status, heredity, white race, and weight (thin women are at greater risk). Menopause secondary to surgical removal of ovaries is especially contributory if the surgery has been performed before the natural age of menopause. Modifiable risk factors for both cardiovascular disease and bone mineral density are decreased physical activity, poor diet, inadequate calcium intake, alcohol consumption, and smoking.

Risk factors for osteoporotic fracture include:

Nonmodifiable:

- Personal history of fracture as an adult
- History of fracture in a first-degree relative
- Caucasian race
- Advanced age

Modifiable:

- Cigarette smoking
- Low body weight
- Estrogen deficiency
- Low calcium intake

- Alcoholism
- Recurrent falls
- Inadequate physical activity

Signs and symptoms: Most patients are symptomatic as they undergo slow reduction in bone density. The most common clinical presentation is back pain related to vertebral compression fractures. Fractures of the hip may be the first indication of significant bone disease. Physically, the patient may have no signs, but kyphosis or loss of height may be seen in some (see Box 14–1).

Diagnostic tests:

Test	Results Indicating Disorder	CPT Code
Dual-energy x-ray absorptiometry (bone density test) (DEXA)	40% or more of bony mass lost; see Appendix A	76075 (axial skeleton) 76076 (peripheral)
Complete blood count	Normal in idiopathic osteoporosis	85025
Calcium	Normal in idiopathic osteoporosis	82310
Alkaline phosphatase	Normal in idiopathic osteoporosis	84075

- Perform evaluation for osteoporosis using bone densitometry on all postmenopausal women who present with fractures.
- Recommend densitometry testing for all women over age 65, regardless of risk factors.
- Recommend bone densitometry testing for postmenopausal women under age 65 who have one or more additional risk factors for osteoporosis.

Box 14–1
Bone Densitometry Testing (Osteoporosis)

Measurements of bone mineral density (BMD) at any skeletal site have value for indicating fracture risk. BMD is expressed as a relationship to two norms: the expected BMD for the patient's age and sex and/or the norm for a "young normal" adult. The difference between the patient's score and the norms will be reported.

BMD testing techniques:

- Dual energy x-ray absorptiometry (DEXA) can be used to measure BMD in spine, hip, or wrist. Scanning is completed in a few minutes with radiation exposure one-tenth that of a standard chest x-ray.
- Single energy absorptiometry measures BMD in the forearm or finger and sometimes the heel.
- Radiographic absorptiometry (RA) is a technique used in a standard x-ray of the hand.
- Quantitative computed tomography measures trabecular and cortical bone density at several sites in the body. It may be used as an alternative to DEXA scanning for vertebral measurements.
- Ultrasound densitometry assesses bone in the heel, tibia, patella, or other sites where bone is relatively superficial. Ultrasound measurements are not as precise as DEXA or single scans but accurately predict fracture risk.

- Women who are considering medication for the prevention of osteoporosis may find testing helpful in decision-making.

Differential diagnosis:

- Vitamin A deficiency (low blood levels)
- Metastatic carcinoma (radiologic examination)
- Multiple myeloma
- Cortisol excess, either intrinsic (Cushing's disease) or from use of exogenous steroids.
- Osteoarthritis (which may cause back pain, but has a different clinical course and X-ray picture)

Treatment: The treatment of osteoporosis includes calcium, exercise, alendronate (nontoxic, nonhormone therapy capable of stabilizing osteoporotic bone), and HRT.

- Calcitonin, a naturally occurring polypeptide, acts to suppress osteoclast activity and subsequent bone resorption. For many years, calcitonin in injection form was used to treat osteoporosis. Recently, the FDA has approved calcitonin in an intranasal form. The medication is administered in doses of 200 IU daily in the form of one puff in one nostril daily (alternating nostrils). Calcitonin should be used with calcium and vitamin D.
- Oral sodium fluoride works to stimulate bone formation by increasing the number of osteoblasts, and has been used in Europe for many years. This should also be used with calcium and vitamin D.
- Biphosphonates act to decrease bone resorption and to prevent bone loss. Biphosphonates can now be taken once per week. They should be taken with calcium and vitamin D.
- Women who have undergone premature surgical oophorectomy should receive estrogen replacement. Patients with carcinoma of the breast in a first-degree relative are at risk for carcinoma, and consultation is necessary.
- Maintenance of an adequate calcium intake (>1.0 gram/day) may have some protective factor, and is unlikely to do harm. The addition may be in the form of increased intake of dairy products or use of over-the-counter calcium supplements (500mg/dose). This should begin well before menopause.
- Supplemental vitamin D 400 IU every day is recommended in conjunction with calcium; the elderly get very little natural vitamin D.

Follow-up: Preventive interventions should be addressed at health-care maintenance visits, but further follow-up for symptomatic patients should be individualized.

Sequelae:

- Fractures of the femoral neck with mild or minimal trauma
- Other fractures, including vertebral compression fractures
- Breakthrough bleeding from estrogen therapy

Prevention/prophylaxis: Primary prevention of bone loss seems to be more effective in preventing symptoms than treatment after pain or fractures have occurred. All women should be encouraged to exercise regularly, not to smoke, to take supplemental calcium, and not to drink to excess. These measures will help prevent bone loss. Maintenance of moderate physical activity with aging may help preserve bony mass. Weight-bearing exercise is most beneficial.

Referral:

- For all patients with symptomatic back pain related to compression fractures
- Young patients with osteoporosis
- Bleeding before the twelfth day of progestogen therapy
- Suspicion of multiple myeloma

Education:

 Clinical Pearl: Counsel all women on risk factors for osteoporosis.

- Weight bearing physical exercise 3 times per week
- Calcium intake 1000 to 1500 mg per day in divided doses of 500 mg at a time with 400 IU supplement of vitamin D
- Healthy lifestyle behaviors of: no smoking, decreased alcohol intake, healthy diet
- Wearing good shoes to limit tripping hazards

CONTRACEPTIVE CONCERNS FOR PERIMENOPAUSAL WOMEN

Pregnancy is possible when women are ovulating irregularly. During the perimenopausal period, contraception should be discussed.

- The diaphragm may cause irritation because of vaginal dryness during mid-life.
- Condoms may be uncomfortable because of lack of lubrication. (Condoms may be necessary, however, if the woman is at risk for human immunodeficiency virus [HIV].)
- The intrauterine device (IUD) may be an acceptable contraceptive method, but it must be removed before uterine atrophy occurs.
- Oral contraceptives can be used by many perimenopausal women. If a woman is healthy and nonsmoking, low-dose oral contraceptives can be considered.
- Progestin-only contraceptives can be used. They can produce amenorrhea, which may be helpful in women with irregular bleeding.

ALTERNATIVES TO HYSTERECTOMY

Description: Hysterectomy involves the removal of the entire uterus (a total hysterectomy) through an abdominal incision. Hysterectomy can also be performed via laparoscopy. (The uterus is removed in pieces via the vagina.) The laparoscopic approach creates less postoperative discomfort, shorter hospital stay, and quicker recovery.

Etiology: Hysterectomy is performed most commonly for fibroids, dysfunctional uterine bleeding, prolapse, and endometriosis. For discussion of treatment options for these conditions, see Chapter 15.

Occurrence: Hysterectomy is the second most frequently performed operation in the United States. The United States has the highest rate of hysterectomy in the world, with about five out of 1,000 women per year having the surgery (Centers for Disease Control and Prevention, 2002).

Age: Not significant.

Ethnicity: Not significant.

Contributing factors: Experts agree that hysterectomy is necessary for invasive cancer of the uterus, cervix, or ovaries, and for uterine hemorrhage. Cancer accounts for approximately 15% of hysterectomies performed. Other reasons for hysterectomy require discussion of other therapies.

Options Concerning Hysterectomy

- If the ovaries are removed, which happens in one half of hysterectomies, the loss of estrogen creates menopausal symptoms. Careful consideration of removal of healthy ovaries should be discussed if hysterectomy is chosen as the treatment method.

- Leaving the cervix behind following hysterectomy reduces the risk of infection. It also reduces the chance of decreased sexual response after hysterectomy.

- Myomectomy is an option for women with fibroids. The fibroid is removed, and the uterus remains intact. The operation has a higher risk of complications than a hysterectomy. The surgeon must be familiar with methodology for the surgery. Fibroids can grow back after myomectomy. Of women who have had myomectomy, 25% need further surgery. Myomectomy preserves fertility in women who desire future pregnancies.

- Uterine fibroid embolization is a minimally invasive procedure that blocks the arteries carrying the blood to fibroids. In this procedure, an interventional radiologist threads a small catheter from the groin into the uterine artery. Dye is injected followed by embolic agents. This procedure is performed under local anesthesia.

- Endometrial ablation can be used to treat excessive uterine bleeding. The endometrium, along with any fibroids and polyps within the endometrium, are destroyed in this procedure. Ablation can be performed in one of three ways. *Cryotherapy* destroys the uterine lining with freezing. In *thermal ablation,* a balloon is inserted into the uterus and filled with hot water that burns and destroys the endometrium. The endometrium can also be destroyed with *electricity.* About 50% of women who undergo ablation will never menstruate again; 25% will have a reduction in flow. Local anesthesia can be utilized with the new methods of endometrial ablation.

Procedure	CPT Code
Hysterectomy	58150 (total; abdominal approach) 58210 (radical; abdominal) 58260 (vaginal hysterectomy; <250 grams) 58262 (vaginal with removal of tubes and/or ovary; <250 gm) 58275 (vaginal with total or partial vaginectomy) 58285 (vaginal; radical) 58290 (vaginal; >250 grams) 58291 (vaginal; with removal or tubes and/or ovary; >250 gms) See CPT code book for other specific procedures not listed.
Laparoscopic hysterectomy	58550
Oophorectomy	58940 58951 (with total hysterectomy)
Supracervical	58180
Myomectomy	58140 (abdominal approach; 1–4 removed) 58145 (vaginal approach) 58146 (abdominal with 5 + removed) 58545 (laparoscopic; 1–4) 58546 (laparoscopic; 5+)
Uterine fibroid embolization	58340
Endometrial ablation	58353

For more information on alternatives to hysterectomy:

National Women's Health Network *www.womenshealthnetwork.org*
National Women's Health Information Center *www.4woman.gov*
National Uterine Fibroids Foundation *www.nuff.org*
Endometriosis Association *www.endometriosisassn.org*

ALTERNATIVE THERAPY

Of respondents to a 1998 survey conducted by the American Medical Association, 40% reported using alternative therapies to improve their health (Astin, 1998). The most common use was chiropractic, followed by diet, exercise, and relaxation therapies. Only 4% of the respondents used alternative therapy alone. Most combined alternatives with traditional medicine. Of the people who used alternative medicine, more were highly educated than poorly educated. Clearly, alternative therapies are not alternatives at all. They are adjuncts. Providers of health care should be informed and open-minded about nonmedical therapies for peri-menopause and postmenopause. The National Menopause Society states that one of three women with menopausal symptoms tries alternatives for symptom relief (Wilbur et al, 1998). Menopausal women in the United States spent $600 million dollars in 1999 purchasing alternative thera-pies for menopausal symptoms.

Exercise, dietary changes, and cognitive techniques may all be consid-ered "alternatives" to medical therapy.

The following is a list of a few of the more common alternative thera-pies employed by perimenopausal and postmenopausal women.

- Black cohosh is an herb native to Eastern North America that can be used to relieve hot flashes, vaginal dryness, anxiety, and depression. Black cohosh is a source of natural plant estrogen. The recommended dose is 40 mg daily. The safety profile of black cohosh is positive—low toxicity, few to mild side effects, and good tolerability.

- Phytoestrogens are naturally occurring compounds found in plants that are structurally similar to estradiol. Soy is an example of a plant estrogen. A daily dose of soy to reduce menopausal symptoms has not been established. Soy was found to be superior to a placebo for treatment of hot flashes when ingested at a rate of 60 gm per day. There are some indications that soy prevents osteoporosis.

- Flax seeds are a source of a substance similar to plant estrogen. Flax seeds can help treat hot flashes and vaginal dryness. Taking two tablespoons a day reduces these symptoms.

- Progesterone can be found in wild yams. A significant improvement in vasomotor symptoms has been seen with natural progesterone. Natural progesterone can be placed in a cream form and applied topically for relief of perimenopausal symptoms.

- Evening primrose oil, in a double-blinded placebo-controlled pilot study, did not show any benefit over the placebo in treating hot flushes.

- *Gingko biloba,* possibly the best researched herb used for therapy, shows a small but significant effect on anxiety and depression, memory and dementia.

- Aromatherapy, the use of smells, has demonstrated a decrease in anxiety.

- Chiropractic techniques have not demonstrated a role in the treatment of menopausal symptoms.

- Yoga reduces stress, decreases heart rate and blood pressure, and improves physical fitness, and therefore has been found to be helpful to many patients with menopausal symptoms.

- Vitamin E can be utilized for hot flashes and breast tenderness. It may also treat vaginal dryness. Recommended dose is 400 to 600 IU daily. Vitamin E is also a powerful antioxidant and plays a role in the prevention of atherosclerosis.

- Calcium supplementation was shown to reduce long bone fractures in adults age 65 and over. Daily doses of 1200 to 1500 mg of calcium should be enhanced with 700 IU of Vitamin D daily.
- Vitamin B plays a role in the prevention of osteoporosis and cardiovascular disease, by converting an amino acid that is toxic to vascular endothelium into a harmless substance.
- Magnesium should be kept in balance with calcium with a 2:1 ratio. 600 mg daily achieves this ratio, approximately. Deficiency of this mineral is believed to be connected to coronary artery disease. Adequate intake of magnesium is also required to prevent osteoporosis.

Natural or alternative medicines were perceived by perimenopausal and menopausal women to be safer and "somewhat effective" in surveys. Personal control of menopausal symptoms was a major issue for surveyed women. Menopausal women expressed a desire to feel in control of their health. A need for informed choice of treatments was clearly demonstrated in a survey published in the *Canadian Family Physician* (Seidl and Stewart, 1998). It is important to ask your patients if they are using alternative therapies owing to the potential for interactions with other medications. Remember that using alternative therapies is only a "perceived" safety because they may have the same potential interactions as the pharmacologic drugs we use every day.

SUMMARY

Perimenopausal and postmenopausal women require comprehensive care that includes a complete history, thorough physical examination, risk factor assessment, age-appropriate screening, and education.

Women may not be well informed about menopause. A Harris survey indicated that only one half of working women of menopausal age were able to name any long-term health concerns related to the postmenopausal years. Of those who could, 27% mentioned osteoporosis and only 6% mentioned heart disease. A study published by the American College of Obstetricians and Gynecologists showed that only 1 in 40 women interviewed knew about an increased risk of heart disease after menopause (American College of Obstetricians and Gynecologists, 1996).

There is need to explain "changes" that occur in a woman during the perimenopausal and postmenopausal years. Reassurance and education may be the only therapy required in many cases.

A one-size-fits-all therapeutic regimen clearly will not work for women in mid-life. There is a great variety in symptomatology and risk factors. Plans of care must be individualized and should include health promotion strategies, screening, and therapies such as HRT and/or herbal remedies.

The final decision for health maintenance and promotion rests with the woman. Guidance is provided based upon current symptoms and personal and family history. . A better job of education and explanation is needed, as is creating a long-term partnering in the health-care relationship with mid-life women. Women wish to make informed choices about the health management of mid-life. HRT or not? Surgery or not? Alternatives or not? Forming a health-promotion strategy is needed for all mid-life women. The practitioner and the woman working together and exploring all options for increasing the quality and longevity of life are ideal.

REFERENCES

Allen, K, and Phillips, J: Women's Health Across the Lifespan. Lippincott, Philadelphia, 1997.

American College of Obstetricians and Gynecologists: Guideline for Women's Health Care. ACOG, Washington, DC, 1996.

Astin, J: Why patients use alternative medicine. JAMA 279(19):1548, 1998.

Baker, A, et al: Sleep distribution and mood changes associated with menopause. J Psychosom Res 3(44):359, 1997.

Barile, L: Theories of menopause. J Psychosoc Nursing Mental Health Serv 35(2):36, 2002.

Brown, W, et al: Changes in physical symptoms during the menopause transition. Int J Behav Med 9(1), 2002.

Bren, L: Alternatives to hysterectomy. FDA Consumer 35(6), 2001.

Burkman, R: Reproductive hormones and cancer. Obstet Gynecol Clin North Am 29(3), 2003.

Calaf, I, and Alsina, J: Benefits of hormone replacement therapy. Int J Fertil Women's Med 42(suppl 2):329, 1997.

Cholerton, B, et al: Estrogen and Alzheimer's disease. Drugs and Aging, 19(6), 2002.

Clark, A, et al: Sleep disturbances in mid-life women. J Adv Nursing 22(3):562, 1995.

Cooper, G, and Sandler, D: Age at natural menopause and mortality. Ann Epidemiol 8(4):229, 1998.

Cornell University Medical College, The Center for Women's Healthcare: Women's Health Advisory, September, 1998.

Cowan, B, et al: Interventional magnetic resonance imaging cryotherapy of uterine fibroid tumors. Am J Obstet Gynecol 186(6), June 2002.

Damewood, M: Hormonal strategies of the menopause. Maryland Med J 46(8):415, 1997.

Elmore, J, et al: Ten year risk of false positive screening mammograms and clinical breast examination. N Engl J Med 338(16):1089, 1998.

Ewes, A: A comprehensive approach to the menopause. JOGNN 56(10), 2001.

Hall, S: Psychological intervention and antidepressant treatment in smoking. Arch Gen Psychiatry, 2002.

Hammond, C: Management of menopause. Am Fam Physician 55(5):1667, 1997.

Hoole, A J, et al: Patient Care Guidelines for Nurse Practitioners. (5th edition) Lippincott Williams & Wilkins, Philadelphia, 1999.

Hulley, S, et al: Randomized trial of estrogen plus progestin for secondary prevention of coronary heart disease in postmenopausal women. JAMA 280:605, 1998.

Kessenich, C: Update on pharmacologic therapies for osteoporosis. Nurse Pract 21(8):19, 1996.

Knopman, D: Pharmacotherapy for Alzheimer's disease. Clin Neuropharmacol March/April, 2003.

Kuh, DL, et al: Women's health in midlife: The influence of the menopause, social factors and health in earlier life. Br J Obstet Gynecol 104(8):923, 1997.

Lewis, J, and Bernstein, J: Women's Health. Jones and Bartlett, Sudbury, MA, 1996.

McDonough, P: The randomized world is not without its imperfections: Reflections on the Women's Health Initiative Study. Fertil Steril 78(5), 2002.

McKenna, D, et al: Black cohosh: efficacy, safety, and use in clinical and preclinical applications. Alternative Therapies in Health and Medicine 7(3), 2001.

Parker, W: Total laparoscopic hysterectomy. Obstet Gynecol Clin North Am 27(2), 2000.

Pelisser, A: Menopause, hormone replacement therapy (HRT), stomatologic pathologies. Contraception Fertil Sexual 26(6):439, 1998.

Robins, J, and Lui, J: Alternatives to hysterectomy. Intern J Clin Practice 54(4), May 2000.

Rodgers, M, and Miller, J: Adequacy of hormone replacement therapy for osteoporosis prevention. Br J Gen Pract 47(416):161, 1997.

Rymer J, and Morris, E: Extracts from the clinical evidence: Menopausal symptoms. Brit Med J 321(7275), 2000.

Seidl, M, and Stewart, D: Alternative treatments for menopausal symptoms. Can Fam Physician 44:1271, 1998.

Shaver, J: Beyond hormonal therapies in menopause. Exper Gerontol 29, 1994.

South, P: Osteoprosis. Part 1: Evaluation and assessment. Am Fam Physician 63(5), March 2001,

Waldman, T: Menopause: When hormone replacement therapy is not an option. J Women's Health 7(5):559, 1998.

Wilbur, J, et al: Sociodemographic characteristics, biological factors, and symptom reporting in mid-life women. Menopause 5(1):43, 1998.

Chapter 15

REPRODUCTIVE DISORDERS

BACTERIAL VAGINOSIS

SIGNAL SYMPTOM▶   vaginal discharge

Vaginosis, bacterial	ICD-9-CM: 616.60

Definition: Bacterial vaginosis (BV) is a bacterial infection of the vagina.

Etiology: Overgrowth of the anaerobes *Gardnerella* and *Mycoplasma hominis* is the core of bacterial vaginosis.

Occurrence: BV is the most common vaginitis in women of childbearing age. BV causes 40%–50% of symptomatic vaginal infections. Up to 50% of women who are asymptomatic for vaginitis will culture positive for the organisms that cause BV.

Age: Sexually active women ages 15–44.

Ethnicity: Three times more black women than white women present with a symptomatic BV infection.

Contributing factors: The number of sexual partners.

Symptoms: Of women infected with BV, 50% either have no symptoms or mild discomfort as the only symptom; 50% of women report increase in vaginal discharge that is foul-smelling. They also report swelling, burning, and itching.

Diagnostic tests:

Test	Results Indicating Disorder	CPT Code
Vaginal pH	pH > 4.5	83986
Vaginal discharge	Thin, gray, milky homogeneous discharge	Observation
Whiff test (add 10% potassium hydroxide [KOH] to secretions on a glass slide)	Positive	87210
Wet mount	Clue cells present on wet mount (clue cells are epithelial cells coated with bacteria)	87210

Differential diagnosis:

- Gonorrhea (yellow to green discharge; culture to isolate the organism)
- *Chlamydia* infection (thick, cloudy discharge; culture to isolate organism)
- Herpes (itching, fever, tingling sensation 24 hours before eruption)
- Condylomata (fleshy warts)
- Allergy (soaps, sprays, contraceptive foam, cream, or jelly)
- Foreign body (lost tampons, condoms)
- Atrophic vaginitis (due to lack of estrogen, labia less prominent)

Also see Table 15–1.

Treatment: The organisms that create BV can be present in culture without symptoms. BV is treated if symptoms are present.

 Clinical Pearl: If the woman is pregnant, BV is treated with or without symptoms.

Treatment includes:

- Metronidazole 2 g stat (85% effective) or metronidazole 500 mg bid for 7 days (recommended during pregnancy after first trimester)
- Oral clindamycin 300 mg bid for 7 days or clindamycin cream h.s. for 7 days
- Metronidazole gel (Metrogel) 0.75% intravaginally once daily for 5 days

Follow-up: Recurrent BV dictates partner treatment.

Sequelae: Infection following abortion, infection following hysterectomy, preterm labor, pelvic inflammatory disease (PID). *Mycoplasma* infection is associated with endometritis, low-birth-weight infants, habitual abortion, and infertility.

Prevention/prophylaxis: Use of condoms.

Referral: Consultation is required for ineffective therapy and recurrent infection.

Table 15–1 Comparison of Bacterial Vaginosis, Candidiasis, and Trichomoniasis

	Bacterial Vaginosis	*Candidiasis*	*Trichomoniasis*
Source	Bacterial infection	Yeast infection	Parasitic infection
Symptoms	Asymptomatic or foul-smelling discharge	White vaginal discharge; vaginal itching and burning	Yellow-green discharge; vaginal itching and irritation
Findings	pH > 4.5; gray discharge; positive Whiff test and clue cells on wet mount	pH < 4.5; thick, white discharge; erythema, edema, and excoriation; hyphae and spores on wet mount	pH between 5 and 7; yellow-green discharge; "strawberry" cervix; motile trichomonads and leukocytes on wet mount
Treatment	Antibiotic; treat partner(s)	Antifungal medication; partner(s) need not be treated	Antibiotics; treat partner(s)

Education: Encourage proper use of medication. Recommend follow-up examination if symptoms do not resolve after therapy. Instruct the patient not to consume alcohol with metronidazole. Metronidazole should not be taken in the first trimester of pregnancy. The results of clinical trials indicate that a woman's response to therapy and the possibility of relapse or recurrence are not affected by treatment of her sex partner; therefore, routine treatment of the woman's partner is not recommended.

CANDIDIASIS OF THE VULVA AND VAGINA

SIGNAL SYMPTOMS vaginal itching; vaginal burning; pain with intercourse; thick, white vaginal discharge

Candidiasis	ICD-9-CM: 112.1

Definition: *Candida* infection, commonly called a "yeast" infection, is a fungal infection that occurs in the vagina.

Etiology: *Candida albicans* is responsible for 80%–90% of all *Candida* infections. The remaining infections are related to *C. glabrata* and *C. tropicalis.*

Occurrence: 75% of women report at least one episode of *Candida* infection; 20%–25% of all symptomatic vaginal infections are related to *Candida.*

Age: After menarche and prior to menopause.

Ethnicity: Not significant.

Contributing factors: Depressed immunity, high blood glucose level, administration of antibiotics, use of oral contraceptives, low pH prior to menses.

Signs and symptoms: Itching; burning; dysuria; dyspareunia; and thick, white vaginal discharge.

Diagnostic tests:

Test	Results Indicating Disorder	CPT Code
pH indicator	pH of 4.5 or below	83986
Vaginal discharge	Presence of thick, white adherent discharge	Observation
Appearance of vulva	Erythema, edema, and excoriation of the vulva	Observation
Yeast culture	Positive	87106
Wet mount (visualization can be enhanced with 10% KOH)	Positive for hyphae and spores	87210

Differential diagnosis:

Hypersensitivity, allergic or chemical reaction, and contact dermatitis.

See Table 15-1: Comparison of Bacterial Vaginosis, Candidiasis, and Trichomoniasis.

Treatment: Clotrimazole, miconazole, butoconazole, tioconazole, or terconazole in cream form used for 3–7 days h.s. is 80% effective.

Nystatin may also be used. Oral fluconazole can be used for recurrent infections if the woman is not pregnant.

Follow-up: Follow-up appointments are necessary only if infection is not resolved with treatment. No need to treat partners.

Sequelae: Recurrent candidiasis.

Prevention/prophylaxis: Use of antibiotics only as appropriate, good control of diabetes.

Referral: Consultation is needed for unresolved vaginitis.

Education: Instruct the patient to complete the medication regimen prescribed. Teach the patient to dry the vaginal area as completely as possible after bathing and before dressing. Loose underwear that permits airflow decreases the incidence of recurrent candidiasis.

TRICHOMONIASIS VAGINAL INFECTION

SIGNAL SYMPTOMS green-yellow vaginal discharge, vaginal and vulvar irritation

Trichomoniasis	ICD-9-CM: 131.01

Definition: Trichomoniasis is a vaginal infection caused by the organism *Trichomonas vaginalis.*

Etiology: *T. vaginalis,* a flagellated protozoan, acts in a parasitic relationship with the vaginal mucus. Transmission is by sexual contact.

Occurrence: Of all symptomatic vaginal infections, 15%–20% are related to *Trichomonas. Trichomonas* organisms may also be found in the urethra.

Age: After puberty and before menarche

Ethnicity: Not significant

Contributing factors: Number of sexual partners (see Box 15–1).

Box 15–1
Sexual History

Sexual history should include the following:
- Demographic history: gender, race, culture, religion, education, employment
- Sexual orientation
- Medical and surgical history
- Childhood sexual experiences: wanted and unwanted
- Sources of sex education
- Reproductive data
- Contraceptive data
- Sexually active?
- Significant relationship(s)
- Quality of relationship(s)
- Level of sexual desire
- Sexual fears
- Satisfaction with sexual interaction

Signs and symptoms: Dysuria, yellow-green vaginal discharge, itching, dyspareunia, and vaginal and/or vulvar irritation.

Diagnostic tests:

Test	Results Indicating Disorder	CPT Code
Vaginal discharge	Presence of thin, yellow-green vaginal discharge	Observation
pH	5.0–7.0	83986
Vulvar examination	Vulvar irritation and edema	Observation
Examination of the cervix	Strawberry cervix—petechial hemorrhages on the cervix	Observation
Saline wet mount	Motile trichomonads and leukocytes seen on saline wet mount (50%–60% sensitive)	87210
Vaginal or cervical culture	Positive for trichomonads (90% sensitive)	87070
Pap smear	Positive for trichomonads (60%–70% sensitive)	88142

Differential diagnosis:

- Bacterial vaginosis (foul-smelling vaginal discharge, positive Whiff test, wet mount positive for clue cells)
- Gonorrhea (yellow-to-green discharge; culture to identify organism)
- *Chlamydia* infection (thick, cloudy discharge; culture to isolate organism)
- Herpes (itching, fever, tingling sensation 24 hours before eruption)
- Condylomata (fleshy warts)
- Foreign body (tampons, condoms)
- Allergies (soaps, sprays, contraceptive foam, jelly or cream)

Also see Table 15–1.

Treatment:

- Metronidazole 2 g stat (80%–88% effective).
- Metronidazole 500 mg bid for 7 days (95% effective).
- Partner(s) must be treated simultaneously (30%–70% of partners are also infected by trichomonads).

Follow-up: For unresolved infection.

Sequelae: Premature rupture of membranes and post-hysterectomy cellulitis have been associated with trichomoniasis.

Prevention/prophylaxis: Use of condoms.

Referral: Consultation is required for unresolved infection.

Education: Instruct patient to complete the medication regimen. Inform the patient that all partners must be treated. Intercourse should be avoided until the woman and her partner(s) have been treated. Instruct the patient to avoid alcohol when taking metronidazole. Instruct the patient not to take metronidazole in the first trimester of pregnancy.

CHLAMYDIA INFECTION

SIGNAL SYMPTOMS vaginal discharge, postcoital bleeding, pain with intercourse, pain with urination

Chlamydia	
Inflammatory disease of uterus	ICD-9-CM: 615.0
Cervicitis	ICD-9-CM: 616.0

Definition: *Chlamydia* infection is a parasitic disease of the mucous membranes that may infect the genital and/or urinary tracts.

Etiology: *Chlamydia trachomatis* (CT) is the causative organism. Transmission is by sexual contact.

Occurrence:

Clinical Pearl: *Chlamydia trachomatis* is responsible for close to 4 million cases of genital and urinary tract infections in the United States per year.

Age: Adolescents and young women.

Ethnicity: CT is seen more often in black women than in Hispanic or white women.

Contributing factors: Age under 21 years, new sexual partner, multiple partners, partner with multiple partners; 30%–50% of the time gonorrhea is present with CT (see Box 15–1: Sexual History).

Signs and symptoms: Symptoms depend on area of infection; 75% of infected women have cervical infection; in 50%, the urethra is infected; and in 33%, the endometrium is infected. Infected women may be asymptomatic; they may have mucopurulent discharge, postcoital bleeding, and/or dyspareunia, lower abdominal discomfort, vaginal bleeding, and dysuria.

Diagnostic tests:

Test	Results Indicating Disorder	CPT Code
Culture of the endocervix with a DNA probe	Positive for CT	83896
Urine-based testing—urinary ligase chain reaction	Positive for CT	81099
Vaginal discharge	Presence of mucopurulent discharge	Observation
Cervical changes	Ectropy and/or edema: friability of the cervix	Observation
Bimanual examination	Uterine or adnexal tenderness	Included in exam code

Differential diagnosis:

- Gonorrhea (yellow-to-green discharge; culture needed to identify organism)
- Cystitis (dysuria, frequency, urinary urgency)

- PID (lower bilateral pelvic/abdominal pain, vaginal discharge, spotting, dyspareunia, dysuria)

Treatment: Doxycycline 100 mg bid for 7 days or Azithromycin 1g orally in a single dose. Treatment of partners prevents reinfection. Frequent coinfection with gonorrhea indicates need for treatment of both diseases simultaneously. Sexual partners with exposure 60 days prior to diagnosis should be evaluated, tested, and treated.

Follow-up: Women do not need to be retested for chlamydial infection after finishing therapy unless symptoms persist or you suspect reinfection.

Sequelae: PID, ectopic pregnancy, and infertility

Prevention/prophylaxis: All sexually active teenage women and women 20–24 years of age should be routinely screened for CT.

Referral: Consultation is recommended for unresolved infection.

Education: Reinforce the importance of completing the medication regimen. Inform the patient that douching should be avoided in all women with CT because it increases the incidence of PID. Partners should be referred for treatment. Advise the woman to abstain from intercourse until she completes the therapy.

GONORRHEAL INFECTION

SIGNAL SYMPTOMS ▶ vaginal discharge, pelvic pain

Gonorrhea	ICD-9-CM: 098.20

Definition: Gonorrhea is a sexually transmitted bacterial infection. The causative organism is *Neisseria gonorrhoeae*.

Etiology: *Neisseria gonorrhoeae* is a gram-negative diplococcus that is transmitted sexually by direct contact with infected mucosa to the cervix and endocervix, the urethra, Bartholin's glands, Skene's glands, the rectum, or the pharynx. The most common site of infection is the cervix.

Occurrence: 600,000 cases of gonorrhea are reported to the Centers for Disease Control and Prevention (CDC) each year.

Age: The most common ages for women who develop gonorrhea are 15–29.

Ethnicity: Gonorrhea is diagnosed more often in black than in white women.

Contributing factors: Multiple sexual partners (see Box 15–1: Sexual History).

Signs and symptoms:

 Clinical Pearl: The woman can be asymptomatic.

The woman may present with vaginal discharge, dysuria, dysmenorrhea, pelvic pain, dyspareunia, menorrhagia, intermenstrual bleeding, fever, chills, or abdominal pain. Vaginal discharge may be apparent on examination. Adnexa may be tender on bimanual examination.

Diagnostic tests:

Test	Results Indicating Disorder	CPT Code
Culture with a DNA probe (one swab is used in the cervix for both CT and gonorrhea)	Positive	83896
Urine test	Positive for gonococcal nucleic acid	81099
Vaginal discharge	Presence of mucopurulent discharge	Observation
Bimanual examination	Uterine and adnexal tenderness	Included in exam code

Differential diagnosis:

- *Chlamydia trachomatis* (thick, cloudy discharge, dyspareunia, postcoital bleeding in women, positive culture)
- Bacterial vaginosis (fishy, musty odor, clue cells on wet mount, gray discharge)
- Trichomoniasis (foul-smelling, frothy discharge, trichomonads on wet mount)
- Candidiasis (white, cottage cheese discharge, musty odor, may be taking antibiotics or oral contraceptives, KOH prep positive)

Treatment: Azithromycin 1 g orally in a single dose, cefixime 400 mg in a single dose, or ceftriaxone 125 mg IM, or ciprofloxacin 500 mg PO once, or ofloxacin 400 mg PO once and doxycycline 100 mg bid for 7 days. Ceftriaxone is recommended for pharyngeal gonorrhea. Doxycycline or azithromycin is recommended by the CDC to eliminate *Chlamydia trachomatis* that often occurs simultaneously with gonorrhea. All sexual partners within the last 30 days of diagnosis require evaluation and treatment.

Follow-up: Depends on the severity of the disease; follow-up can be within 24–72 hours. Culture should be repeated following completion of therapy.

Sequelae: PID, infertility, increased rate of ectopic pregnancy.

Prevention/prophylaxis: Use of condoms.

Education: Stress the need for all women infected with gonorrhea to be tested for HIV and syphilis. Stress the importance of the patient's taking all of the medication. Inform the patient that all partners should be treated. Advise the patient to abstain from intercourse until therapy is completed.

PELVIC INFLAMMATORY DISEASE (PID)

SIGNAL SYMPTOMS ▶ lower abdominal pain, vaginal discharge

| PID | ICD-9-CM: 614.9 |

Definition: Pelvic inflammatory disease (PID) is a spectrum of diseases that includes endometritis, salpingitis, oophoritis, tubo-ovarian abscess, and pelvic peritonitis.

Etiology: The two most common organisms causing PID are *Neisseria gonorrhoeae* and *Chlamydia trachomatis*. Other possible organisms causing infection are *Escherichia coli,* streptococci, *Haemophilus influenzae, Mycoplasma* species, and *Ureaplasma* species.

Occurrence: One million women per year in the United States are reported to have PID.

Age: Adolescents have the highest incidence of any age group for PID; 70% of all cases of PID are diagnosed in women less than 25 years of age.

Ethnicity: Not significant.

Contributing factors: PID is related to a sexually transmitted disease 60% of the time. Multiple sex partners, previous sexually transmitted disease, recent insertion of an intrauterine device (IUD), douching, and cigarette smoking are all contributing factors. It has been suggested that BV may predispose or facilitate the ascent of gonorrhea or *Chlamydia* into the upper genital tract (see Box 15–1: Sexual History).

PID can occur postpartum, post-abortion, or postoperatively.

Signs and symptoms: Symptoms range from almost completely asymptomatic to life-threatening. Symptoms include bilateral lower abdominal pain, bleeding, abnormal discharge, fever, nausea and vomiting, dysmenorrhea, and dyspareunia (see Figure 15–1).

Diagnostic tests:

Test	Results Indicating Disorder	CPT Code
Bimanual examination	Adnexal tenderness, cervical motion tenderness*	With exam code
Temperature	Elevation to more than 101° F	With exam code
Vaginal discharge	Mucopurulent discharge	Observation
Wet mount	WBCs present	87210
Complete blood count (CBC)	High white cell count; elevated erythrocyte sedimentation rate	85025
Vaginal and cervical culture	Positive for gonorrhea and/or *Chlamydia trachomatis* organisms	87070
Transvaginal ultrasound	Thickening of the tubes with or without free pelvic fluid or tubo-ovarian complex	76817
Laparoscopy	Pelvic inflammation	49320
MRI	Changes compatible with inflammatory disease	72195 (without contrast) 72197 (with contrast)

* Lower abdominal tenderness, cervical motion tenderness, and adnexal tenderness are the hallmark symptoms of PID.

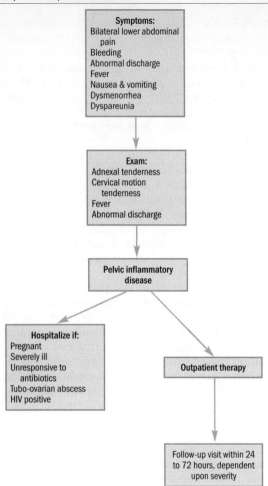

Figure 15–1. Pelvic inflammatory disease.

Differential diagnosis:

- Ectopic pregnancy (lower abdominal pain, bleeding)
- Appendicitis (severe abdominal pain with fast onset, localizes to RLQ)
- Bowel disease (diarrhea and pain in lower abdomen; relieved by defecation)
- Endometriosis (recurrent abdominal pain, dull, burning, stabbing, increased dysmenorrhea, premenstrual spotting)
- Ovarian torsion
- Bleeding from a corpus luteum

- Viral gastroenteritis (crampy, diffuse abdominal pain relieved by vomiting or defecation)

Treatment: No currently available data compare the efficacy of parenteral versus oral therapy. Parenteral therapy can be administered on an outpatient or inpatient basis. The decision to hospitalize is made by the health care providers. Hospitalization is recommended if the woman is pregnant, does not respond to therapy, is severely ill, has a tubo-ovarian abscess, or is HIV-positive. If medical management is conducted on an outpatient basis, follow-up is essential.

Treatment of PID should be initiated in sexually active young women if the following are present: lower abdominal tenderness, adnexal tenderness, and cervical motion tenderness. Additional criteria that support a diagnosis of PID, according to the CDC, are temperature greater than 101° F, abnormal cervical or vaginal discharge, elevated erythrocyte sedimentation rate, elevated C-reactive protein level, and laboratory documentation of infection. Any of these symptoms require treatment for PID.

Medications used for therapy include a parenteral regimen such as cefotetan 2 g IV every 12 hours or cefoxitin 2 g IV q 6 hr plus doxycycline 100 mg IV or orally q 12 hr. An oral regimen such as ofloxacin 400 mg orally twice daily for 14 days plus metronidazole 500 mg orally twice daily for 14 days can be utilized.

Follow-up: The first follow-up visit is within 24–72 hours depending upon severity. Women who do not demonstrate improvement within 3 days after initiation of therapy usually require additional intervention. Sexual partner(s) exposed within 60 days of diagnosis should be treated simultaneously with the woman. Cultures should be repeated in 4–6 weeks.

Sequelae: Chronic pelvic pain, recurrent disease, ectopic pregnancy, and infertility. Older age (over 35) and self-reported drug misuse predict longer hospitalization for women diagnosed with PID.

Prevention/prophylaxis: Screening cultures for at-risk populations, use of condoms.

Referral: A diagnosis of PID always requires a medical consultation.

Education: Stress the importance of partner(s) being examined and treated. Discuss the need for decreased activity and adequate diet and fluid intake during therapy. Emphasize the importance of completing medical therapy. Suggest that the patient use condoms. Recommend HIV testing.

SYPHILIS

SIGNAL SYMPTOM▶   painless ulcer on mucous membrane

| Syphilis | ICD-9-CM: 097.9 |

Description: Syphilis, a sexually transmitted disease that can affect any tissue, has a wide range of signs and symptoms ranging from none to neurologic impairment. Syphilis has periods of active disease and periods of latency.

Etiology: *Treponema pallidum,* a sexually transmitted spirochete.

Occurrence: 50,000 cases of syphilis are reported to the CDC per year, 2.9 per 100,000 women.

Age: The most common age group for this disease is 20–25 years.

Ethnicity: Syphilis is seen more commonly in Hispanics and blacks and in inner-city residents. Rates have remained highest in the South and lowest in the West.

Contributing factors: Gonorrhea infection, HIV infection, and drug abuse are contributing factors (see Box 15-1: Sexual History).

Signs and symptoms: Syphilis occurs in stages.

Primary syphilis: After contact, a chancre, a painless firm ulcer with raised edges, appears in 10–90 days and heals within 3–8 weeks.

Secondary syphilis: Multiple skin lesions appear that last 3–12 weeks.

Latent syphilis: Syphilis for more than 1 year or of unknown duration.

Tertiary syphilis: Latent syphilis for many years; 20%–30% of untreated people with syphilis develop tertiary syphilis.

Diagnostic tests:

Test	Results Indicating Disorder	CPT Code
Rapid plasma reagin (RPR) or Venereal Disease Research Laboratories (VDRL) These tests are 80%–90% accurate in making a diagnosis.	Positive. A positive RPR or VDRL result must be confirmed with a FTA-ABS.	86592
Fluorescent treponemal antibody absorption test (FTA-ABS)	Positive	86255

Differential diagnosis:
- Herpes (itching, fever, dysuria, tingling 24 hours before appearance of lesion)
- Condylomata lata (fleshy warts)
- Lymphogranuloma venereum (ulcerative genital lesions, swelling of groin lymph nodes, headache, fever, malaise)
- Granuloma inguinale (vulvar ulcer)
- Chancroid (*Haemophilus*-created ulceration, papule that increases and ulcerates)

Treatment: Primary and secondary syphilis are treated with penicillin 2.4 million units IM. Latent and tertiary syphilis are treated with three doses of penicillin 2.4 million units IM at 1-week intervals. All confirmed cases of syphilis must be reported to the health department for follow-up. Sexual partners exposed to the disease within 90 days of diagnosis should be treated.

Follow-up: Titers should be repeated and the woman should be re-examined at 1 month, 3 months, 6 months, and 12 months after diagnosis and treatment.

Sequelae: Cardiovascular syphilis, neurosyphilis, congenital syphilis (transplacental transmission occurs during the second and third trimesters).

Prevention/prophylaxis: Use of condoms.

Referral: All cases of latent and tertiary syphilis require consultation with a physician. Pregnant women with syphilis require consultation. HIV-positive women with syphilis require consultation.

Education: Emphasize the need for treatment of partner(s). Explain the disease process to the woman. Stress the importance of follow-up visits. Recommend HIV testing.

LYMPHOGRANULOMA VENEREUM

SIGNAL SYMPTOMS mucous membrane ulceration, tender lymph nodes

Lymphogranuloma Venereum	ICD-9-CM: 099.1

Definition: Lymphogranuloma is a sexually transmitted disease characterized by localized lymphatic infection.

Etiology: *Chlamydia* endemic to tropical areas.

Occurrence: Unknown.

Age: Any sexually active female.

Ethnicity: Lymphogranuloma is a disease from tropical areas of the world.

Contributing factors: Multiple partners; see Box 15-1: Sexual History.

Signs and symptoms:

- Lymphogranuloma has an incubation period of 5–7 days. The first sign of infection is a pustule or papule on the vaginal wall, vulva, or cervix that ulcerates and then heals spontaneously.
- A bubo, that is, a tender, firm, infected lymph node that resolves spontaneously, follows the pustule or papule.
- The third stage is fibrosis of the lymphatic tissue.

Diagnostic tests:

Test	Results Indicating Disorder	CPT Code
Serologic complement fixation test	Titers > 1:64	86171

Differential diagnosis:

- Syphilis (painless ulcer on mucous membrane, positive RPR or VDRL)
- Hodgkin's disease (painless enlargement of the lymph nodes, abdominal pain, fever, enlarged liver, spleen)
- Cat scratch fever (headache, malaise, fever, history of cat scratch, scratches with papule or vesicle)
- Lymphadenitis (swelling of lymph nodes in a region)

Treatment: Doxycycline 100 mg bid for 21 days.

Follow-up: Follow-up is necessary at 1- and 2-week intervals until resolution of symptoms. A 6-month follow-up visit should be scheduled after successful treatment.

Sequelae: Scar formation, fistula formation, and suppuration of lymphatic vessels.

Prevention/prophylaxis: Use of condoms. Avoid intercourse with partners who have open lesions.

Referral: Consultation with a physician for confirmation of diagnosis and treatment.

Education: Instruct the patient that she must complete the full course of medication. Inform the patient that her partner should have an examination. Stress importance of follow-up visits.

TOXIC SHOCK

SIGNAL SYMPTOMS fever, erythematous rash, myalgia, toxic condition out of proportion to local findings

Toxic Shock	ICD-9-CM: 040.82

Definition: Toxic shock is a syndrome in which bacterial growth, plus a toxin that acts as a superantigen, creates a serious systemic infection.

Etiology: Infection with a bacteriophage, a specific strain of *Staphylococcus aureus,* creates a toxin. The toxin plus enterotoxin B enter the circulatory system and create the symptoms.

Occurrence: Unknown.

Age: One of the variables predictive of toxic shock is advancing age. Host factors are important determinants for the development of the disease. Toxic shock can occur in both menstruating and nonmenstruating women.

Ethnicity: Not significant.

Contributing factors: Menses, use of tampons, vaginal infections, vaginal delivery or cesarean birth, or spontaneous abortion. In cases involving menstruation, 99% are associated with tampon use (see Box 15-1: Sexual History).

Signs and symptoms: Temperature of 102° F or more, erythematous rash, hypotension, vomiting, and myalgia.

Diagnostic tests:

Test	Results Indicating Disorder	CPT Code
Bacterial culture of the cervix and vagina	Positive for *Staphylococcus aureus*	87070
Titer for toxin TSST−1	< 1:5	
Cytokinins, prostaglandins, leukotrienes	Elevated	84150 (prostaglandins); (cytokinins); (leukotrienes)

Differential diagnosis:
- Shock from another origin
- Meningococcemia (petechial hemorrhages on trunk and extremities)

Treatment: Hospitalization including treatment with large doses of penicillin or clindamycin.

Follow-up: After hospitalization, follow-up requires close monitoring for resolution of symptoms. Medication management is required.

Sequelae: Toxic shock syndrome rapidly leads to multisystem organ failure with serious morbidity and mortality.

Prevention/prophylaxis: Appropriate use of tampons.

Referral: All cases of toxic shock syndrome require medical consultation.

Education: Inform the patient that, following diagnosis of toxic shock, she should discontinue the use of tampons.

ENDOMETRIOSIS AND ADENOMYOSIS

SIGNAL SYMPTOM ▶ pain with menses

Endometriosis of uterus	ICD-9-CM: 617.0
Endometriosis of ovary	ICD-9-CM: 617.1
Endometriosis of fallopian tube	ICD-9-CM: 617.2
Endometriosis of pelvic peritoneum	ICD-9-CM: 617.3
Endometriosis of rectovaginal septum and vagina	ICD-9-CM: 617.4
Endometriosis, other specified sites (e.g., bladder, vulva)	ICD-9-CM: 617.8
Endometriosis, unspecified site	ICD-9-CM: 617.9
Adenomyosis	ICD-9-CM: 258.0

Definitions: Endometriosis is extrauterine growth of the endometrial glands or stroma. Adenomyosis occurs when the boundary between the endometrium and the myometrium is breached.

Etiology: Endometriosis is believed to occur through retrograde menstruation or differentiation of "totipotential" cells, or both. Adenomyosis is endometriosis interna. The normal endometrial lining invades the myometrium.

Occurrence: Of women of reproductive age, 1% to 5% have endometriosis. The most common sites for endometriosis are within the pelvis. Rarely does endometriosis occur outside of the pelvis.

Age: The most common age for the diagnosis of endometriosis is the late 20s. Adenomyosis occurs most commonly in women aged 40–50.

Ethnicity: Not significant.

Contributing factors: Factors leading to endometriosis are unknown. The risk for endometriosis appears to be related to increased exposure to menstruation—shorter cycle length, increase in flow, and reduced parity. Contributing factors for adenomyosis include increased parity, previous cesarean birth, induced abortions, dysmenorrhea, abnormal uterine bleeding, and late menarche.

Signs and symptoms: Common sites for implantation of endometriosis are ovaries, serosal surfaces of uterus, bladder, bowel, and rectovagina. An endometrioma is an ovarian cyst that has formed as a result of endometriosis.

Symptoms are related to the site of implantation. Symptoms may include dysmenorrhea, pelvic pain, infertility, dark vaginal "spotting" before menses, or referred back pain. Sites of implantation bleed during menses and create symptoms in two thirds of the women with endometriosis. One third of women with the disease have no symptoms. The degree of pain is not directly related to the level of involvement in this disease. A woman may have minimal endometriosis and extreme pain with menses, or she may have minimal pain but extensive disease.

In adenomyosis, during menses the lining grows and develops but cannot shed. This causes bleeding into the myometrium, and thus pain occurs during menses. Adenomyosis can cause abnormal vaginal bleeding.

Diagnostic tests:

Test	Results Indicating Disorder	CPT Code
Bimanual examination	Pelvic tenderness on examination. In adenomyosis, the uterus is enlarged, tender, and boggy.	Included in physical exam
Ultrasound of the pelvis	In adenomyosis: enlarged uterus, irregular vascular spaces	76857 (limited) 76856 (complete)
Magnetic resonance imaging (MRI) of the pelvis	In adenomyosis: irregular and indistinct margins in the myometrium	72195 (without contrast) 72196 (with contrast) 72197 (with and without)
Laparoscopy	Sites of endometrial implants visualized	49320
Pathology examination	Adenomyosis is frequently diagnosed on a pathology report following hysterectomy.	88329

Differential diagnosis:

- PID (foul vaginal discharge, fever, lower abdominal pain, dyspareunia)
- Adhesions (history of previous surgeries)
- Ectopic pregnancy (one-sided, lower abdominal pain)
- Fibroids (benign smooth muscle tumor, possible bleeding, pain; MRI confirms diagnosis)

- Ovarian neoplasms (ultrasound, MRI, positive cytology)
- Diverticulitis (left lower quadrant pain and tenderness, cramping, positive CT scan for presence of diverticula)
- Irritable bowel syndrome (diarrhea, pain in lower abdomen relieved on defecation)
- Adenocarcinoma (cytology)
- Leiomyosarcoma (cytology)

Treatment: Endometriosis symptoms can be treated with nonsteroidal anti-inflammatory medications. Oral contraceptives on a continuous regimen can be utilized to suppress menstruation. Gonadotropin-releasing hormone (GnRH) agonists can be utilized to suppress menses. Danazol, a 17-ethinyl testosterone derivative, can be taken daily. Medroxyprogesterone acetate can be taken daily. Surgical therapy to eliminate implantation sites can be utilized.

Hysterectomy can be prescribed for adenomyosis. GnRh can give temporary relief for adenomyosis.

Follow-up: Close follow-up for either medical or surgical therapy is indicated.

Sequelae:

Clinical Pearl: Endometriosis can cause infertility from direct tubal damage, immunologic factors, and increased prostaglandin levels.

Clinical Pearl: Adenomyosis is associated with endometrial cancer and endometrial hyperplasia 20% of the time.

Prevention/prophylaxis: None.

Referral: Every woman with a possible diagnosis of endometriosis or adenomyosis requires consultation with a physician.

Education: Endometriosis is treated with a combination of therapies. Explanations of the disease process and various therapies are an important part of the treatment.

LEIOMYOMAS (FIBROIDS)

SIGNAL SYMPTOMS▶   often asymptomatic; uterine bleeding, infertility and/or pain (10 to 40%); menorrhagia

Leiomyomas (uterus)	ICD-9-CM: 218.9
Interstitial/intramural	ICD-9-CM: 218.1
Submucous	ICD-9-CM: 218.0
Subperitoneal/subserous	ICD-9-CM: 218.2

Definition: Leiomyomas are benign tumors of the reproductive tract in women.

Etiology: Leiomyomas arise from the uterine musculature, grow slowly, and diminish rapidly at menopause.

Occurrence: Fibroids, a common condition of the female genital tract;

occurs in one out of every four or five women. They are usually found in the uterus but may appear in the vulva or vagina. One in five women will be diagnosed with a fibroid tumor.

Age: Fibroids are most commonly diagnosed in the fifth decade of life.

Ethnicity: One out of three women of African American descent will be diagnosed with leiomyomas. When risk factors are controlled, there is a higher rate of fibroids in premenopausal black women. The average age at diagnosis for black women is 37.5 years. For white women, the average age is 41.6 years.

Contributing factors: Age at first birth, history of infertility

Signs and symptoms: Menometrorrhagia, lower abdominal pain, anemia, and constipation. Symptoms can increase in the perimenopausal period. Symptoms decrease with menopause.

Diagnostic tests:

Test	Results Indicating Disorder	CPT Code
Pelvic examination	Large, firm, irregularly shaped uterus	Included in exam code
Ultrasound of the pelvis	Location, degree of calcification of the fibroid(s)	76857 (limited) 76856 (complete)
Hysteroscopy	Visualization of submucosal myomas	58555
MRI	Distinguishes uterine from ovarian masses	72195 (with and without contrast) 72196 (with contrast) 72197 (without contrast)

Differential diagnosis: The vast majority of smooth muscle tumors are leiomyomas. The occurrence of leiomyosarcomas is very infrequent. Great care must be taken to differentiate between the two at the time of diagnosis.

Treatment: Medical treatment consists of progesterone and GnRH agonists. When medical treatment fails, surgical treatment—myomectomy or hysterectomy—is performed. Transcatheter bilateral uterine artery embolization, an interventional radiological procedure, is a relatively new modality that is being offered more and more as an alternative to surgery for the treatment of fibroids.

Follow-up: Fibroids are generally asymptomatic and do not require intervention. Careful monitoring for growth is recommended. Medical therapy requires follow-up for resolution of symptoms. Surgical therapy requires follow-up.

Sequelae:

 Clinical Pearl: Fibroids require special management in cases of infertility, pregnancy, and menopause.

Prevention/prophylaxis: None.

Referral: Diagnosis of fibroid requires consultation with a physician.

Education: Stress the benign nature of fibroid "tumors." Inform the patient that uterine myomas are frequently-occurring tumors that require treatment only if they are symptomatic. Explain about the possible therapies if appropriate.

CANCERS OF THE GENITAL TRACT

CERVICAL CANCER

SIGNAL SYMPTOM none

Cervical malignancy	ICD-9-CM: 180.9
Benign cervical neoplasm	ICD-9-CM: 219.0
Cervical cancer in situ	ICD-9-CM: 233.1
Cervical dysplasia	ICD-9-CM: 622.1

Description: In virtually all cases, intraepithelial neoplastic changes precede invasive squamous cervical cancer. These changes have been called dysplasia, cervical intraepithelial neoplasia (CIN), squamous intraepithelial lesion (SIL), and carcinoma in situ. Cells in the cervical epithelium develop the capacity to divide repeatedly rather than mature in a controlled fashion.

Etiology: A specific agent likely to be responsible for cervical cancer is human papilloma virus (HPV), the cause of most venereal warts. HPV of genotypes 16 and 18 shows a significant presence in women with cervical cancer.

Occurrence: In the year 2000, an estimated 12,800 women developed cervical cancer. For any American woman, the lifetime probability of developing cervical cancer is 0.7%. The incidence of carcinoma in situ is more than three times that of invasive disease.

Age: The overall incidence of cervical cancer for any age group is 4 per 100,000. Carcinoma in situ can occur in women aged 25–29. However, a peak in incidence occurs in women aged 30–45, with 6 per 1000 women developing carcinoma in situ. Another peak occurs in women older than 60, with 5 per 1000 developing carcinoma in situ. Prevalence of invasive carcinoma is highest in older age groups, rising precipitously after age 50.

Ethnicity: Not significant.

Contributing factors: First intercourse before age 20, multiple sex partners, sexual partner who has multiple partners, history of HPV or sexually transmitted disease, smoking, exposure to diethylstilbestrol (DES) in utero, lack of barrier contraception, immunosuppression, and lack of screening (see Box 15–1: Sexual History).

Signs and symptoms:

 Clinical Pearl: The classic symptom of cervical cancer is intermenstrual bleeding following intercourse or douching.

This symptom occurs late in the course of the disease. The mean duration of a detectable asymptomatic period is approximately 10

years for carcinoma is situ and approximately 5 years for invasive carcinoma.

Diagnostic tests:

 Clinical Pearl: Early detection of this disease improves prognosis.

The Pap smear is a screening device for cervical cancer. All women who are or have been sexually active or who have reached the age of 18 years should have an annual Pap smear (CPT code: 88142) and pelvic examination. After a woman has had three consecutive satisfactory normal evaluations, she may have Pap tests less frequently at the discretion of her health-care provider (see Table 15–2; Figures 15–2 and 15–3; and Box 15–2).

Table 15–2 Management of Abnormal Pap Smear Results

Result	Interpretation
Unsatisfactory for evaluation	Repeat smear in 6 weeks.
Fungus consistent with *Candida*	*Candida* colonization is not dangerous to women or their partners. If no complaints are offered by the woman or she has been treated, the Pap smear should be repeated at the regular interval.
Trichomonas vaginalis	Treat on the basis of the Pap smear finding.
Predominance of coccobacilli consistent with shift in vaginal flora	This finding suggests bacterial vaginosis. Treat or further evaluate for treatment with wet mount.
Bacteria morphologically consistent with *Actinomyces*	This result refers to anerobic bacteria that may cause pelvic inflammatory disease (PID). This finding requires evaluation of the woman.
Reactive cellular changes associated with inflammation	This result dictates benign metaplasia, irritation, post-traumatic repair, *Chlamydia* or gonorrhea, viral infection, or cervical cancer. Presistent presentation of this finding leads to colposcopic referral.
Atrophy with inflammation	This result suggests estrogen deficiency. Treatment is necessary only if the woman is symptomatic.
Atypical squamous cells of undetermined significance (ASCUS)	Abnormal, yet not consistent with SIL.
ASC-H	Atypical cells more likely to be precancerous; colposcopy needed.
Low-grade SIL	Colposcopy is indicated.
High-grade SIL	Refer for colposcopy.
Endometrial cells, cytologically benign in a postmemopausal woman	Refer for endometrial sampling.
A typical glandular cells (AGC)	Refer for colposcopy and endometrial biopsy.

Technology (liquid-based cervical cytology versus cells placed onto a slide) is taken into consideration.
SIL = squamous intraepithelial lesion.

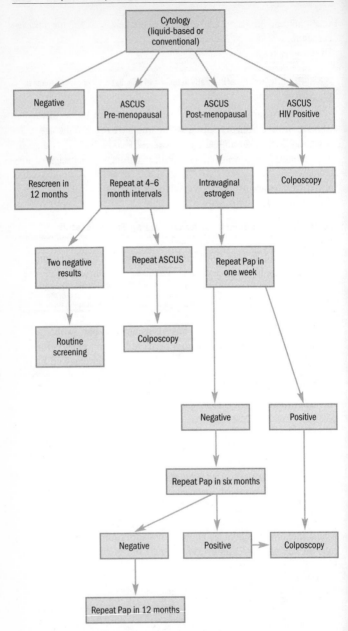

Figure 15–2. Management of women with ASCUS-Repeat cytology.

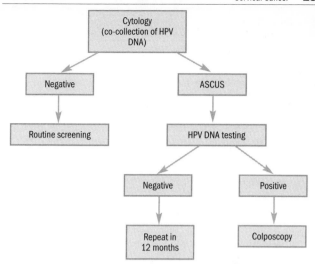

Figure 15–3. Management of women with ASCUS-HPV DNA Testing.

Box 15–2
The Bethesda System For Reporting Cervical/ Vaginal Cytologic Diagnosis

FORMAT OF THE REPORT
A. Statement of the adequacy of the specimen for evaluation
B. A general categorization, which may be used to assist with clerical triage (optional)
C. The descriptive diagnosis

ADEQUACY OF THE SPECIMEN
- Satisfactory for evaluation
- Satisfactory for evaluation, but limited by (specify reason)
- Unsatisfactory for evaluation (specify reason)

GENERAL CATEGORIZATION (OPTIONAL)
- Within normal limits
- Benign cellular changes: see descriptive diagnoses
- Epithelial cell abnormality: see descriptive diagnoses

DESCRIPTIVE DIAGNOSES
Benign cellular changes
Infection:
- *Trichomonas vaginalis*
- Fungal organisms morphologically consistent with *Candida* spp.
- Predominance of coccobacilli consistent with shift in vaginal flora
- Bacteria morphologically consistent with *Actinomyces* spp.
- Cellular changes associated with herpes simplex virus
- Other

(Continued on following page)

Box 15–2 (Continued)
The Bethesda System For Reporting Cervical/ Vaginal Cytologic Diagnosis

Reactive changes
Reactive cellular changes associated with:
- Inflammation (includes typical repair)
- Atrophy with inflammation ("atrophic vaginitis")
- Radiation
- Intrauterine contraceptive device
- Other

Epithelial cell abnormalities
Squamous cell
- Atypical squamous cells of undetermined significance: Qualify*
- Low-grade squamous intraepithelial lesion encompassing human papillomavirus† or mild dysplasia/CIN‡

High-grade squamous intraepithelial lesion encompassing
- Moderate and severe dysplasia
- CIS/CIN2 and CIN3
- Squamous cell carcinoma

Glandular cell
- Endometrial cells, cytologically benign, in a postmenopausal woman
- Atypical glandular cells of undetermined significance: Qualify*
- Endocervical adenocarcinoma
- Endometrial adenocarcinoma
- Extrauterine adenocarcinoma
- Adenocarcinoma, not otherwise specified (NOS)

Other malignant neoplasms: Specify
Hormone evaluationn (applied to smears only)
- Hormone pattern compatible with age and history
- Hormone pattern incompatible with age and history: Specify
- Hormone evaluation not possible due to: Specify

*Atypical squamous or glandular cells of undetermined significance should be further qualified as to whether a reactive or a premalignant/malignant process is favored.
† Cellular changes of human papillomavirus—previously termed koilocytosis atypia or condylomatous atypia—are included in the category of low-grade squamous intraepithelial lesions.
‡CIN indicates cervical intraepithelial neoplasia.

Women with any risk factors associated with cervical cancer should have annual Pap smears. Women who have been exposed to DES should have their first Pap smear at the onset of menstruation, a baseline colposcopy at first intercourse, and Pap smears every 6–12 months until age 30 and annually thereafter (see Table 15–3).

Differential diagnosis:

- Cervical infection (vaginal discharge, positive culture identifying organism)
- Dysfunctional uterine bleeding (menses at inappropriate times or inappropriate amount)
- Atrophy

Treatment: Surgical excision.

Follow-up: Depends on treatment. If hysterectomy is performed, the woman should have a Pap smear every 3 months for 2 years, every 6 months for 3 years, and yearly thereafter.

Table 15–3 Cancers of the Genital Tract

Type of Cancer	Most Common Type	Most Common Stage	Most Common Symptom	Screening
Vulvar	Squamous	I	Vulvar lesions; changes in pigmentation or thickness	Visualization by provider; vulvar self-examination
Vaginal	Squamous	Rare	None	Pap smear
Cervical	Squamous	I	Intermenstrual bleeding	Pap smear
Endometrial	Adenocarcinoma	I	Postmenopausal bleeding	None
Ovarian	Epithelial	III	Asymptomatic or pelvic pressure; bloating; dull pelvic pain	None

Sequelae: The most important factor affecting prognosis is stage of the disease. Histologic type influences outcome. Lymph node metastasis reduces the 5-year cure rate.

Prevention/prophylaxis: Cervical cancer is the only gynecologic malignancy for which a screening modality is widely accepted. Unfortunately, more than 50% of cervical cancers occur in women who have not been screened optimally.

Referral: All cases of cervical carcinoma require referral to a gynecologist for evaluation and treatment.

Education: The Pap smear is a simple, painless, and cost-effective tool that screens for cervical cancer. Since its inception, the number of deaths from cervical cancer has decreased. Women who adhere to the recommended screening intervals have a survival rate of 95% related to early detection. New technology has been introduced to reduce the Pap smear false-negative rate. Encourage all women to have regular Pap smear screening.

ENDOMETRIAL CANCER

SIGNAL SYMPTOM ▶ postmenopausal bleeding

Endometrial Cancer	ICD-9-CM: 182.0

Description: Cancer of the endometrium is the most common gynecologic malignancy in the United States.

Etiology: Adenocarcinoma of the endometrium of the uterus has a histologic precursor of atypical endometrial hyperplasia.

Occurrence: Endometrial cancer, which is three times more prevalent than cervical cancer, represents 10% of all cancers in women. Although most women with endometrial cancer present with an early stage disease and have an excellent chance of cure, approximately 6600 women in the United States will die of the disease in 2002. The lifetime probability of developing endometrial cancer for all American women is 3%.

Age: Advancing age is the most important risk factor for endometrial cancer; only 5% of these tumors occur before age 40. Most tumors occur in the sixth and seventh decades of life.

Ethnicity: Not significant.

Contributing factors: Obesity and glucose intolerance have been correlated with endometrial carcinoma. Strong evidence exists that estrogen, endogenous or exogenous, has a role in the development of endometrial cancer. There is a high incidence of this cancer in women with polycystic ovarian syndrome. An association exists between menstrual abnormalities and infertility and endometrial cancer. Of women with endometrial cancer, 20%–30% are nulliparous. The use of estrogen after menopause substantially increases the risk of endometrial cancer. A program of estrogen plus progesterone for postmenopausal therapy has not been associated with endometrial cancer. Low parity, late menopause, and hypertension have been associated with endometrial carcinoma.

Signs and symptoms:

 Clinical Pearl: Postmenopausal bleeding is by far the most common symptom associated with endometrial carcinoma.

See Table 15–3: Cancers of the Genital Tract.

Diagnostic tests:

Test	Results Indicating Condition	CPT Code
Transvaginal pelvic ultrasound	Endometrial thickness >5mm indicates need for biopsy	76817
Endometrial biopsy	Positive histology	58100
Dilatation and curettage (D&C)	Verifies diagnosis of endometrial cancer	58120
Hysteroscopy with endometrial biopsy, with or without D&C	Verifies diagnosis of endometrial cancer	58558

Differential diagnosis:

- Infection (positive culture, vaginal discharge)
- Atrophy

Treatment: Surgical excision.

Follow-up: Operative and histologic findings assign the risk for recurrence. Radiation therapy is used for women with intermediate or high risk. Hormonal therapy and chemotherapy may be used for advanced disease.

Sequelae: Various factors influence the prognosis, including histologic differentiation, depth of invasion, and lymph node metastases. Histologic type also influences the outcome.

Prevention/prophylaxis: None

Referral: All cases of suspected endometrial cancer must be referred to a gynecologist for evaluation and treatment. Endometrial sampling should be discussed with a gynecologist for those women at risk for endometrial cancer.

Education: Explain the significance of postmenopausal bleeding to every woman at the time of menopause. Estrogen should not be taken without progesterone in the postmenopausal period.

OVARIAN CANCER

SIGNAL SYMPTOM ▶ none—most women asymptomatic until the disease has metastasized

Ovarian Cancer	ICD-9-CM: 183.0

Description:

Clinical Pearl: Cancer of the ovary is the most lethal of pelvic malignancies in women.

Etiology: Unknown.

Occurrence: More than 23,000 new cases of ovarian cancer are diagnosed annually, making ovarian cancer the fifth most common malignancy among U.S. women. For women in the United States, the overall risk for developing ovarian cancer is 1.4% to 1.8%. 12,000 women die annually of the disease. The lifetime probability of developing the disease is 1 in 70 for American women. Late diagnosis is the primary reason for the poor prognosis. Reliable screening for this disease has not yet been developed.

Age: 80% to 90% of ovarian cancers occur after age 40. Fewer than 1% of ovarian cancers occur in women under 20 years of age. The peak incidence of invasive ovarian cancer is age 60. Hereditary ovarian cancers occur approximately 10 years earlier.

Ethnicity: The incidence of ovarian cancer is highest in the United States, Europe, and Israel, and lowest in Japan and in the developing countries. Ovarian cancer incidence is higher in Caucasian women than in women from African-American or Asian descent.

Contributing factors: Increasing age and family history are the most important risk factors for ovarian cancer.

The most significant risk factor for ovarian cancer is family history of the disease. The risk depends upon the number of affected first- and second-degree relatives as well as their ages at diagnosis with ovarian and breast cancer. This holds true for relatives on both the maternal and paternal side. Families with BRCA-1 and BRCA-2 mutations are at risk for breast and ovarian cancer. Overall lifetime risk for women with this genetic mutation for ovarian cancer is as high as 30%. There are also individuals who are at risk for ovarian cancer as part of their colorectal cancer genetic risk.

 Clinical Pearl: Only about 5 to 10% of ovarian cancers are familial.

Late menopause may be associated with a slightly higher incidence of ovarian cancer. An increase in ovarian cancer risk among nulliparas is consistently reported.

Signs and symptoms: Ovarian cancer may be totally asymptomatic. The woman may experience pelvic pressure, bloating, dull pelvic pain, or bladder pressure. Ovarian cancer may be related to ovarian enlargement (see Table 15-3).

Diagnostic tests:

Test	Results Indicating Disorder	CPT Code
Annual pelvic examination	ASCUS or abnormal result	Included in exam code
Rectovaginal exam	Ovarian enlargement	Included in exam code
Transvaginal ultrasound with Doppler	Visualization of masses	76830

Annual pelvic examination is recommended after age 18 for all sexually active women. Rectovaginal examination may be necessary to detect ovarian enlargement. Ovarian enlargement cannot always be palpated, making pelvic examination a limited diagnostic test.

Transvaginal ultrasonography with the use of color Doppler images improves the sensitivity for diagnosis of ovarian cancer.

 Clinical Pearl: Laparoscopy is the gold standard tool for diagnosis of ovarian cancer.

There is a great deal of interest in cancer antigen (CA) 125 as a diagnostic tool. Sensitivity of the test currently is between 9% and 96%. Specificity is higher in postmenopausal women and lower in women who have not yet experienced menopause. Many women screened for ovarian cancer with this testing methodology receive false positives. CA 125 level fluctuates with the menstrual cycle and is elevated in ovarian cysts, fibroid tumors, pregnancy, endometriosis, and PID.

Differential diagnosis:

- Stool-filled sigmoid colon (constipation, feeling of fullness)
- Distended bladder (fullness, bloating, pain, discomfort)
- Pelvic kidney, diverticular abscess (pain, tenderness, fever)
- Cysts (dermoid, functional, cystadenoma) (midcycle, sharp abdominal pain, bleeding or spotting)
- Tubo-ovarian abscess (pain that may come and go, fever)

Treatment: Surgical excision.

Follow-up: Frequently chemotherapy and radiation therapy follow surgery. Bone marrow transplants are recommended in selected cases.

Sequelae: On diagnosis, three out of four cases of ovarian carcinoma have spread beyond the ovary. Ovarian cancer is less common than breast cancer but has the highest case-fatality rate. Ovarian cancer is the fifth leading cause of cancer mortality in women, with 14,000 deaths annually. More women die from ovarian cancer than for all the other gynecologic malignancies combined.

Prevention/prophylaxis: Use of the oral contraceptive pill reduces the risk of ovarian cancer by 35%–50%. Women reduce their risk of ovarian cancer by 40% and 60% by taking oral contraceptives for four to eight years respectively.

Any pregnancy reduces the risk by 50%; increasing the number of pregnancies further reduces the risk.

Tubal ligation and possibly hysterectomy appear to reduce the risk of ovarian cancer.

Referral: Women with a significant family history of ovarian cancer and/or breast cancer should be referred for genetic counseling. Women with a significant family history should be referred to a gynecology oncologist for discussion of prophylaxis.

Education: Routine screening for women without family history of ovarian cancer is not currently recommended. Stress the importance of an annual pelvic examination for all women.

VULVAR CANCER

SIGNAL SYMPTOM ▶ lesion(s) on the vulva

Vulvar cancer (malignant/primary site)	ICD-9-CM: 184.4
Malignant/secondary site)	ICD-9-CM: 198.82
In situ	ICD-9-CM: 233.3
Benign	ICD-9-CM: 221.2
Uncertain	ICD-9-CM: 236.3
Unspecific	ICD-9-CM: 239.5

Description: The most common premalignant condition of the vulva is vulvar intraepithelial neoplasia (VIN).

Etiology: VIN has been associated with HPV. The vulva can develop carcinoma with the potential to become invasive.

Occurrence: Vulvar cancer comprises 5% of all cancers of the genital tract.

Age: VIN is most commonly associated with women in the 20–30-year age group. Squamous cell carcinoma occurs in women more than 45 years of age. Granular cell carcinoma occurs in women aged 30–40. Basal cell carcinoma occurs in women older than 70.

Ethnicity: Granular cell carcinoma occurs more often in African-American women.

Contributing factors: VIN is associated with immunocompromised women, smoking, and HPV.

Signs and symptoms: Changes in pigmentation, thickness, or symmetry of the vulva can indicate carcinoma. Mild whitening of the epithelium can be noted, but lesions that are tan or brown can also indicate cancer (see Table 15–3: Cancers of the Genital Tract).

Diagnostic tests:

Test	Results Indicating Disorder	CPT Code
Colposcopy	Carcinoma of vulva	57452
Vulvar biopsy with colposcopy	Diagnostic for cancer	57454

Differential diagnosis:
- Condylomata (fleshy warts)
- Vulvar infection (vaginal discharge, itching, positive culture for the organism)

Treatment: Surgical excision.

Follow-up: After surgery, vulvar cancer is followed every 3 months for the first year and every 6 months for the second year.

Sequelae: Depends on the extension of the excision.

Prevention/prophylaxis: Treatment of HPV; avoiding cigarette smoke

Referral: Any suspicious lesion on the vulva should be referred to a physician for biopsy.

Education: Encourage vulvar self-examination.

OTHER DISORDERS

SECONDARY AMENORRHEA

SIGNAL SYMPTOM ▶ interruption in normal menstrual pattern

| Absence of menstruation | ICD-9-CM: 626.0 |

Description: Primary amenorrhea is defined as failure to menstruate at puberty. Secondary amenorrhea is defined as the cessation of menses after it has been established; that is, an interruption in normal menstruation.

Etiology: Reasons for lack of menses include pregnancy, menopause, insufficient body fat, use of hormones for contraceptive reasons, thyroid disease, pituitary tumor, polycystic ovarian syndrome, premature ovarian failure, and Asherman's syndrome. Cervical stenosis can cause secondary amenorrhea (see Box 15–3).

Occurrence: The incidence of secondary amenorrhea is 3.3% in the population of menstruating American women.

Age: Secondary amenorrhea can occur in any woman after menses have been established during puberty.

Contributing factors: Situational stress, dieting, concurrent illness, increased exercise, and drugs.

Signs and symptoms: Cessation of menses for 3 or more months in a woman with formerly regular menses.

Diagnostic tests: Menstrual history must be taken carefully. Information must be obtained on contraceptive history and medications. Physical examination must include weight and general appearance,

---

Box 15–3
Causes of Amenorrhea

- Hypothalmic dysfunction
  - Mild—related to stress, dieting, exercise, drugs
  - Severe—related to anorexia nervosa; concurrent illness; excess androgen; prolactin, or cortisol
- Pituitary disease
- Ovarian
  - Menopause
  - Premature ovarian failure
  - Polycystic ovarian syndrome
  - Uterine
    - Asherman's syndrome
    - Cervical scarring
  - Endocrine disease
    - Thyroid
    - Cushing's
- Pregnancy

including hirsutism and virilization, palpation of the thyroid, and breast examination (particularly for evidence of discharge). Speculum examination should be performed, noting atrophy, and bimanual examination, noting enlarged uterus or adnexa. Lab data must include serum HCG, serum prolactin, and thyroid-stimulating hormone (TSH) levels and Pap smear.

After pregnancy has been ruled out, giving the patient a trial of progesterone is a common diagnostic test. The woman is given 10 mg of medroxyprogesterone (Provera) daily for 5 days. She will or will not have withdrawal bleeding after the completion of the progesterone trial.

Differential diagnosis:

- Pregnancy (positive pregnancy test)
- Menopause (hot flashes, depression, FSH level > 100mIU/ml)
- Insufficient body fat (low BMI, history of anorexia, history of significant changes in behavior, weight, exercise pattern)
- Use of hormones for contraceptive reasons (history of hormonal birth control)
- Thyroid disease (thyroid panel, lab values decreased or increased depending on the condition, thyroid scan)
- Pituitary tumor (radiologic evaluation)
- Polycystic ovarian syndrome (hirsutism, obesity, underdeveloped breasts, palpable enlarged cystic ovaries)
- Premature ovarian failure
- Asherman's syndrome (amenorrhea, absence of secondary sexual characteristics, hysterosalpingography or hysteroscopy for diagnosis)
- Cervical stenosis can cause secondary amenorrhea.

Treatment: Hormone replacement, bromocriptine, and surgery are possible treatments for secondary amenorrhea. Treatment depends on diagnosis (see Figure 15-4).

Follow-up: Medical or surgical therapy requires close follow-up for evaluation of menstrual patterns.

Prevention/prophylaxis: Avoidance of excessive dieting and exercise

Sequelae: Secondary amenorrhea can be treated successfully in most cases by a gynecologist. Reproductive endocrinology consultation is required for serious disease.

Referral: Consultation with a reproductive endocrinologist is necessary for secondary amenorrhea related to hypothalamic, pituitary, or ovarian dysfunction, as well as for thyroid disorders.

Education: Reassure any women with amenorrhea following the use of oral contraceptives about future fertility. If the desire for pregnancy is not immediate, advise the patient regarding methods of contraception because spontaneous ovulation can and does occur. Stress the importance of proper evaluation and treatment in women who require referral.

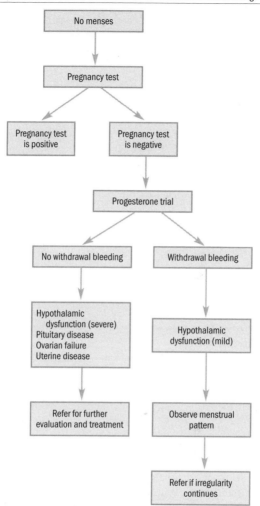

Figure 15–4. Secondary amenorrhea.

ABNORMAL BREAST DISCHARGE

SIGNAL SYMPTOM▶   breast discharge

Abnormal breast discharge	ICD-9-CM: 611.79

Description: The third most common symptom of breast disease is fluid emission from the mammary nipple. Discharge is symptomatic of disease in only 8%–10% of evaluated women.

Etiology: Pregnancy, stimulation of the breast, trauma to the chest, exercise, and stress can all cause breast discharge. Many medications cause breast discharge, including antipsychotic medications, oral contraceptives, and antiemetics. Tumors of the breast, pituitary, or hypothalamus can cause breast discharge. Infections cause discharge.

Occurrence: Of all women with breast symptoms, 5%–8% report discharge.

Age: Breast discharge can occur at any age.

Contributing factors: Sexual activity, exercise programs, thyroid disease

Signs and symptoms: Breast discharge can be unilateral or bilateral, clear or cloudy, dark or light, or bloody. Watery and bloody discharge can be associated with carcinoma.

Diagnostic tests:

Test	Results Indicating Disorder	CPT Code
Pap smear of the breast discharge	Microscopic inspection to rule out infection	88142
Serum prolactin level	> 25 ng/ml	84146
Mammogram	Rule out malignancy of the breast	76090 (unilateral)
Ductography or galactography	Benign intraductal papilloma or cancer	76086 (single duct) 76088 (multiple ducts)

Differential diagnosis:
- Thyroid disease (thyroid panel, lab values decreased or increased depending on the condition, thyroid scan)
- Drug-induced galactorrhea (history of ingestion of drugs that cause breast discharge)
- Pituitary tumor (radiologic evaluation)
- Intraductal papilloma (mammogram, cytology)
- Intraductal carcinoma (mammogram, cytology)
- Galactocele (palpable mass, ultrasound, cytology)

Treatment: Bromocriptine, a medication that inhibits the secretion of prolactin, can be given. Pituitary tumors are surgically removed, as are intraductal papillomas and carcinomas. Galactocele can be aspirated.

Follow-up: Bromocriptine treatment requires a follow-up visit every 2–3 months. Surgical therapy is followed up at the discretion of the surgeon.

Prevention/prophylaxis: None.

Sequelae: Resolution can be achieved for all benign conditions causing breast discharge.

Referral: Consultation with a physician is required for breast discharge related to medication, tumor, or infection.

Education:

Clinical Pearl: Inform the patient that breast discharge in nonlactating women should be reported to a health-care provider for diagnosis and treatment.

INFERTILITY

SIGNAL SYMPTOM ▶ inability to conceive

Female infertility, associated with adhesions; peritubal	ICD-9-CM: 614.6
Female infertility, anovulation	ICD-9-CM: 628.0
Female infertility, endometriosis	ICD-9-CM: 617.0
Infertility, Stein-Leventhal syndrome	ICD-9-CM: 256.4
Infertility, fallopian tube anomaly	ICD-9-CM: 628.2
Infertility, tubal occlusion or block	ICD-9-CM: 628.2

Definition: The definition of infertility is unprotected sexual intercourse for 1 year without conception. The 1-year length is related to the rate of conception in fertile couples of 50% in 3 months, 75% in 9 months, and 90% in 1 year.

Etiology: The etiology of infertility is discussed in terms of male and female. Male factor relates to azoospermia or oligospermia. The etiology can be gonadal, gonadotropic, obstructive, or functional. Female infertility is emphasized in this chapter, including:

- *Disorders of ovulation,* accounting for 20%–40% of female factors. Hypothalamic dysfunction, polycystic ovarian syndrome, premature ovarian failure, hyperprolactinemia, androgen excess, Turner's syndrome, hypothyroidism, uncontrolled diabetes mellitus, and hypercortisolism can cause lack of ovulation (see also Figure 15–5).
- *Tubal damage,* accounting for 25%–40% of female factors. Tubal damage is caused by pelvic adhesions related to PID or endometriosis.
- *Uterine pathology,* accounting for 5% of female factors. Uterine pathology is caused by fibroids, endometriosis, septate uterus, duplication of cervix and uterus, exposure to DES, and intrauterine adhesions (Asherman's syndrome).
- *Cervical abnormalities,* accounting for 3%–5% of female factors. Cervical abnormalities are caused by cervical incompetence, cervical stenosis related to prior surgery on the cervix, or abnormalities of cervical mucus.
- *Vaginal factors,* such as an intact hymen, a vaginal septum, or vaginal infection.
- *Luteal phase defect*, as defined by decreased progesterone secretion.
- *Recurrent fetal loss* (three or more spontaneous abortions) is classified as infertility.

Occurrence: In the United States, 10%–15% of couples are diagnosed as infertile.

- One third of infertility is related to male factor.
- One third of infertility is related to female factor.
- One third of infertility is related to both male and female or cause is unknown.

Age: Childbearing age. Infertility increases with age, most significantly from the late 30s forward.

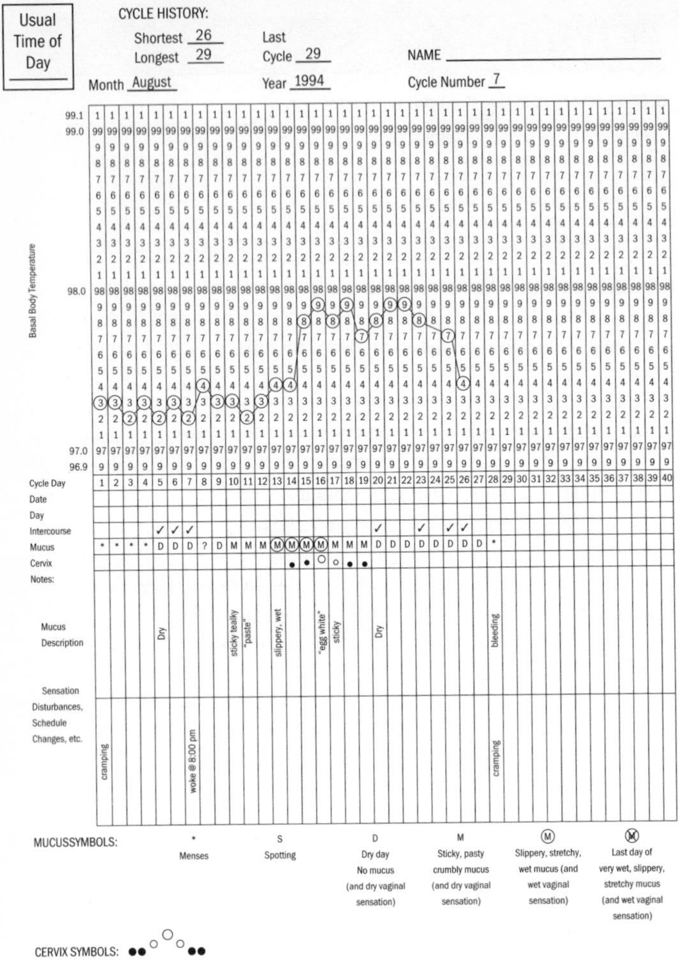

Usual Time of Day

CYCLE HISTORY:

Shortest 26 Longest 29

Month August

Last Cycle 29

Year 1994

NAME _____

Cycle Number 7

Basal Body Temperature

(temperature grid ranging 96.9 to 99.1)

Cycle Day: 1 2 3 4 5 6 7 8 9 10 11 12 13 14 15 16 17 18 19 20 21 22 23 24 25 26 27 28 29 30 31 32 33 34 35 36 37 38 39 40

Date

Day

Intercourse: ✓ ✓ ✓ (day 7-9) ✓ (21) ✓ (23) ✓ ✓ (25-26)

Mucus: • • • D D D ? D M M M Ⓜ Ⓜ Ⓜ M M M D D D D D D • D

Cervix: • • ○ ○ • •

Notes:

Mucus Description: cramping / Dry / sticky tacky "paste" / slippery, wet / "egg white" sticky / Dry / bleeding

Sensation

Disturbances, Schedule Changes, etc.: cramping / woke @ 8:00 pm / cramping

MUCUS SYMBOLS:

•	S	D	M	Ⓜ	Ⓧ
Menses	Spotting	Dry day No mucus (and dry vaginal sensation)	Sticky, pasty crumbly mucus (and dry vaginal sensation)	Slippery, stretchy, wet mucus (and wet vaginal sensation)	Last day of very wet, slippery, stretchy mucus (and wet vaginal sensation)

CERVIX SYMBOLS: •• ○ ○ ○ ••

Figure 15–5. Sample basal body temperature (BBT) form. Adapted from the Fertility Awareness Manual: An Instructional Guide for Clients. James Bowman: San Francisco.

Contributing factors: Aging, reduced frequency of intercourse, timing of intercourse, use of lubricants with spermicidal properties, douching, exposure to occupational hazards (chemicals, radiation), exposure to environmental hazards (heat, smoking, alcohol, drug abuse), excessive weight loss, psychologic stress (see Box 15–1: Sexual History).

Signs and symptoms: Pregnancy does not occur after 1 year of unprotected regular intercourse (see Box 15–4).

Diagnostic tests:

Test	Results Indicating Disorder	CPT Code
Male history and physical examination	History of signs of infertility	Included in history and physical exam code
Pap smear	Presence of cervical cancer or infection	88142
Serum pregnancy test	Negative	84702
Ovulation prediction kit and basal body temperature	No ovulation present	84830
Endometrial biopsy late in cycle after pregnancy test	Verify ovulation and rule out luteal phase defect	85100
Semen analysis	See Table 15-4: Normal Semen Analysis	89320
Female history: emphasis on menstrual and reproductive history	History of signs of infertility	Included in history code
Female physical exam	Enlarged thyroid gland, positive secondary sex characteristics, obesity and hirsutism	Included in physical exam code
Pelvic exam	Lack of mobility, pelvic masses, enlargement, thickening, tenderness	Included in physical exam code
Vaginal and cervical cultures for gonorrhea, Chlamydia, Mycoplasma, Ureaplasma organisms	Positive cultures	87850 Gonorrhea 87110 Chlamydia 87109 Mycoplasma 87070 other
Urine culture	Positive for infection	87088
Serum prolactin	Increased	84146
Follicle-stimulating hormone (FSH)—[Days 21–23]	Decreased	80426
Luteinizing hormone (LH)—[Day 21–23]	Decreased	80426
Serum progesterone—[Days 21–23]	Decreased	84144
Thyroid panel (TSH, T_3, T_4, and T_7)	Indicating thyroid disease	84443 (TSH) 84436 (T_4) 84439 (free T_4) 84479 (thyroid uptake) 84480 (T_3)
Postcoital test	Cervical mucus for sperm, ferning and spinnbarkeit at ovulation (none)	89300 (Huhner test) 87210 (wet prep)
Hysterosalpingogram (injection of dye through the cervix, performed in radiology)	Presence of tubal obstruction or abnormalities of the uterine cavity	58752
Hysteroscopy (injection of dye through the cervix, performed in OR)	Irregularities, adhesions, endometriosis, fibroids seen	58558
Laparoscopic surgery	Diagnose and treat adhesions, endometriosis, fibroids, or polycystic ovaries	58545

Hysteroscopy and laparoscopy can be performed simultaneously.

Box 15-4
History for Women with Infertility

- Age
- Menstrual history (irregular menstrual bleeding, hypothermia, amenorrhea)
- Obstetric history
- Previous contraceptive methods
- Symptoms of ovulation
- Dysmenorrhea
- Dyspareunia
- Premenstrual spotting
- Frequency of intercourse
- Medical history (PID)
- Surgical history
- Family history
- Drug use
- Galactorrhea
- Hirsutism
- Heat and cold intolerance
- Medication history
- Alcohal or cigarette use

See also Figure 15-6.

Differential diagnosis:

- Anorexia nervosa (history of weight loss, low BMI, history of eating disorder)
- Bulimia (self-induced vomiting, use of laxatives, diuretics, excessive exercise, discoloration of teeth from vomiting)
- Psychiatric disorders (history of depressive disorder)

Treatment: Infertility can be treated medically or surgically. Ovulation can be induced medically. Tubal disorders and uterine pathology are usually treated surgically. Multiple therapies can be implemented. Both partners may require treatment.

Follow-up: Infertility evaluation and treatment are often lengthy and require commitment of time, energy, and finances.

Prevention/prophylaxis: Prevention of PID would reduce the incidence of infertility.

Sequelae: Successful diagnosis and treatment of infertility result in pregnancy.

Table 15-4 Normal Semen Analysis

Characteristic	Results
Volume	2–6 mL
Concentration	> 20 million/mL
Viscosity	Liquefaction in < 30 min
pH	7.2–7.8
Motility	> 50%
Morphology	> 50% normal
Leukocytes	< 1 million/mL

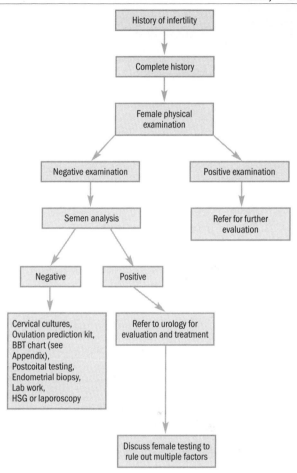

Figure 15–6. Infertility.

Referral: Of couples diagnosed with infertility, 44%–96% go on to conceive without treatment. The reason for infertility may resolve itself. Watchful waiting is in many cases a reasonable suggestion to couples. Referral, if indicated, should be to a reproductive endocrinologist.

Education: Counseling for infertility is necessary no matter what the cause. Resolution or adaptation must be facilitated. Infertile couples may choose to wait and watch, treat, adopt, employ a surrogate, or live without children. Couples who choose waiting should be educated about the timing of ovulation, the findings of their infertility "workup," and the prevention of sexually transmitted diseases.

PELVIC RELAXATION

SIGNAL SYMPTOMS sense of heaviness, fullness in the pelvis, sense of "dragging" in the pelvis, backache

Cystocele/rectocele (without uterine prolapse)	ICD-9-CM: 618.0
With uterine prolapse	ICD-9-CM: 618.4
Complete	ICD-9-CM: 618.3
Incomplete	ICD-9-CM: 618.2
In pregnancy	ICD-9-CM: 654.4
Obstructing labor	ICD-9-CM: 660.2

Description: The pelvic floor is composed of the anterior, middle, and posterior compartments. When there is a disorder in one, there is often a disorder in another. Cystocele is the most frequent disorder of the anterior compartment. Uterine prolapse is more frequent in the middle compartment, whereas rectocele occurs more often in the posterior compartment.

Etiology: Most pelvic floor dysfunction relates to childbirth trauma and progresses with age. A small number of pelvic floor dysfunctions are congenital or hereditary.

Occurrence: Unknown.

Age: Over 35 years of age.

Contributing factors: Childbirth, aging, and atrophy.

Signs and symptoms: Mild prolapse will create minimal symptoms. Significant prolapse can produce a range of complaints.

Uterine prolapse: Uterine prolapse produces low back pain, "pressure," and "aching," prior to and during menses; dysmenorrhea; and dyspareunia.

> *First degree:* Cervix descends nearly to the introitus.
> *Second degree:* Cervix descends and protrudes through the introitus.
> *Third degree:* Total prolapse with evagination of the cervix and uterus.

Cystocele: herniation of posterior bladder into the anterior vagina. The herniation can be minimal, moderate, or large. The primary symptom with cystocele is urinary incontinence.

Rectocele: outpouching of the anterior rectal wall into the posterior vagina. This outpouching can be minimal, moderate, or large. The primary symptom is inability to evacuate without straining. Some women with rectocele must insert digital pressure onto the posterior vagina in order to evacuate.

Diagnostic tests:

Test	Results Indicating Disorder	CPT Code
Pelvic examination	Prolapse of the cervix, bladder, rectum	Included in exam code
Pelvic ultrasound	Pelvic floor muscle relaxation	76857 (limited) 76856 (complete)

Test	Results Indicating Disorder	CPT Code
MRI	Distinguish fascial and muscular layers of pelvic support	72195 (without contrast) 72196 (with contrast) 72197 (without and with contrast)
Urodynamic investigation	Stress incontinence	51792

Differential diagnosis:

- Urinary tract infection (positive culture)
- Herniation of the peritoneum into the posterior cul-de-sac (radiologic evaluation)
- Multiple sclerosis (muscle weakness, visual changes)
- Parkinson's disorder (rigidity, tremor, slow movement)
- Senile atrophy

Treatment: Uterine prolapse can be treated with a pessary. If a pessary is fitted for the woman, she must be able to remove it, clean it, and replace it. Uterine prolapse can also be treated with vaginal hysterectomy. Cystocele and rectocele are treated with Kegel exercises. Both can also be treated with surgery.

Follow-up: Surgical therapy requires follow-up for monitoring of healing and resolution of symptoms. Nonsurgical therapy requires frequent follow-up for resolution of symptoms.

Sequelae: Stasis of the urine in a large cystocele can lead to chronic or recurrent cystitis.

Prevention/prophylaxis:

 Clinical Pearl: Kegel exercises, to be performed on a daily basis after vaginal delivery.

Referral: Second- and third-degree uterine prolapse and cystocele and rectocele unresponsive to Kegel exercises should be referred to a physician for evaluation and treatment.

Education: Teach Kegel exercises to women with mild cystocele and/or rectocele. When a pessary is prescribed, demonstrate its use.

ABNORMAL VAGINAL BLEEDING

SIGNAL SYMPTOM▶ menses at inappropriate times and/or inappropriate amount of flow

Abnormal Vaginal Bleeding	ICD-9-CM: 623.8

Description: Normally in the absence of implantation of a fertilized egg, the ovarian corpus luteum undergoes regression 9–11 days after ovulation. The normal menstrual cycle ranges from 23–39 days. The menstrual period lasts 2–7 days, with most of the bleeding occurring in the first few days. Normal ovulation may be accompanied by a small amount of midcycle "staining." At times mittelschmerz, pain associated with ovarian follicle rupture and release, accompanies the staining.

Abnormal vaginal bleeding occurs at an inappropriate time or in an excessive amount.

Etiology: Possible causes include malignancy, disturbance in the hypothalamus-pituitary-ovary connection, fibroids, polyps, foreign bodies, pregnancy, and puberty.

- Uterine fibroids are a common cause of abnormal bleeding, representing about one third of the presenting cases. Fibroids that are submucosal can lead to heavy bleeding. The location, not necessarily the size, of the fibroids creates abnormal bleeding.
- Postcoital bleeding and intermenstrual spotting are characteristic of cervical carcinoma.
- Polyps can create intermenstrual spotting, seen especially after intercourse.
- Infection is a common cause of vaginal bleeding. Postcoital, intermenstrual, or heavy menstrual bleeding can be related to cervical or endometrial infection.
- Foreign bodies such as IUDs can cause endometrial irritation and resultant bleeding. Tampons can irritate the vaginal mucosa and create bleeding.
- Ectopic pregnancy can present as a delay in menses followed by spotting and pain. Delayed menses followed by vaginal bleeding and cramping characterize pregnancy loss.
- Oral contraceptives create "breakthrough bleeding," indicating that the balance of estrogen and progesterone is incorrect for the woman.
- Anovulatory cycles are seen in puberty and perimenopause, and can create irregular vaginal bleeding.
- Postmenopausal bleeding can indicate endometrial carcinoma.
- Polycystic ovarian syndrome creates chronic anovulation and thus irregular vaginal bleeding.
- Hypothalamic dysfunction creates oligomenorrhea or amenorrhea.

Occurrence: Depends on etiology.

Age: Abnormal vaginal bleeding can occur in any menstruating female and in postmenopausal women.

Contributing factors: Situational stress, weight loss, exercise training, iron deficiency anemia, chronic illness.

Signs and symptoms: Variation from the woman's normal menstrual pattern. Menses occur at an inappropriate time or in an excessive amount.

Diagnostic tests: History and physical examination are the cornerstones of diagnosis for abnormal vaginal bleeding (see Figure 15–7).

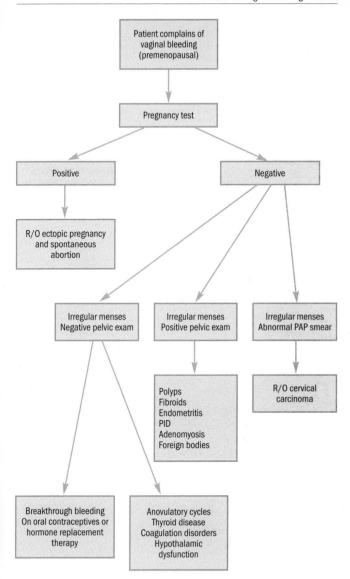

Figure 15–7. Abnormal vaginal bleeding.

History: A careful and detailed menstrual history must be obtained. The woman's usual menstrual pattern must be identified. Method of contraception, symptoms of pregnancy, presence of premenstrual symptoms, intensity of the bleeding (measured in use of pads and tampons), duration of the bleeding, as well as time in the cycle of the bleeding must be elicited. Presence of vaginal discharge, bleeding related to intercourse, and presence of pain should be described. Recent emotional stress and/or weight loss should be determined. Medication use should be reviewed. In postmenopausal women, any history of bleeding, even minimal bleeding, can be evidence of malignancy.

Physical examination: Speculum and bimanual examination should be performed, looking for discharge, erosion, polyps, tenderness, and signs of pregnancy. Examination of the postmenopausal woman should note friability of the vaginal mucosa and cervix.

Diagnostic testing:

Test	Results Indicating Disorder	CPT Code
Pregnancy test	Assist in diagnosis	84702
CBC	Assist in diagnosis	85025
Pelvic ultrasound	Assist in diagnosis; diagnostic for endometrial carcinoma in the postmenopausal woman	76857 (limited) 76856 (complete)
Pap smear	Assist in diagnosis	88142
Cervical culture	Assist in diagnosis	87070
FSH level	In perimenopausal bleeding, confirmatory (a level of more than 40 suggests ovarian failure)	83001
D and C hysteroscopy	Diagnostic for endometrial carcinoma in the post-menopausal woman	58558

Differential diagnosis: See Figure 15–7.

Treatment: The diagnosis determines whether a surgical or medical approach is more appropriate.

Follow-up: Organic pelvic pathology, hormone-related dysfunction, systemic problems, endocrine causes, and disorders of pregnancy all require close follow-up after diagnosis.

Sequelae: Monthly menses should occur after medical therapy.

Prevention/prophylaxis: Abnormal uterine bleeding is a frequent complaint. Making an accurate diagnosis and ruling out serious causes are essential.

Referral: Consultation with a physician for evaluation and treatment is essential. Prompt referral is necessary in cases of heavy vaginal bleeding or possible ectopic pregnancy.

Education: Inform the patient that abnormal menstrual bleeding can affect a woman at any age. A health-care provider should investigate stress to the patient that causes irregular or heavy vaginal bleeding.

REFERENCES

Vaginal infections

Adad, S, et al: Frequency of *Trichomonas vaginalis*. São Paulo Med J 119(6), 2001.

Caillouette, J, et al: Vaginal pH as a marker for bacterial pathogens and menopausal status. Am J Obstet Gynecol 176(6):1275, 1997.

Centers for Disease Control and Prevention: Guidelines for Treatment of Sexually Transmitted Diseases. MMWR 51, 2002.

Jonsson, M, et al: The associations between risk behavior and reported history of sexually transmitted diseases among young women: A population based study. Int J STD AIDS 8(8):501, 1997.

Marrazzo, JM, et al: Community-based urine screening for *Chlamydia trachomatis* with a ligase chain reaction assay. Ann Intern Med 127:796, 2000.

Oakeshott, P, et al: Opportunistic screening for chlamydial infection at time of cervical smear testing in general practice. Br Med J 31:316, 1998.

Page, D, et al: Bacterial vaginosis and preterm birth. J Nurse Midwifery 43(2):83, 1998.

Quan, M: Vaginitis. Clinical Cornerstone 3(1): 2000.

Sanchez, S, et al: Rapid and inexpensive approaches to managing abnormal vaginal discharge or lower abdominal pain. Sexually Transmitted Infections 1:S85, 1998.

Sobel, J: Vaginitis. N Engl J Med 26:(337):1896, 1997.

Thorsen, P, et al: Few microorganisms associated with bacterial vaginosis may constitute the pathologic core. Am J Obstet Gynecol 178(3):580, 1998.

Pelvic Inflammatory Disease

Blythe, M: Pelvic inflammatory disease in the adolescent population. Semin Pediatr Surg 7(1):43, 1998.

Benaim, J, et al: Adolescent girls and pelvic inflammatory disease. Arch Pediatr Adolesc Med 152(5):449, 1998.

Munday, P: Clinical aspects of pelvic inflammatory disease. Hum Reprod 12(11 Suppl):121, 1997.

Price B, and Martens, M: Outpatient management of pelvic inflammatory disease. Current Women's Health Reports 1(1), 2001.

Risser, W, et al: Pelvic inflammatory disease in adolescents. Texas Medicine 98(2), 2002.

Ross, J: An update on pelvic inflammatory disease. Sexually Transmitted Infections 78(1), 2002.

Toxic Shock

Herzer, C: Toxic shock syndrome: Broadening the differential diagnosis. J American Board Fam Pract 14(2), 2001.

Hyns, G, et al: Understanding sepsis: from SIRS to septic shock. Dynamics 13(1), 2002.

Issa, N, and Thompson, R: Staphylococcal toxic shock syndrome. Postgraduate Medicine 110(4), 2001.

Endometriosis and Adenomyosis

Arumugam, K, and Lim, J: Menstrual characteristics associated with endometriosis. Br J Obstet Gynecol 104(8):948, 1997.

Duleba, A: Diagnosis of endometriosis. Obstet Gynecol Clin North Am 24(2):331, 1997.

Eskenazi, B, and Warner, M: Epidemiology of endometriosis. Obstet Gynecol Clin North Am 24(2):235, 1997.

Howard, F: Pelvic Pain: Lippincott Williams & Wilkins, Philadelphia, 2000.

Parazzini, F, et al: Risk factors for adenomyosis. Human Reprod 12(6):1275, 1997.

Vavilis, D, et al: Adenomyosis at hysterectomy. Clin Exp Obstet Gynecol 24(1):36, 1997.

Fibroids

Braude, P, et al: Embolization of uterine leiomyomata. Human Reproduction Update 6(6), 2000.

Hutchins, F: Uterine fibroids: Diagnosis and indications for treatment. Obstet Gynecol Clin North Am 22(4):659, 1995.

Kjerulkk, K, et al: Uterine leiomyomas. J Reprod Med 41(7):483, 1996.

Prayson, R, and Hart, W: Pathologic considerations of uterine smooth muscle tumors. Obstet Gynecol Clin North Am 22(4):637, 1995.

Walker, W, et al: Fibroid embolization. Clin Radiol 57(5), 2002.

Malignancies of the Genital Tract

American College of Obstetricians and Gynecologists: Guidelines for Women's Health Care. ACOG, Washington, DC, 1999.

Collins, W, et al: Screening strategies for ovarian cancer. Curr Opin Obstet Gynecol 10(1):33, 1998.

Copas, P, et al: Basal cell carcinoma of the vulva. J Reprod Med 41(4):283, 1996.

Foulks, MJ: The Papanicolaou smear: Its impact on promotion of women's health. JOGNN 27(4):367, 1998.

Gupta, J, et al: Ultrasonographic endometrial thickness for diagnosing endometrial pathology. Acta Obstetrica et Gynecologia Scandanavica 81(9), 2002.

Holschneider, C, and Berek J: Ovarian cancer: Epidemiology, biology and prognostic factors. Semin Surg Oncol 19(3):3, 2000.

Lea, J, and Miller, D: Optimum screening interventions for gynecologic malignancies. Texas Med 97(2):49, 2001.

Mitchell, M, et al: Colposcopy for diagnosis and treatment of squamous intraepithelial lesions: A meta-analysis. Obstet Gynecol 91(4):626, 1998.

Paley, P: Ovarian cancer screening: are we making any progress? Curr Opini Oncol 13(5):399, September, 2001.

Plaxe, S, and Saltzstein, S: Impact of ethnicity on the incidence of high risk endometrial carcinoma. Gynecol Oncol 65:8, 1997.

Porter, S: Endometrial cancer. Semin Oncol Nurs 18(3), 2002.

Seltzer, V, and Pearse, W: Women's Primary Health Care. McGraw-Hill, New York, 1995.

Simone, J, et al: Granular cell tumor of the vulva. J Louisiana State Med Soc 148(12):539, 1996.

Secondary Amenorrhea

Goroll, A, et al.: Primary Care Medicine. Lippincott, Philadelphia, 1995.

Youngkin, E, and Davis, M: Women's Health. Appleton & Lange, East Norwalk, CT, 1994.

Abnormal Breast Discharge

Rongione, A et al: Ductography is a useful technique in evaluation of abnormal nipple discharge. Amer Surg 62(10), 1996.

Pelvic Relaxation

Bernier F, and Jenkins, P: The role of vaginal estrogen in the treatment of uro-genital dysfunction in postmenopausal women. Urol Nurs 17(3), 1997.

Koduri, S, and Saand, P: Recent developments in plevic organ prolapse. Curr Opini Obstet Gynecol 12(5), 2000.

Pandit, I, and Ouslander J: Postmenopausal atrophy and atrophic vaginitis. Amer J Med Sci 314(4), 1997.

Strohbehn, K, et al: Pelvic organ prolapse in young women. Obstet Gynecol 90(1):33, 1997.

Name	Address and Telephone	E-mail or Web site
800 Cocaine Information	Summit, NJ 1-900-262-2463	
Academy for Eating Disorders	1-703-556-9222	www.acadeatdis.org
AIDS Hotline	Atlanta, GA 1-800-551-2728	
Alcoholics Anonymous		www.alcoholics-anonymous.org/
American Academy of Dermatology	930 N. Neacham Rd, PO Box 4014 Schaumburg, IL 60168 1-800-462-DERM 1-312-856-8888	www.aad.org/ www.coppertone.com
American Cancer Society	1599 Clifton Road Atlanta, GA 1-800-227-2345	www.cancer.org
American Lung Association	1740 Broadway New York, NY 10019-4371 1-800-LUNG-USA	www.lung.usa.org
American Pseudo-Obstruction & Hirschsprung's Disease Society	P.O. Box 772 Medford, MA 02155 1-617-395-4255	
American Sleep Disorder Association	1610 14th St., NW, Suite 300 Rochester, MN 55901 1-507-287-6006	www.asda.org
BASH—Bulimia Anorexia Self-Help	St Louis, MO 1-800-227-4785	
Bladder Health Council	300 W. Pratt St. Suite 401 Baltimore, MD 21201 1-800-242-2393	www.afud.org
Canadian Women's Health Network		www.cwh.ca/resource
Centers for Disease Control and Prevention		www.cdc.gov

Name	Address and Telephone	E-mail or Web site
Centers for Disease Control Division of Bacterial and Mycotic Diseases Disease Information		www.cdc.gov/ ncidod/dbmd/ diseaseinfo
Eating Disorders Awareness and Prevention, Inc.	1-800-931-2237	www.edap.org
Epilepsy Foundation of America	4351 Garden City Dr. Landover, MD 20785 1-800-332-1000	www.efa.org
Food Allergy Network	4744 Holly Ave. Fairfax, VA 22030-5647 1-800-929-4040	www.foodallergy.org
Food and Drug Administration		www.fda.org
FoodNet		www.cdc.gov/ncidod/ dbmd/foodnet
Gateway to Government Food Safety Information		www.foodsafety.gov
Internet Public Library: Women's Health		www.ipl.org
JAMA Women's Health Information Center		www.ama-assn.org
Medic Alert Foundation	Turlock, CA 1-800-344-3226	www.medicalert,org
Medscape OB/GYN and Women's Health		www.medscape.com
National Association for Continence	P.O. Box 8310 Spartanburg, SC 29305 1-800-BLADDER	www.nafc.org
National Asthma Educational Program National Heart Lung/Blood Institute	1-301-251-1222	
National Breast Care Coalition	P.O. Box 66373 Washington, DC 20035 1-800-935-0434	www.nat/bcc/org
National Center for Education in Maternal and Child Health	38th and R St., N.W. Washington, DC 20057 1-202-625-8400	
National Council on Alcoholism and Drug Dependence	1-800-622-2255	
National Council on the Aging		www.ncoa.org
National Herpes Hotline	1-919-361-8488	
National Inhalant Prevention Coalition		www.inhalants.org/
National Institute on Drug Abuse	1-800-662-4357	
National Institutes of Health		www.nih.gov
National Multiple Sclerosis Information Hotline	New York, NY 1-800-227-3166	

Name	Address and Telephone	E-mail or Web site
National Scoliosis Foundation	72 Mount Auburn St. Watertown, MA 02172 1-617-926-0397	www.nichcy.org
National STD Hotline	1-800-227-8922	
Office of National Drug Control Policy (ONDCP)		www.whitehousedrug policy. gov/
Overeaters Anonymous	World Service Office P.O. Box 44020 Rio Rancho, NM 87174-4020 1-505-891-2644	
Partnership for Food Safety Education		www.fightbac.org
Planned Parenthood	1-800-230-7526	
Stingray Bay Sun Protection	1-800-969-4SUN	www.stingrayby.com
United States Department of Agriculture(USDA) **Foodborne Illness Education Information Center**		www.nal.usda.gov/ fnic/foodborne/ foodborn.htm
USDA Food Safety and Inspection Service		http://www.fsis.usda. gov
Women with Disabilities		www.4women.gov
Women's Health Information Center	240 Elm St., Somerville, MA 02144	www.4woman.gov

Web Sites for Women's Health Nurse Practitioners

Name	Web Sites
American Academy of Nurse Practitioners	www.aanp.org/
American College of Nurse-Midwives	www.midwife.org/
American Nurses Association	www.ana.org/
Association of Women's Health, Obstetric and Neonatal Nurses (AWHONN)	www.awhonn.org/
Centers for Disease Control and Prevention	www.cdc.gov/
National Association of Neonatal Nurses	www.nann.org/
National Association of Pediatric Nurse Associates and Practitioners	www.napnap.org/
National Council of State Boards of Nursing	www.ncsbn.org/
National Institutes of Health	www.nih.gov/
March of Dimes	www.modimes.org/

Appendix ***B***
HANDOUTS

NUTRITION FOR WOMEN

Diet plays an important role in health. Studies have shown that coronary artery disease, stroke, diabetes, and some types of cancer have nutrition-related risks. Proper nutrition and weight control are important preventive health measures.

Recommendations from the U.S. Department of Agriculture, the U.S. Department of Health, and the U.S. Surgeon General are as follows:

- Eat a variety of foods.
- Maintain a healthy weight.
- Choose a diet low in fat and cholesterol.
- Eat adequate vegetables, fruits, starch, and fiber.
- Use sugar in moderation.
- Avoid excessive salt.
- Consume no alcohol or alcohol in moderation.
- Approximately 2200 calories per day are needed by the average nonpregnant woman.
- Total fat intake should not exceed 30% of the calories consumed in the diet.
- Calcium requirements are 1200 mg daily for adolescent girls, at least 800 mg daily for adult women, 1200 mg daily for pregnant women, and 1200 to 1500 mg per day for menopausal and postmenopausal women.
- Menstruating women should include iron-rich food in their diet and take an iron supplement daily.

Cancer research provides the following dietary recommendations for women:

- Avoid obesity.
- Decrease fat intake.
- Increase intake of whole-grain foods.
- Increase intake of dark green, deep yellow, and orange vegetables.
- Eat smoked and cured foods in moderation.
- If alcohol is used, use it in moderation.

GUIDELINES FOR ADDING CALCIUM TO YOUR DIET

The typical American diet includes 600 mg of calcium daily. About 75% to 80% of calcium consumed in American diets is from dairy products. Before menopause, healthy women need 1200 mg of calcium daily. After menopause, they need 1200 to 1500 mg daily.

Sources of Calcium

- Milk   300 mg per 8 ounce serving
- Yogurt   400 mg per 8 ounce serving
- Cheese   200 mg per 1 ounce serving
- Sardines   370 mg per 3 ounce serving
- Oysters   270 mg per cup
- Canned salmon   160 mg per 3 ounce serving
- Tofu   120 mg per 3 ounce serving

Vitamin D

Vitamin D plays a major role in calcium absorption and bone health. Vitamin D is found in vitamin D–fortified milk (400 IU per quart) and cereals (50 IU per serving), egg yolks, saltwater fish, and liver. A regular intake of 400 to 800 IU daily is recommended for bone health.

Medications

Drugs that interfere with calcium absorption are anticonvulsants, steroids, tetracycline, diuretics, and aluminum-containing antacids.

Calcium Supplements

Calcium carbonate has the highest amount of calcium per tablet—40%. Calcium lactate and calcium gluconate have only about 10% of each tablet containing calcium.

ADDING IRON
TO YOUR DIET

FOODS HIGH IN IRON CONTENT

Meats, Poultry, Fish, Dry Beans, Eggs, Nuts

Beef liver
Clams
Oysters
Beef
Black-eyed peas
Chickpeas
Lentils
Lima beans
Pinto beans
Soybeans

Sugar

Molasses, black
Sugar, brown

Vegetables

Avocado
Potato (baked with skin on)
Spinach

Fruits

Dried figs
Prunes
Raisins

Breads, Cereals, Rice, Pasta

Bran flakes
Cream of wheat
Enriched pasta
Wheat flakes

MAMMOGRAM

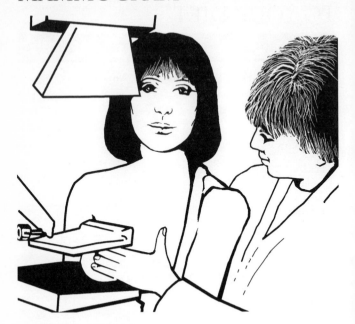

Figure H1–1. Mammogram.

What Is a Mammogram?

A mammogram is a low-dose x-ray of the breasts. This procedure detects tumors that are too small to be felt by breast self-examination. Mammograms are performed in an outpatient setting, such as a radiology center or a doctor's office. A technician who has been trained in mammography performs a mammogram, and a radiology physician interprets the results.

What Can I Expect During a Mammogram?

You are asked to undress from the waist up, remove necklaces, and wear an examination gown that opens in the front. You are then asked to stand in front of a mammogram machine. Two plastic plates are used to compress one breast at a time while films are taken. Compression is used to enhance the films taken and to reduce radiation exposure. After the films are taken, you are asked to wait a few minutes before dressing while the technician develops the films to make sure that they can be read by the radiologist. Results of the mammogram can be given shortly after the test. In some settings, results will not be forwarded to you until several days after the test.

How Do I Prepare for a Mammogram?

To prepare for a mammogram, do not apply powder, cream, or deodorant on the day of the test. These substances may appear on the x-ray film and lead to false positives (indications of problems when there are none).

There is temporary discomfort with the compression needed to perform the test. To minimize the discomfort, the test should be performed during the week after menses when breasts are least tender. Discomfort occurs only with compression, and ceases as soon as the plates are removed.

When Should I Have a Mammogram?

Your first mammogram should be performed between the ages of 35 and 40. Mammograms should then be performed every year or every other year until age 50 and once a year thereafter.

BREAST SELF-EXAMINATION

Breast Self-examination

Breast self-examination should be performed on a regular monthly basis beginning at age 20. Breast self-examination should be performed after menses when breasts are the least tender. If you are not menstruating on a monthly basis, breast self-examination should be performed on the same day each month. If you are lactating, breast self-examination should be performed when the breasts are empty.

Remember:

- Breast self-examination is just one of three examinations that promote early detection of breast cancer. The other two equally important examinations are mammogram and clinical breast examination.
- The vast majority of changes noted during breast self-examination are NOT cancers.
- The following technique should also be used if you have breast implants.

Steps in the Breast Self-examination

Step 1 Begin by looking at your breasts. Look in a mirror noting the shape, size, color, and texture of each breast. Observe the breast with your hands at your sides, with your hands over your head and with you hands on your hips. When your hands are on your hips, press them in slightly.

Step 2 Observe the breasts while you are leaning forward somewhat with your hands on your hips. You are looking for any puckering of the breast or changes from the last inspection.

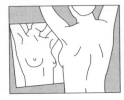

Step 3 Next fold a small towel and place it under your shoulder while you are lying down on your back. Your arm should be placed out, up and over your head at an angle.

Step 4 Feel the entire breast — arm pit to breast bone and collar bone to bra line. Use three fingers to palpate the finger.

Step 5 Use the pads of the fingers making small dime size circles in each area of the breast. Do not take your hand off the breast while examining because you may miss an area. Make three small circles in each area - one light, one deeper and one deeper yet so that you feel all the layers of the breast. Cover the entire breast ending with the breast tissue in the armpit area.

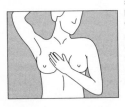

Step 6 Move the folded towel to the opposite shoulder and examine the other breast. You are looking for a lump or thickening that feels different from the rest of the breast.

Breast self-examination takes just a few minutes each month, is easy to perform and very important for every woman's health.

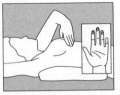

Figure H1–2. Breast self-examination.

Chapter 2

HANDOUTS

PAINFUL MENSES

Painful menses is a crampy feeling in the lower abdomen (belly) that occurs with a menstrual period. Cramping with periods is diagnosed typically in adolescents. The pain starts before the period begins but is most severe during the first day of bleeding. The pain is usually confined to the lower abdomen, but can extend to the thighs and back. At times fatigue, nausea, or vomiting accompany the cramping.

The first choice for relief is ibuprofen: 200–400 mg every 4 to 6 hours to relieve the hypercontractions of the uterus and relieve the pain. (This medication should be taken with food.)

In women who do not desire contraception and have severe cramping with their periods, birth control pills are indicated. This form of birth control provides relief from painful menses for 90% of women. Other pain-relief methods include:

- Exercise
- Increased fiber in the diet
- Increased water intake
- Heating pads or warm baths
- Relaxation techniques

In women who did not have painful menses as young adults but begin to experience them in the third and fourth decades of life, the cramping may indicate a pelvic problem. An appointment is required with a health-care provider to address this problem.

WOMEN AND HEADACHE

There are many kinds of headaches, but the most common ones that plague women are tension headaches and migraines.

Tension Headaches

What causes tension headaches is poorly understood. Ninety percent of women's headaches fall into this category. These headaches usually occur during times of stress and tension. When they occur on a daily basis, they are often associated with depression and require treatment for depression for relief of the headaches. Usually no diagnostic tests are indicated for tension headache. The history of the headache makes the diagnosis.

Tension headaches are not associated with any negative consequences. Ibuprofen is the drug of choice for relief.

Migraine Headaches

Migraine headaches are recurrent and may be accompanied by visual or gastrointestinal disturbance. In this type of headache, spasms in vessels of the head cause the pain. Migraine produces unilateral throbbing pain (on one side only), often accompanied by nausea, and often there is discomfort in bright light. Frequently women with migraine headache have a family history of migraines.

There is a range of medication prescribed for migraine. Some women require medication to prevent migraine "attacks." Stress or certain foods can trigger migraines.

Factors related to headache in women:

Diet: Although unrelated to tension headache, diet is related to migraine headache.

Family history: This factor is positive for migraine headache, but negative for tension headache.

Menses: Migraine can be strongly related to menstrual patterns. Of female migraine sufferers, 60% to 70% have migraines around the time of menses, and 50% have a reduction of migraines during pregnancy.

Headache prior to menses can be related to falling estrogen levels, allowing migraine inducers to create a headache.

GENITAL HERPES

Genital herpes is caused by a virus. There are two different types of the virus, but both are spread by direct skin contact, including genital-genital contact and oral-genital contact. Anyone who is sexually active can get herpes. You can get it if you have only one partner who happens to be infected. Many people do not know that they have herpes; they infect others without realizing they are doing so. Using a condom can prevent the spread of genital herpes and other sexually transmitted diseases.

The only way to tell for sure that you have herpes is to visit a health-care provider. Herpes can look like many things, including simple irritation. It is important to report to the practitioner any redness or sores in the genital area.

A first outbreak of genital herpes can occur in 2–21 days after sex with an infected partner. Some women have severe symptoms, whereas others have mild symptoms. Herpes symptoms include:

- Pain or itching in the genital area or buttocks
- Burning during urination
- Unusual vaginal discharge
- Swelling and reddening
- Small bumps in the genital area
- Bumps become painful sores that open up, crust over, and eventually heal.
- Fever, chills, muscle aches, tiredness, headache

If not treated, a first outbreak can last for about 3 weeks. Most people experience repeated outbreaks that are less severe and last for a shorter time. The interval between outbreaks varies from woman to woman.

After the virus has infected someone, it remains with that person for life. There is no cure, but it can be treated and outbreaks reduced.

GENITAL WARTS

What Are Genital Warts?

Genital warts are small growths that appear on or inside the genitals of both men and women. They are spread from person to person by close physical contact during vaginal, anal, or oral sex.

Where Do they Appear?

Genital warts look and feel like bumps. They are usually painless but can cause itching and burning. In women, they occur inside and outside the vagina and on the cervix (the opening to the uterus). They can also occur on the rectum (anus) and in the throat.

The warts can be seen and/or felt if they are on the outside of the body. Warts inside the vagina and on the cervix can be detected only by a health-care provider. An abnormal Pap smear may mean that you have genital warts.

What Causes Genital Warts?

A virus causes genital warts. The virus is contagious and can be passed to someone else during sex. Warts can take weeks to appear after the virus has been contracted. The virus remains in the body even after the warts are removed.

How Are Genital Warts Treated?

Treatment depends on how many warts are present and if they are inside or outside of the body. Some warts can be removed with a medicine that is applied to them. Some can be frozen or burned off. Some need to be removed by surgery. Warts can return after they have been removed because the virus remains in the body.

There are several "wart" viruses. Most are not associated with cancer, but a few are associated with cancer of the cervix. If genital warts are discovered on the cervix, follow-up Pap smears are very important.

What About My Sex Partner(s)?

Your partner should be examined and treated when you are diagnosed with genital warts.

How Do I Prevent Getting Genital Warts?

- Examine your partner before having sex.
- Use latex condoms every time you have sex. Condoms can protect you from sexually transmitted diseases, including genital warts.
- Do not have sex with a person you think might have a sexually transmitted disease.
- Do not use drugs or alcohol before having sex.

PUBIC LICE

What Are Pubic Lice?

A species of human lice causes a common sexually transmitted disease. Another name for pubic lice is "crabs." Body and head lice do not usually affect the pelvic area. Pubic lice, however, have been found in beards, eyelashes, and eyebrows.

How Do I Get Pubic Lice?

The crab louse requires human blood to survive. Off the body, the lice die quickly. Direct contact must occur for lice to be "caught."

Itching is the primary symptom. Itching leads to scratching, redness, and irritation.

How Do I Get Rid of Pubic Lice?

Lice are treated with over-the-counter or prescription medication. Some medications may not be used during pregnancy. Follow the manufacturer's directions for use carefully.

- Wash with hot water, dry-clean, or run through the dryer all contaminated clothing, towels, and bedclothes to destroy the lice.
- Spray couches, chairs, and items that cannot be washed or dry-cleaned with an over-the-counter product.
- Sexual partner(s) should be treated simultaneously.

BLADDER INFECTIONS IN WOMEN

Urine is sterile—that is, without any bacteria—in the normal state. The urethra (the opening where the urine comes from), the bladder, or the kidneys can be infected with bacteria. The bacteria will be apparent in the urine when the bladder or kidneys are infected. Bladder infections are experienced by 10% to 25% of women.

Where Do the Bacteria Come From?

Bacteria normally reside in the bowel. Many infections of the bladder in women are caused by bacteria normally found in the intestinal tract.

Sexual activity places women at risk. The risk for infection of the bladder increases specifically with vaginal intercourse. Any manipulation of the urethra through oral sex or masturbation can also increase the risk. The vagina is not sterile; it houses organisms that can produce bladder infections.

What Are the Symptoms of Bladder Infection?

- Frequency of urination
- Urgency of urination (must urinate immediately)
- Pain (burning) with urination

How Can I Avoid Bladder Infections?

- Void after intercourse.
- Avoid intercourse with a partner who has burning on urination.
- Do not delay urinating when the urge occurs.
- Drink 6 to 8 glasses of water per day.
- Avoid the use of a diaphragm for birth control.

How Are Bladder Infections Treated?

Bladder infections must be treated promptly with an antibiotic. It is possible for bladder infection to progress to kidney infection, a more serious illness.

URINARY INCONTINENCE

Urinary incontinence is the involuntary passing of urine. It can affect both men and women, especially middle-aged and elderly persons. It frequently goes untreated because people are too embarrassed to seek treatment and/or assume that incontinence is part of the aging process. Television ads can reinforce the idea that incontinence is part of the aging process.

Incontinence in women occurs when the pelvic muscles have been damaged or stretched or when pressure is applied to the bladder. There is an "urge" to urinate and an inability to reach a toilet "in time." Urine can be lost during laughing, coughing, sneezing, or lifting heavy objects.

Urinary incontinence can be a symptom of an underlying problem, such as urinary tract infection or neurologic disease. Urinary incontinence can be a result of medication. It can be a result of pregnancy and childbirth or deterioration of the pelvic muscles. In women, an age-related decline in estrogen levels can contribute to urinary incontinence.

If you have problems holding your urine, you should talk to your health-care provider. To help your health-care provider determine the cause of the problem and devise a treatment plan, collect the information requested below before your appointment and bring it along to the visit.

- When did the urine loss start?
- Does it happen during the day, night, or both?
- Does it happen when lying down or sitting still?
- Do you feel a sense of urgency before losing urine?
- When you use the toilet, how much urine do you release?
- Do you have difficulty starting or stopping the flow of urine?
- Do you have pain when urinating?
- Do you lose urine when coughing, sneezing, or straining?
- When you lose urine, how much do you lose?
- Have you had pelvic or bladder surgery?
- Do you have a neurologic disease?
- Are you taking any medications? (If so, take them with you to the visit.)

Ask your health-care provider about available treatments for incontinence. Treatments may include bladder training, Kegel exercises, biofeedback, medication, or surgery. The first step in curing the problem is to discuss it with a health-care provider.

PREVENTION OF HEPATITIS

Chronic liver disease is the tenth most common cause of death in the United States. Viral hepatitis, in all of its forms, is the most common cause of chronic liver disease.

Hepatitis A infects up to 200,000 Americans each year. Hepatitis A is caused by a highly contagious virus that attacks the liver. This virus is transferred from person to person via the gastrointestinal tract.

Hepatitis B is caused by a virus with a core made of DNA plus an antigen.

This virus is transferred from one person to another.

- Via mother–infant contact at the time of birth
- Sexually (Sexual activity is the most common method of transmission of Hepatitis B in North America.)
- Horizontally (by sharing razors, toothbrushes, etc.)
- Through instruments that are not sterile (e.g., those used for tattoos)
- Through intravenous drug use (through shared needles and syringes)
- Via hospital staff through needle sticks

Hepatitis C is caused by a virus. Infection occurs via:

- Infected blood products
- Contaminated dialysis equipment
- Transplanting of infected organs
- Sharing contaminated needles among IV drug users

Hepatitis D is caused by a small RNA virus. Injection drug use is the most common mode of transmission for hepatitis D. In humans, hepatitis D infection occurs in the presence of hepatitis B infection.

OSTEOPOROSIS

What Is Osteoporosis?

Osteoporosis is the most common human bone disease. Osteoporosis means low bone mass, deterioration of bone leading to fragile bones, and an increased risk of fractures (breaks). Osteoporosis affects many women; it is estimated that between 13% and 18% of all women who have experienced menopause have osteoporosis. The consequence of osteoporosis can be a fracture (break) of a bone. The most serious of these is fracture of the hip.

Osteoporosis is preventable and treatable, but there are no warning signs until fracture occurs— osteoporosis is a silent disease.

How Do I Prevent Osteoporosis?

Ensure adequate calcium absorption. All women should maintain an adequate intake of calcium; 1200 mg should be consumed daily, using supplements if necessary. Women at risk for osteoporosis (i.e, elderly, chronically ill, homebound, or institutionalized women) should also consume vitamin D at a level of 400 to 800 IU daily. Calcium and vitamin D reduce the risk of fracture.

Perform regular weight-bearing and muscle-strengthening exercises. Muscle strengthening improves agility, strength, and balance, thus reducing the risk of falls. Weight-bearing exercise increases bone density. Weight-bearing exercise includes walking, jogging, stair climbing, dancing, and tennis.

Avoid tobacco smoking, and reduce alcohol intake. The use of tobacco has a negative effect on health in general and on bones in particular. Alcohol is detrimental to bone health if consumed at more than a moderate level.

How Is Osteoporosis Diagnosed?

Osteoporosis is diagnosed by bone densitometry testing. All women should be screened for osteoporosis after menopause. Women with low body weight, estrogen deficiency, low calcium intake, alcoholism, and a history of recurrent falls or of fractures should also be tested.

Bone density can be measured anywhere on the skeleton. Bone densitometry testing is done by scanning portions of the skeleton. It is not painful and can be completed in a few minutes, with total radiation exposure much less than that of a chest x-ray.

How Is Osteoporosis Treated?

Osteoporosis is treated with hormone replacement therapy, calcium supplementation, and medications that prevent bone loss and thereby reduce the risk of fracture.

PREMENSTRUAL SYNDROME

Premenstrual syndrome (PMS) refers to a variety of symptoms that a woman may have prior to her period. The most common symptoms of PMS are tension and irritability, weight gain, headache, and depression. Other symptoms include breast tenderness, lower abdominal cramping, fatigue, and anxiety.

PMS always occurs prior to menses and improves once the period has started. The timing of the symptoms is central to distinguishing between PMS and other disorders. In PMS, the symptoms are followed by at least one symptom-free week, and the pattern of symptoms tends to remain constant from month to month.

Keeping a careful daily diary of symptoms is important to the diagnosis of PMS. This record of symptoms should be kept for at least three cycles. The diary or symptom calendar should be discussed with a health-care provider familiar with the diagnosis and treatment of PMS. Many treatment options exist. Medications that target the most bothersome symptoms can be prescribed.

The following treatment for PMS can be initiated without a practitioner:

- Try to minimize stressful situations during the time that you have PMS.
- Reduce refined sugar in your diet during PMS.
- Avoid caffeine found in coffee, tea, chocolate, and cola.
- Take daily B$_6$ supplements, up to 50 mg.
- Get regular outdoor exercise.

A visit to a health-care provider is needed for further treatment options.

Month ____
Name ____

Date of Birth ____

LMP ____

Symptom	1	2	3	4	5	6	7	8	9	10	11	12	13	14	15	16	17	18	19	20	21	22	23	24	25	26	27	28	29	30	31
1																															
2																															
3																															
4																															
5																															
6																															
7																															
8																															
9																															
10. Weight each day																															

Day 1 is the first day of menstrual bleeding.
Directions: Write in symptoms in the column labeled 1–10. Mark with either a X or ✔ under the day of the cycle that the symptom occurs. At the end of the cycle, circle the days that each symptom was the most distressing.

Figure H8–1. Menstrual cycle diary.

Chapter 10
HANDOUTS

BENEFITS OF STRESS MANAGEMENT

Various factors contribute to the stressors that women experience and the ways in which women cope with the stressors. Women have practical problems related to everyday existence that men do not experience.

Women cope with stress by evaluating the situation, examining the available resources, and problem solving (coping). The ability to solve or cope with the stressor depends upon the woman. At times, stressors can be avoided or removed. At other times, stressors cannot be dealt with or removed but must be lived with.

When a stressor cannot be removed, coping strategies are necessary. These strategies can include:

Learning about the body. Through health-care providers and/or through reading materials, women can become more aware of their bodies and their function and as a result can help themselves to deal with physical stressors. Learning about the mind's connection with the body can help women to deal with some psychological stressors.

Stress management techniques. These exercises have been designed to assist women in reducing tension in their bodies.

Counseling. Counseling can help the woman examine issues on her mind and thus can help her to deal with real-life dilemmas.

Support groups. These groups can be helpful in assisting women in crisis. The groups are a source of emotional support and they are avenues for discussion about the stressor.

Relaxation Techniques
Guided Imagery
Guided imagery is a way to employ your imagination to create relaxation. Guided imagery focuses on images to put you into a relaxed state and is designed to relieve tension and stress. The elements of guided imagery

include finding a comfortable position, closing your eyes, focusing on your physical sensations, and practicing deep breathing. Listen and allow yourself to follow the directions. Don't force the issue; let it flow freely.

Leave the room and the cares of the day behind... You find yourself walking on a path in beautiful meadow... It's a bright and sunny day, and a gentle breeze is blowing. As you walk along, find a little path to walk on. Let the gentle breeze blow against your body, see the beautiful flowers blowing... As you walk along, find a spot to sit in and put down your stress, all the things that cause you tension, all your worries. Give these tensions shapes and colors. Now set them down on the side of the path. Continue to walk on your path until you come to a big beautiful blue lake. Walk long the sandy beach, feel the warm sand on your feet, feel the warm breeze blowing. Look out across the lake. What do you see? Find yourself a comfortable spot by the lake. Look around; tell yourself that this is your very special place to relax and that you can come here anytime you need to relax. Now come back to the room.

Progressive Relaxation

Progressive relaxation is essential in learning the difference between a muscle that is tense and one that is relaxed. The basic principle used is that when a muscle or group of muscles is tensed, the opposite energy difference is relaxation. Because immediately relaxing the muscle is difficult to do, it is beneficial to begin with tensing a muscle, as a person would do when exercising, and then performing the opposite relaxing response. To obtain an even deeper relaxed state, it is important for you to be aware of the difference in the feeling of your muscles when tensed in contrast to the feeling when they are relaxed. This should give you a better mental understanding of the relaxed state you should obtain.

Take three deep breaths, inhaling as deeply as possible through your nose and exhaling as much air as possible out of your mouth. Then allow your body to breathe at will.

Feet, ankles, and lower legs: Point your toes away from you and feel the areas of tension. Now point your toes toward your head and feel the areas tense. Now relax and allow the lower legs to go limp. Notice how your feet tend to point outward as you relax and allow them to do so. Repeat two times.

Knees and adjoining muscles: Push your heels away from you; feel the tension in the muscle areas. Now relax. Note the difference. Repeat two times.

Thighs and buttocks: Tense your thighs by tensing your complete leg and tightening your buttock muscles. Feel the tension. Now relax. Repeat two times.

Pelvic area and buttocks: Again tighten your buttocks and tense the pelvic area. Feel the tension. Now relax. Repeat two times.

Stomach and lower back: Tense this area by bearing down, but don't strain yourself. Now relax. Repeat two times.

Chest, shoulders, and upper back: Squeeze your upper arms toward your body and slightly arch your back. Feel the tension. Now relax. Repeat two times.

Shoulders: Raise your shoulders toward your head and press them backward. Feel the tension. Now relax. Repeat two times.

Upper arms: Tense your upper arms by bending your arms toward your head. Hold that tension. Now relax. Repeat two times.

Lower arms: Press your hands flat down against whatever surface you are lying on. Feel the tension. Now relax. Repeat two times.

Hands: Make a fist in both hands. Then spread your hands open as far as you can. Now make a fist again. Hold the tension. Now relax. Repeat two times.

Face, jaw, and neck: Bite down with your jaw, push your tongue up toward the roof of your mouth, and press your chin forward against your chest. Now press your lips together and squint your eyes. Feel the tension. Now relax. Repeat two times.

Eyes and forehead: Squint your eyes, make a frown, and wrinkle your forehead. Feel the tension. Now relax.

Complete body tension: Press your head backward, push your heels downward, and press your hands flat against the floor. Tense your complete body. Feel the tension. Now relax. Do not repeat; instead, take three deep breaths, inhaling through your nose and exhaling through your mouth. Try not to move any other parts of your body. Just allow yourself to feel completely relaxed.

Source: Griffith-Kennedy, J: Contemporary Women's Health. Addison-Wesley Publishing Co., Menlo Park, CA, 1986, with permission.

SYMPTOMS OF DEPRESSION

Depression is more than having a bad day. It should not be confused with the "down" days or "blues" we all have. Depression is an illness that affects your body, your mood, and your thoughts.

Depression can occur at any age and at any time. Depression occurs twice as often in women as in men. Depression can be mild, moderate, or severe. Mild depression usually occurs after a trauma in your life. Moderate depression leaves you feeling less energetic and enthusiastic. Job productivity goes down and you wonder if life is worth living. Severe depression creates suffering such that you can hardly function. There is no joy in life and you feel completely powerless to change. Feelings of hopelessness and worthlessness prevail.

Depression can accompany serious medical illnesses. It can also be related to medication. People who are most likely to suffer from depression are those who have suffered from depression previously, have attempted suicide in the past, have recently delivered a child, or are substance abusers.

Symptoms of Depression

- Feelings of sadness and irritability that don't go away
- Loss of interest or pleasure in activities you used to enjoy
- A change in weight or appetite
- Sleep disturbances
- Feelings of guilt, lack of self-worth, or helplessness
- Decreased ability to concentrate
- Fatigue
- Restless or slowed activity
- Thoughts of life not being worthwhile or about suicide or death

Depression can be treated. Depression is not a personal weakness or flaw. Several treatment options are available to those who suffer from depression. Seek help if you have symptoms of depression. Assist someone who is displaying symptoms of depression in seeking help.

WOMEN AND ALCOHOL

Although women currently use, abuse, and become dependent on alcohol and other drugs at a rate less than men, use is quickly becoming similar to that of men. Women experience more devastating physical, emotional, psychological, and social responses and consequences than men do.

Alcohol abuse has a range of presentations, from social drinker to the person who uses alcohol in excess when under stress.

Social drinker: This person consumes alcohol in amounts and circumstances that seem socially acceptable. There may be a problem if social occasions are a reason for overindulging in alcohol.

Heavy social drinker: This is someone who drinks in socially appropriate circumstances but seeks out situations in which to drink and drinks excessively. At least two drinks per day are consumed, and the amount increases over time. This person's work and social routines do not seem to be affected.

Problem drinker: This person engages in heavy drinking and gets drunk on occasion; consequences of alcohol can be seen in the medical, legal, or social arena. Functioning varies, and denial that a problem exists is common.

Alcohol-dependent drinker: This is someone who consumes the same amount of alcohol regardless of mood or situation. Alcohol is given top priority in all situations, including work and social situations. Tolerance to alcohol develops, and withdrawal symptoms can be seen. Drinking at lunch and at "happy hour" is needed to relieve symptoms.

Severely deteriorated drinker: This person maintains a constant state of intoxication, undergoes hospitalization for detoxification, and has medical problems related to alcohol use.

Getting Help

Help for alcohol problems requires a combination of medical interventions, counseling, health education, life skills, and social service. Treatment can be in an inpatient center that deals with women with alcohol problems or on an outpatient basis with a team that works with women to achieve full recovery.

SEXUAL ASSAULT

Who Is at Risk for Sexual Assault?

Any woman is a risk for sexual assault regardless of age, race, socioeconomic status, or education. Women between the ages of 15 and 24 are at the highest risk. Sexual assault can occur in women, children, and men. Anyone can be forced to have unwanted sex by a stranger, friend, relative, or partner.

What Are the Warning Signs?

- Men who see women as sex objects and do not indicate respect for women
- Men who resent women in positions of authority
- Men who continue to touch women even after they have been asked to stop touching
- Men who act aggressively
- Men who expect relationships with women to be on their terms only

How Can I Prevent Sexual Assault?

- Sexual assault cannot always be prevented.
- Communicating desires and limits *clearly* may help to prevent sexual assault by an acquaintance.
- If you are feeling uncomfortable in a situation with a man, pay attention to that feeling.
- Be alert for warning signs.
- Using alcohol or drugs increases the risk for sexual assault. For many young women who report rape, alcohol and/or drug use by the victim and the perpetrator was involved.

If I Am Threatened with Sexual Assault, What Should I Do?

- Try to stay calm.
- Be assertive.
- Try leaving the situation.
- Trust your feelings about the situation. Sometimes submission will decrease the chance of injury.

If I Am Sexually Assaulted, What Should I Do?

- Do not blame yourself.
- Seek medical help.
- Seek help from a rape crisis center via a hotline and/or call the police.

CONTRACEPTIVE OPTIONS

How to Use a Male Condom Correctly: Instructions for Women

- Make sure that your partner uses a new condom every time you have sex. Never reuse a condom.
- Do not open the condom package until you are ready to use the condom (the condom can dry out and possibly tear during use).
- Handle condom carefully. Avoid damaging it with teeth or fingernails.
- Have your partner put the condom on his penis after it is erect, but before it touches your body.
- Make sure that there is adequate space left between the end of the condom and the tip of the penis.
- Check to make sure that no air is trapped in the tip of the condom.
- Lubricate the condom if desired after it is put on. Use only water-soluble lubricants such as K-Y jelly. Do not use oil-based lubricants such as Vaseline, cooking oils, or massage lotions.
- Make sure you are adequately lubricated for intercourse.
- Use a spermicidal foam, cream, or jelly.
- Make sure that your partner holds the condom firmly against the base of his penis when pulling out so that the condom does not slip off. He should withdraw his penis when it is still erect to be sure that no semen leaks out of the top of the condom.

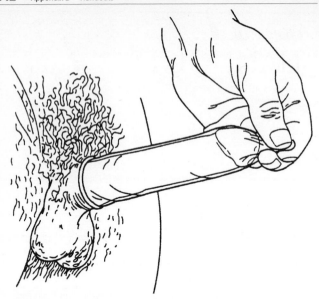

Figure H11–1. Using a male condom. Leave a half-inch empty space at the tip. (Adapted from standard forms currently in use by Planned Parenthood Association of Bucks County, PA)

Using a Female Condom

- A female condom has been approved by the Food and Drug Administration and is now available in drugstores. The female condom is a thin polyurethane sheath that lines the vagina and has a ring at both ends.
- The female condom is inserted much like a tampon or diaphragm. Squeeze the inner ring at the closest end of the pouch and insert it into the vagina, placing the ring behind the pubic bone so that it covers the cervix.
- Carefully follow the manufacturer's directions for insertion.
- The female condom can be inserted up to 8 hours before intercourse, during foreplay, or prior to intercourse.
- You do not have to use spermicide with the female condom, but you may if you like.
- Female condoms are prelubricated.
- Like the male condom, it can be used for only one act of intercourse.
- Unlike the male condom, it can be used only for vaginal sex.
- Unlike the male condom, it is available in only one size.
- Like the male condom, maximum prevention of pregnancy and STDs depends upon correct use.

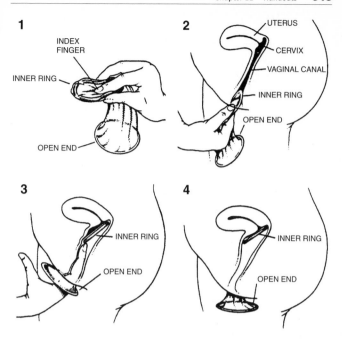

Figure H11–2. Using a female condom: four-step insertion. (Adapted from standard forms currently in use by the Planned Parenthood Association of Bucks County, PA)

USING A CERVICAL CAP

Instructions for Insertion and Removal

- Spermicide may be placed in the cap prior to insertion. If utilized, the spermicide should fill approximately one third of the cap.
- Choose a position for insertion—stand with one foot on a chair, lying down or squatting.
- Locate your cervix with one finger.
- Squeeze the cap rim and insert the cap while separating the labia with the other hand.
- Slide the cap into the vagina and push it up onto the cervix.
- Place the rim around the cervix, creating suction. Sweep a finger around the cap to make sure that the cervix is completely covered.
- The cap must stay in place for 8 hours after intercourse.
- To remove the cap, push the rim away from the cervix to break the suction and pull the cap out.
- Do not leave the cap in place for longer than 48 hours.
- Do not use the cap during menses.

Guidelines for Use

Cervical caps may not be for all women. For some, their cap size is unavailable or insertion is too difficult. Women with abnormal Pap smears cannot be fitted with a cap until the reason for the abnormal test result is resolved. Women with a history of toxic shock syndrome should not use a cervical cap. Inflammation of the cervix or previous surgery to the cervix may make fitting impossible.

Contact the nurse practitioner if any of the following occur:

- Sudden high fever with vomiting and diarrhea, weakness, a sunburn-like rash
- Pain or burning with urination
- Discomfort when the cap is in place
- Unusual vaginal discharge
- Irregular vaginal spotting or bleeding

Source: Text adapted from standard forms currently in use by Planned Parenthood Association of Bucks County, PA.

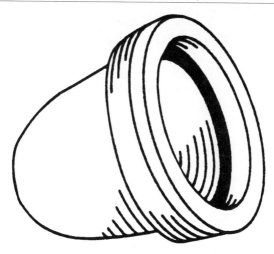

Figure H11–3. Cervical Cap (From Contraceptive Technology, ed. 16, Irvington Publishers, New York, 1994).

USING A DIAPHRAGM

Instructions for Insertion and Removal

- Urinate prior to inserting the diaphragm.
- The diaphragm may be inserted up to 2 hours prior to intercourse.
- Place approximately 1 teaspoon of contraceptive jelly or cream designated for use with a diaphragm in the center of the diaphragm and around the rim. The contraceptive cream or jelly is placed in the diaphragm on the side that will be next to the cervix.
- Choose a position for inserting—standing with one leg on a chair, lying down, or squatting.
- Pinch the rim of the diaphragm together with the cream or jelly inside. Separate the labia with the other hand and insert the diaphragm into the vagina.
- Push the diaphragm up and as far back as possible, making sure that the cervix is covered.
- Feel your cervix to make sure that it is covered by the dome of the diaphragm.
- Leave the diaphragm in place for 6–8 hours after intercourse.
- Urinate after intercourse, leaving the diaphragm in place.
- If intercourse is repeated or occurs more than 2 hours after insertion, leave the diaphragm in place and insert another application of contraceptive cream or jelly.
- To remove the diaphragm, pull the diaphragm down and out using one finger.
- Do not leave the diaphragm in place for more than 24 hours.

Guidelines for Use

Diaphragms should be refitted after a full-term pregnancy, pelvic surgery, or weight gain or loss of 10 pounds or more. Women who have poor vaginal muscle tone or a history of toxic shock syndrome or bladder infection should use diaphragms with caution.

Contact the nurse practitioner if any of the following occur:

- Sudden high fever with diarrhea and vomiting, weakness, a sunburn-like rash
- Pain and burning with urination
- Discomfort when the diaphragm is in place
- Unusual vaginal discharge
- Irregular vaginal spotting or bleeding

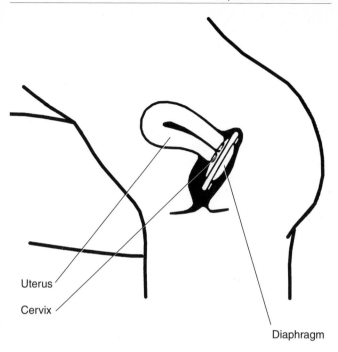

Uterus

Cervix

Diaphragm

Figure H11–4. Diaphragm.

Source: Adapted from standard forms currently in use by Planned Parenthood Association of Bucks County, PA.

NORPLANT INFORMATION

Norplant is a device consisting of thin tubes made of a soft material that have a man-made hormone in them. After insertion of the tubes into the body, usually the arm, a small amount of the hormone is released into the body all the time. Norplant works by keeping eggs from being released and making the mucus from the cervix (opening to the uterus) thick. Norplant prevents pregnancy. For every 100 women who use Norplant, there will be less than one pregnancy per year.

Norplant lasts for 5 years. There is no medicine to take every day, and there is nothing to do before sex to prevent pregnancy.

Norplant should *not* be used if you are pregnant or have serious liver disease, bleeding from the vagina that is not menses, cancer of the breast, or had recent blood clots in the legs or lungs. Discuss the use of Norplant with your practitioner if you have heart disease or stroke, diabetes, abnormal liver tests, depression, or epilepsy.

Some women have experienced one or more of the following problems when they use Norplant:

- Acne, skin rash
- Weight gain
- Change in coloring of the skin over the implant site
- Cysts of the ovaries
- Depression
- Hair loss or increased hair
- Nausea and dizziness
- Nervousness
- Sore breasts

The danger signs to watch for when using Norplant are:

- Sudden, severe headache
- Dizziness, fainting, numbness
- Sharp, crushing chest pain
- Pain in the arm or calf of the leg
- Severe pain in the stomach or belly
- Yellowing of the skin or eyes
- Severe depression
- Unusually heavy vaginal bleeding
- No period after having had a period every month
- Lump in the breast
- Pus, bleeding, or pain at the insertion site
- Norplant coming out

Call your practitioner if any of these signs occur.

Norplant Instructions

- For a few days you may notice tenderness and swelling of the skin around the implants. Bruising and discoloration of the skin may last a week or two.

- Try not to bump the area for a few days. Keep the area clean and dry. Keep the bandage on for 24 hours. Keep the tape on for 3 days.
- You can do normal activities right away. Do not lift heavy objects for a few days.
- After healing, do not worry about bumping the area. You can touch or wash the area as usual.

Return to the office:

- In 72 hours
- In 3 months
- Once a year for checkups

Call the office if you:

- Have questions about Norplant
- Think that you might be pregnant
- Want the Norplant capsules removed

OR if you:

- Have a delayed period after having regular periods
- Experience unusually heavy bleeding
- Have arm pain
- Observe pus or bleeding at the insertion site
- Notice a capsule has come out
- Experience severe headache

Source: Adapted from standard forms currently in use by Planned Parenthood Association of Bucks County, PA.

INTRAUTERINE DEVICES

What Is an Intrauterine Device?

An intrauterine device (IUD) is a small plastic device that is inserted into the uterus to prevent pregnancy.

Are There Different Types of Intrauterine Devices?

Yes, many different kinds of IUDs are used all over the world. Two types of IUDs are currently available in the United States: one has copper and the other contains the female hormone progesterone. Both are shaped like the letter "T" and are about $1\frac{1}{4}$ inches tall. Each IUD has a thread or string on the end, which allows you to check that the IUD is in place; it also makes it easier for the practitioner to remove the IUD.

The copper IUD has copper wire coiled around the stem and arms. The copper IUD can be used for up to 10 years. The progesterone device has a hollow stem that contains the hormone progesterone. The hormone is continuously released into the uterus and acts locally, so there are no hormonal effects throughout the body. This IUD must be replaced once a year.

How Does the Intrauterine Device Work?

All the ways an IUD can prevent pregnancy are not fully understood. The most recent studies suggest that IUDs work mainly by preventing fertilization, interfering with the normal development of the egg and the sperm's ability to reach the egg.

How Effective Are Intrauterine Devices?

IUDs are the most effective form of nonpermanent birth control. The copper IUD is about as effective in preventing pregnancy as sterilization. For every 100 women using the copper IUD, fewer that one per year will get pregnant. With the hormone-containing IUD, about three women per year will get pregnant.

Are There Side Effects?

With the copper IUD, the most common side effects are increased menstrual flow and cramps. Cramps can be relieved by the use of over-the-counter pain medication, such as ibuprofen. These side effects usually lessen after the first few months as the uterus gets used to the IUD. With the hormonal IUD, bleeding may also occur between menstrual periods, although there is less total blood loss and there are fewer painful periods than with the copper IUD.

Are Intrauterine Devices Safe?

Intrauterine devices are a safe and effective method of birth control when used by the right women. Although one of the early IUDs used in the 1970s was associated with an increased risk of pelvic infection, this IUD has been off the market for over 25 years.

Who Can Use an Intrauterine Device?

Women at low risk of STDs are good candidates for using IUDs. The IUD is best for a woman who is in a steady and faithful relationship with a partner who is faithful and who does not have any sexually transmitted infections.

Intrauterine devices do not protect against STDs. STDs can increase a woman's risk of becoming infertile. If you are using an IUD and believe you may be at risk of getting an STD, use a latex condom to help protect yourself. You may also want to discuss with your doctor or nurse whether the IUD is still a good choice for birth control.

What Are the Benefits of Intrauterine Devices?

IUDs are safe, effective, easy to use, and less expensive than most other forms of contraception over the long run. There is no need to remember to use the method every day or with every act of sex. The copper IUD can last for up to 10 years. In addition, because any hormone in the IUD does not affect the entire body, women do not get side effects such as nausea, breast tenderness, or headache.

What if I Get Pregnant?

Overall, the copper IUD protects women against having a pregnancy outside the uterus compared with women not using contraception. However, if you are using an IUD and suspect you are pregnant, you should see a practitioner promptly to rule out ectopic pregnancy.

How Much Does an Intrauterine Device Cost?

Prices for IUDs themselves vary, but range between $100 and $300. The clinic or health-care provider also charges for the medical visit and insertion of the device. About 90% of Planned Parenthood family planning clinics in the United States offer the IUD. In government-funded family planning clinics, about 50% offer the IUD to low-income women. Your insurance policy may or may not cover the cost of the IUD and the insertion visit. Check your health plan.

Source: The Contraceptive Report, November 1998, with permission.

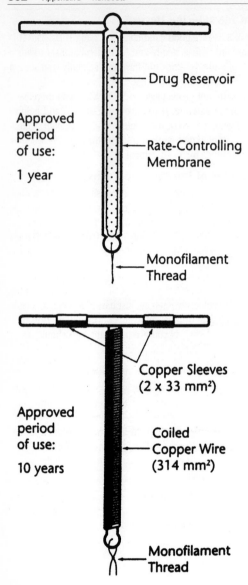

Drug Reservoir

Rate-Controlling Membrane

Approved period of use:

1 year

Monofilament Thread

Copper Sleeves (2 x 33 mm²)

Approved period of use:

10 years

Coiled Copper Wire (314 mm²)

Monofilament Thread

Figure H11–5. IUDs: (1) Progesterone T IUD and (2) Copper T 380A IUD. (Adapted from standard forms currently in use by Planned Parenthood Association of Bucks County, PA)

EMERGENCY CONTRACEPTION

What is Emergency Contraception?

Emergency contraception is a dose of pills that can be taken up to 72 hours after intercourse. Emergency contraception is most effective if taken within 24 hours after intercourse.

How Does it Work?

Emergency contraception pills contain one or two hormones commonly found in birth control pills. Just like birth control pills, emergency contraception prevents sperm from fertilizing an egg and stops or delays ovulation.

How Effective Is it?

The sooner the medication is taken, the more effective it is. The pills can be taken up to 72 hours after intercourse, but the pills are more effective if taken within the first 24 hours post intercourse.

Emergency contraception is not as effective in preventing pregnancy as using regular birth control. Do not rely on this method for ongoing birth control.

How Safe Is Emergency Contraception?

Emergency contraception pills are very safe. The Food and Drug Administration reviewed the evidence and concluded that the treatment is safe and effective.

Are There Women Who Shouldn't Use Emergency Contraceptive Pills?

The World Health Organization confirmed pregnancy as the only reason not to use emergency contraceptive pills.

Information on Emergency Contraception

A toll-free number for information on emergency contraception is 1–888-NOT-2-LATE. This hotline provides 24-hour automated information on emergency contraception methods and a national directory of where to obtain emergency contraception.

VOLUNTARY STERILIZATION

Healthy women are fertile until ages 50 to 51. Healthy men are fertile throughout their life. Because many couples have all the children that they wish to have before the natural end of their reproductive capabilities, they seek sterilization. Voluntary sterilization is a very popular method of birth control in America. It is a very safe and cost-effective method to prevent pregnancy.

Ideally, a couple should consider both vasectomy and female sterilization. They are both comparable in effectiveness, and both are intended to be permanent. If both are acceptable to the couple, vasectomy is the medically preferred procedure.

Female Sterilization

Sterilization for women involves mechanically blocking the fallopian tubes to prevent the sperm and the egg from uniting. This is a safe procedure with a low failure rate. Sterilization can be performed without increasing the risk after the delivery of a baby.

Female sterilization involves the application of clips or bands or burning of the fallopian tubes (the tubes that carry the egg from the ovary to the uterus). The tubes are reached via the abdomen using a small incision, or at the time of cesarean birth or abdominal surgery.

Advantages of female sterilization:

- Permanence
- Effectiveness
- Cost-effectiveness (over time)
- Nothing to buy or remember
- No long-term side effects
- No interruption in lovemaking

Disadvantages of female sterilization:

- Permanence
- Reversibility difficult and expensive
- Surgery required
- Expensive when performed
- Low failure rate, but failure can mean a pregnancy in the tube
- No protection against sexually transmitted diseases

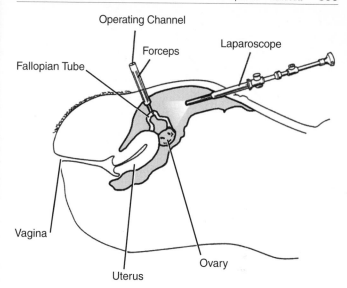

Figure H11–6. Female sterilization.

Male Sterilization

Vasectomy is male sterilization through surgery. This operation blocks the tubes that carry the sperm into the ejaculatory fluid. Vasectomy is very effective. Male sterilization involves exposing the tubes that carry sperm and cutting or burning them.

Advantages of male sterilization:

- High effectiveness
- Inexpensive over time
- Permanence
- Safety
- Quick procedure

Disadvantages of male sterilization:

- Protection for the male, not the female who can become pregnant
- Surgery required
- Expensive in the short term
- Permanence
- No protection against sexually transmitted diseases

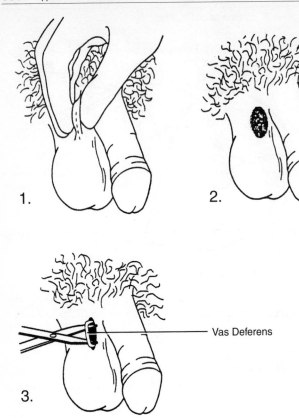

Vas Deferens

Figure H11–7. Male sterilization.

Chapter 12

HANDOUTS

FACTORS TO BE CONSIDERED PRIOR TO PREGNANCY

Immunizations

Appropriate and timely immunizations should be received prior to pregnancy. Rubella, a major cause of birth defects, can be immunized against prior to pregnancy. Women should wait at least one month to become pregnant after rubella vaccination.

Nutrition

- Adequate protein intake
- Adequate calories
- Adequate calcium intake
- Adequate iron
- Additional folic acid: 400 mg daily

Rh Factor

An Rh-negative woman must prevent "sensitization" with the Rh factor. Sensitization is prevented through a drug called RhoGam. RhoGam must be given after the birth of every child, after every miscarriage, and after every abortion.

Infection

Sexually transmitted diseases can create scar tissue within the pelvis that can prevent pregnancy.

Certain viral infections can cause congenital defects. Proper handwashing, particularly for those who work with urine, saliva, and respiratory secretions, can help prevent these infections.

Prior to pregnancy, screening for cytomegalovirus (CMV) and human immunodeficiency virus (HIV) should be performed.

Endometriosis

Early treatment of endometriosis reduces difficulty with conception.

Radiation

Exposure to radiation may affect an early pregnancy. Radiation to the pelvis should be avoided by shielding the abdomen during x-rays. If the pelvis must be exposed, a pregnancy test should be performed prior to testing.

Medications

Drug use—both street and prescription drugs—can affect fertility and can severely affect developing embryos.

Any prescription medication taken on a regular basis should be evaluated by an obstetrician or midwife prior to conception. Some medications affect conception, and some affect the developing fetus. Substitute medications and changes in dose should be considered in these cases.

Avoid over-the-counter (OTC) drugs unless absolutely necessary. If you use an OTC drug, use one with a single ingredient.

Alcohol and Drugs

Women who consume alcohol run the risk of delivering a baby with fetal alcohol syndrome. Reduction in consumption of alcohol should occur prior to pregnancy.

Avoid marijuana, cocaine, and other illicit substances entirely *prior* to pregnancy. Illicit drugs affect fertility and can lead to serious growth and development problems and birth defects for the unborn baby.

Smoking

Smoking affects the developing fetus in a negative way. Smoking creates lower birth weight and a reduction in oxygen available to the developing fetus. The effects are dose-dependent. Stop smoking prior to pregnancy.

Contraception

Any woman taking the pill should use an alternate method of birth control for at least one cycle prior to conception.

Employment

Many women face hazards in their occupations. The most hazardous jobs for women related to pregnancy are nursing, x-ray technicians, hairdressers, and lab personnel.

Avoid exposure to potentially hazardous substances prior to pregnancy. Agents that can affect pregnancy are anesthetics, carbon monoxide, ethylene oxide, lead, mercury, pesticides, radiation, and solvents. If possible, avoid these substances. If possible, use protective garb including gloves, masks, gowns, and ventilation hoods. Wash hands meticulously. Discuss how to reduce the risk of exposure with your obstetrician or midwife prior to pregnancy.

GENETIC SCREENING DURING PREGNANCY

History is the most valuable tool for identifying couples at risk for a child with a genetic abnormality. When you begin pregnancy care, the obstetrician or midwife will ask many questions about your and your partner's family health histories. These questions help to detect health-related abnormalities that may be genetic in origin. Be sure to bring to the practitioner's office health information about your parents, siblings, children, grandparents, uncles, aunts, nephews, nieces, and first cousins. Your and your partner's ethnic backgrounds are important in assigning risk for genetic disease.

Your age also affects the risk for genetic abnormalities. If you are over age 35, genetic counseling will be recommended.

Common Genetic Tests

Amniocentesis

Amniocentesis is a safe procedure in which fluid from around the unborn baby is collected and analyzed. The fluid contains cells shed by the baby. These cells can be examined for genetic abnormalities. The fluid is obtained with a needle under ultrasound guidance.

Chorionic Villous Sampling

Chorionic villous sampling (CVS) can be performed earlier than amniocentesis. In this test, cells from the placenta (afterbirth) are collected and analyzed for genetic defects. This procedure is performed under ultrasound guidance.

Triple Screen

Triple screen is a blood test that combines three different measures to evaluate for certain genetic defects.

Ultrasound

Ultrasound performed during pregnancy screens for genetic defects.

TRIPLE SCREEN

Triple screen is a blood test designed to screen for particular genetic defects. There are three tests involved in a triple screen—thus its name. The first test is called alpha-fetoprotein (AFP), the second is human chorionic gonadotropin (hCG), and the third is an estrogen level. AFP is excreted by the fetus (unborn baby) into the fluid surrounding the baby and into the pregnant woman's bloodstream. The function of AFP is unknown, but the levels that are expected to be present in the mother's blood at each week of pregnancy are known. The function of hCG is to maintain pregnancy; therefore, hCG is the basis for pregnancy tests. hCG is produced by the unborn baby and released into the mother's bloodstream at rates dependent upon the number of weeks of pregnancy. Estriol is the type of estrogen measured as part of the screen. These three levels are determined from a sample of a pregnant woman's blood and calculated with the age of the pregnant woman, her ethnicity, and certain health factors to predict her risk for certain genetic diseases. Triple screen is performed at 16 to 18 weeks of pregnancy.

The results of a triple screen are reported as a "risk" for one of the many defects that are associated with an abnormal test. High levels indicate a risk for some genetic defects, and low levels indicate a risk for other genetic defects. Of all tested pregnant women, 5% have an abnormal test result.

Many more than 5% of pregnant woman have an unusual test result the first time blood is drawn. The reason for this is that the test is very sensitive to the number of weeks of pregnancy. Many pregnant women are not aware of how many weeks of pregnancy have passed prior to their giving blood for the test. Approximately 12% of women will have abnormal test results related to inaccurate reporting of the number of weeks of pregnancy.

When a triple screen indicates risk, correction for error must be determined by accurate reporting of the number of weeks of pregnancy. This is accomplished by ultrasound. Ultrasound will correctly determine the number of weeks of pregnancy, and the test can be repeated. Ultrasound can also rule out many genetic abnormalities suggested by an abnormal triple screen.

If, after adjustment for weeks of pregnancy, the triple screen is still showing increased risk for genetic defects, the obstetrician or midwife will schedule further testing to rule out or verify genetic abnormalities.

The triple screen is just as its name implies—a screen. Further testing must be done for verification of a genetic abnormality. Testing may include an ultrasound by a perinatologist, a specialist in the health of unborn babies, or an amniocentesis in which cells are retrieved from the fluid around the unborn baby.

The triple screen is a useful test, but not a perfect one. Its sensitivity, i.e., its level of accuracy in screening, is approximately 80%. In statistical terms, 80% is far from 100% accurate. Approximately 1 in 30 women with an abnormal triple screen is actually carrying a baby with a problem. The other 29 are carrying a normal baby. In other words, many women will have a triple screen that is abnormal but are carrying a healthy baby. An abnormal triple screen indicates a need for further testing and little else.

MEDICATIONS DURING PREGNANCY

Prescription and over-the-counter (OTC) drugs, including alcohol and cigarettes, have the potential to affect unborn babies. They can affect the unborn baby's growth and development and/or create injury.

The first rule to be applied to medication and pregnancy is: *Discuss any medication with your obstetrician or midwife before taking it.* This includes both prescription and OTC drugs.

Although much has been learned about which drugs can and cannot be taken safely during pregnancy, many new drugs being released have not been tested, and many combinations of drugs have not been tested. It is wise to consult with your midwife or obstetrician before consuming any drug.

It is not just what is taken, but when it is taken and in what quantity. The most dangerous time for the unborn baby to be exposed to drugs is in the first few weeks of pregnancy. It is, therefore, wise to consult your practitioner about drugs while trying to conceive. Remember that you are a few weeks' pregnant when the test becomes positive. During this time, the unborn baby should not be exposed to any drugs, alcohol, or cigarettes.

If there is a prescription medication that you must take to maintain your health, discuss this medication with your obstetrician or midwife prior to becoming pregnant. Risks to the unborn baby may be reduced by a change in the type of medication or the dose of medication.

Revisit an obstetrician or midwife to begin care as soon as you know that you are pregnant.

Take medication while pregnant or attempting to conceive only when absolutely necessary. When you must use an OTC drug, choose one that has a single ingredient. This greatly reduces the chance of its causing a problem for the unborn baby, and it makes the consultation with your obstetrician or midwife more accurate.

Alcohol and cigarettes are hazardous to unborn babies and should not be consumed. Talk to your practitioner about ways to quit smoking and ways to give up alcohol.

A partial list of medications that affect unborn children is:

- Anesthetics
- Androgens
- Anticancer drugs
- Benzodiazepines
- Carbamazepine (Tegretol)
- Warfarin (Coumadin)
- Diethylstilbestrol

- Valproic acid (Depakote)
- Iodine
- Isotretinoin (Accutane)
- Lithium
- Phenytoin (Dilantin)
- Quinolones
- Tetracyclines
- Thyroid agents

NUTRITIONAL REQUIREMENTS DURING PREGNANCY

Category	Food	Number of Servings per Day
Protein	Meat, poultry Beans Eggs	4
Milk Products	Milk Yogurt Cheese Tofu	4
Grains	Bread and rolls Macaroni, rice, noodles, cereal Wheat germ	6
Vitamin C Fruits and Vegetables	Oranges and grapefruits Tomatoes Green peppers Broccoli and cauliflower Cabbage	2
Green Leafy Vegetables	Brussels sprouts Asparagus Greens and lettuce Watercress	1–2
Vitamin A Fruits and Vegetables	Apples Carrots Green beans Bananas Sweet potatoes	3
Fats and Oils	Butter and margarine Salad dressing Cream cheese	3

EXERCISE DURING PREGNANCY

Guidelines for Exercise During Pregnancy

- Exercise on a routine, 3-to-4-time weekly basis.
- Drink water before, during, and after the exercise.
- Do not exercise when ill.
- Do not exercise outdoors in hot and humid weather.
- Take 5 to 10 minutes prior to exercise to warm up and/or stretch and 5 to 10 minutes after exercise to cool down.
- Keep your heart rate under 140 bpm.
- Restrict the most intense portion of the exercise (heart rate at 140 bpm) to 15 to 20 minutes.
- Avoid high-impact exercises.
- Avoid sit-ups and leg raises or other exercises that make use of abdominal muscles.
- Avoid exercises that require uncomfortable positions.
- Do not lie on your back for longer than a few minutes at time.
- Get up slowly.
- Stop exercising if you experience pain related to the specific exercise, bleeding, dizziness, back pain, or pelvic pressure.

Sports to Avoid During Pregnancy

- Skiing—snow or water
- Scuba diving
- Skating—ice or roller
- Any sport performed at high altitudes

Saunas, hot tubs, and whirlpools commonly used after exercise should be avoided during pregnancy. Dizziness can result from the change in circulation due to the high temperatures.

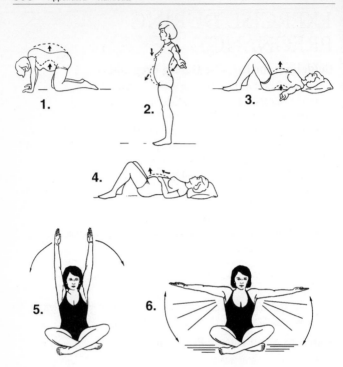

Figure H12–1. Pregnancy Exercises. Pregancy rocking (1, 2, and 3) relieves low back ache. Abdominal breathing (4) aids relaxation and lifts abdominal wall from uterus. Flying exercise (5 and 6) promotes relaxation and reduces discomforts such as heartburn and shortness of breath. (Source: Bobak, Jensen, and Zalar: Maternity and Gynecologic Care: The Nurse and the Family. CV Mosby, St. Louis, 1989)

DANGER SIGNALS DURING PREGNANCY

- Visual disturbance: blurred vision, spots, or double vision
- Swelling of the face
- Severe headache
- Severe muscle irritability or seizures
- Severe stomach ache
- Persistent vomiting
- Fluid discharge from the vagina
- Fever
- Burning upon urination
- Severe diarrhea
- Pain in the abdomen
- Change in fetal movements: any change in usual movement pattern

PREGNANCY AND WORK

In general, women can work until delivery if they have an uncomplicated pregnancy and if the number of hazards in the workplace is low. Every woman should inform her employer about her pregnancy as soon as possible so that modifications in her work can be considered.

Work Modifications Needed During Pregnancy

- The woman should not work longer than 8 hours per day.
- The woman should take two 10-minute breaks per day and one meal break.
- The woman should have a place to rest in a reclining position and she should have a place to elevate her legs.
- A pregnant woman who must sit or stand for most of her workday should be permitted a short time every hour or two to walk.
- The pregnant woman should avoid smoking, chemical fumes, extremes in temperature, and any activities that require good balance or could risk trauma to the abdomen.
- Lifting should be limited to 10 lb–15 lb, and proper lifting techniques should be implemented.
- Several physical conditions associated with pregnancy can create the need for further work modifications. Discuss your work environment with your obstetrician or midwife.

KEGEL EXERCISES

The Kegel exercise is designed to strengthen the muscle group that forms the pelvic floor. The exercise is prescribed for women who have stress incontinence, experience pelvic relaxation, have recently delivered a child vaginally, or have poor vaginal muscle tone.

In order to perform the exercise, the woman must first locate the muscle group. There are two ways to identify the muscle group. One involves stopping the flow of urine by contracting the muscle. The other involves placing a finger or fingers into the vagina and squeezing those fingers with the muscle. These techniques should be used only to identify the muscle, not to perform the exercise itself.

Once the muscle has been identified, the woman contracts the muscle; holds it contracted for a least the count of *one, two;* and then relaxes the muscle for the count of five to ten. This exercise requires concentration so that the muscles being contracted are the correct ones and not the abdominal or the gluteal muscles. Breath-holding is not a part of this exercise.

At the start of an exercise regimen, Kegel exercises should be performed 10 times at least twice daily. In time, the length of time the muscles are held contracted can be increased and the number of repetitions and sessions per day can be increased.

PERINATAL LOSS

The loss of a pregnancy leaves a woman struggling to regain her emotional balance at the same time her body is healing. The following is a list of suggestions for emotional support for women who have experienced the loss of a pregnancy.

Love of a child cannot be measured by time the parent has with the child. There is no less right to grieve for infants than for older children.

The parent will never be "over it." The pain never completely leaves. Grieving continues throughout life for the child who could have been with us. The death of a child at any age or under any circumstances is a tragic, life-changing event. Time eases the pain, but it never goes away.

Sleeping pills or alcohol do not help resolve the pain. Grieving is delayed by medication. The work of grieving should not be delayed.

Having another baby does not decrease the grief. Another child never replaces the lost child. Another baby can add more pressure to the grieving process. Women should be careful not to become pregnant too soon after the death of a child.

Support groups can be helpful. People who understand the depth of the pain are those who have experienced it. Support groups are a safe place for parents to go and share their pain with others who have experienced the same feelings.

Many couples find rituals helpful in mourning. Ceremonies can help bring the grief out into the open, allowing people to share their feelings. People choose different kinds of ceremonies, depending on their belief system. Some people find comfort in traditional religious services while others prefer quiet meditation or the symbolism of planting a tree.

Many people who have experienced the death of a child feel like they are "going crazy." The intensity and array of emotions can be overwhelming and frightening. Some people find work impossible. Others become overly absorbed in work. Reassurance that grieving people are not crazy people can be helpful.

Resources:

Resolve HelpLine: 617-623-0744
    http://www.resolve.org
Compassionate Friends HelpLine: 708-990-0010

Chapter *13*
HANDOUTS

POSTPARTUM EXERCISES

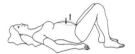

Abdominal breathing. Lie on back with knees bent. Inhale deeply through nose. Keep ribs stationary and allow abdomen to extend upwards. Exhale slowly but forcefully while contracting the abdominal muscles; hold for 3 to 5 seconds while exhaling. Relax.

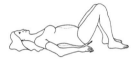

Combined Abdominal Breathing and Supine Pelvic Tilt (Pelvic Rocks). Lie on back with knees bent. While inhaling deeply, roll pelvis back by flattening lower back on floor bed. Exhale siowly but forcefully while contracting abdominal muscles and tightening buttocks. Hold for 3 to 5 seconds while exhaking. Relax.

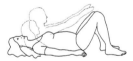

Reach for the knees. Lie on back with knees apart. While inhaling deeply lower chin onto chest. While exhaling, raise haed and shoulders slowly and smoothly and reach for knees with arms outstreached. The body should only rise as far as the back will naturally bend while waist remains on floor or bed (about 6 to 8 inches). Slowly and smoothly lower head and shoulders back to starting position. Relax.

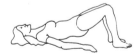

Buttocks Lift: Lie on back with arms at sides, knees bent and feet flat. Slowly raise buttocks and arch back. Return slowly to starting position.

Figure H13–1.

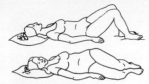

Double Knee Roll. Lie on back with knees bent. Keeping shoulders flat and feet stationary, slowly and smoothly roll knees over to the left to touch the floor or bed. Maintaining a smooth motion, roll knees back over to the right until they touch the floor or bed. Return to starting position and relax.

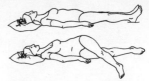

Single Knee Roll. Lie on back with right leg straight and left leg bent at the knee. Keeping shoulders flat, slowly and smoothly roll left knee over to the right to touch the floor or bed and then back to starting position. Reverse position of legs. Roll right knee over to the left to touch floor or bed and return to starting position. Relax.

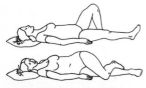

Leg Roll. Lie on back with legs straight. Keeping shoulders flat and legs straight, slowly and smoothly lift left leg and roll it over to touch the right side of floor or bed and return to starting position. Repeat, rolling right leg over to touch left side od floor or bed. Relax

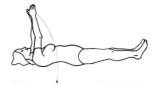

Arm Raise. Lie on back with arms extended at 90º angle from back. Raise arms so they are perpendicular and hands touch. Lower siowly.

Figure H13–1. (Contd.)

Source: Bobak, Jensen, and Zalar: Maternity and Gynecologic Care: The Nurse and the Family. CV Mosby, St. Louis, 1989.

AFTER-DELIVERY GUIDELINES

There is so much to remember once you and the baby are home after delivery.

Checklist before Leaving the Hospital

- Know how to take care of yourself; include care of the vaginal discharge and breast care.
- Know how to care for the infant; include bathing, feeding, and nurturing.
- Know the danger signs that should alert you to call your obstetrician or midwife.
- Discuss birth control methods and when and how to use them.
- If you are breastfeeding, be comfortable with the method, and identify support systems to call if needed.
- Develop a support system for cooking, cleaning, shopping, and so forth.
- Know whom to call, day or night, if you have questions or concerns.
- Schedule a follow-up appointment for yourself and for your baby.

Danger Signs for New Mothers

- Fever
- Foul-smelling or irritating discharge
- Excessive vaginal discharge
- Bright red vaginal bleeding after the discharge has been brown
- A swollen area on the leg that is painful, red, or hot
- Burning upon urination
- Pelvic pain

MENOPAUSE

What is Menopause?

Menopause is the stage at which menstrual periods cease. The ovaries no longer produce eggs and the female hormones decrease. Menopause marks the end of the childbearing years. Menopause is a normal process that can take place over 2 or 3 years.

When Does Menopause Occur?

The average age for menopause is 50–51 years. The age at which menopause occurs does appear to run in families. Your periods will likely end around the same age your mother's did.

What Are the Signs of Menopause?

Lack of menses: For some women, menstruation stops abruptly. For others, there is gradually diminishing flow. For most women, the periods become irregular. The number of days of flow and the length of time between periods varies, with no pattern seen.

Vaginal dryness: With the decrease in estrogen, the vaginal walls become thinner, dryer, and less elastic. Lubrication for intercourse is not produced as easily during sexual stimulation. Intercourse can become painful.

Increased urination: The urethra (where the urine comes from) may become thinner, and women may need to urinate more often.

Hot flashes: A hot flash is an intense feeling of heat that generally starts at the waist and moves up to the head. You may or may not perspire with a hot flash. Some women experience hot flashes at night, "night sweats," and are awakened from sleep, finding themselves wet with perspiration. Hot flashes are not harmful but are annoying.

Other symptoms of menopause: Nervousness, sadness, insomnia, breast tenderness, heavier menses, weight gain, forgetfulness, and lack of interest in sex are all symptoms of menopause.

When Can I Stop Using Birth Control?

Continue to use your birth control method until 1 year has passed without a menstrual period.

What Can I Do to Stay Healthy?

- Examine your breasts every month and have a mammogram as recommended by your health-care provider.
- Maintain good dental health.
- Eat a healthy diet that is high in carbohydrates and low in fat.
- Supplement your diet with calcium.
- Begin a daily exercise routine to strengthen your bones, heart, and lungs. Walking for 30 minutes 3–5 times weekly is a common exercise routine.
- Keep your pelvic muscles strong with Kegel exercises.
- If you smoke, stop.
- Have regular pelvic examinations and checkups.
- Minimize alcohol consumption.

NUTRITION AND MENOPAUSE

Vitamin and Mineral Daily Requirements

Calcium—1200–1500 mg daily
Vitamin D—400–800 IU daily
Vitamin E—200–600 IU daily
B-complex vitamin—daily

Nutritional Guidelines

Breads and grains—6–11 servings/day
Fruits and vegetables—5 servings/day
Protein—2–3 servings/day
Dairy products—2–3 servings/day
Low fat consumption

Some foods have been associated with hot flashes and night sweats. They are:

- Garlic
- Onions
- Cayenne
- Oranges
- Grapefruit
- Tomatoes

Chapter 15
HANDOUTS

MANAGING MENSES

The age at which menses appears has decreased in recent years; the average time at which menses begins is now age 12 or 13 years. In a small number of normal girls menses may occur as early as 10 years of age or as late as 16 years of age. Puberty is a broad term meaning the entire transition from childhood to sexual maturity. The appearance of menses is just one sign of puberty.

The time between menses is usually 28 days, although there is considerable variation among women. Different variations do not indicate infertility (inability to become pregnant).

The menstrual flow usually lasts from 4–6 days, but duration between 2 and 8 days is considered normal. For each woman, the duration of flow usually remains similar from cycle to cycle. The menstrual discharge consists of shed fragments of the lining of the uterus mixed with blood. Usually the blood is liquid, but if the rate of flow is excessive, blood clots of various sizes may be seen. The amount of blood loss per cycle is about $^{1}/_{2}$–1 cup.

There are five main stages to the menstrual cycle. They are as follows:

1. Menstruation
2. Postmenstrual reorganization under the influence of estrogen
3. Ovulation—rupture of an egg
4. Secretion of glands under the influence of estrogen and progesterone
5. Preparation for menses

Menses can produce a cramping feeling. Ibuprofen is very effective for relieving the discomfort in most women.

Suggestions for tampon use:

• Avoid deodorant tampons.
• Avoid "superabsorbent" tampons.

- Do not use more than one tampon at a time.
- Avoid tampon use at the end of a menstrual period (when the flow is light and the vaginal walls are dryer).
- Reduce overall tampon use by using sanitary pads some of the time—perhaps at night.
- Women who experience a high fever, vomiting, or diarrhea from using tampons should not use them.

VULVAR SELF-EXAMINATION

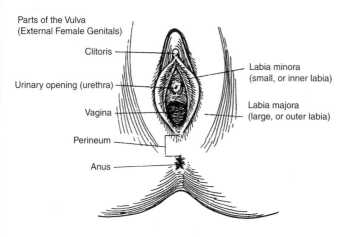

Parts of the Vulva
(External Female Genitals)

Clitoris

Urinary opening (urethra)

Vagina

Perineum

Anus

Labia minora
(small, or inner labia)

Labia majora
(large, or outer labia)

Figure H15–1.

How to Perform Vulvar Self-Examination (VSE)

Where to Look

Position: Find a comfortable, well-lighted place to sit, such as a bed or a carpet. Hold a mirror in one hand. Then, use the other hand to separate and expose the parts of the vulva surrounding the opening to the vagina. Once you have a good viewing position, examine the main parts of the vulva as follows:

Check the "mons pubis" (the area above the vagina around the pubic bone where the pubic hair is located). Carefully look for any bumps, warts, ulcers or changes in skin color (pigmentation, especially newly developed white, red, or dark areas). Then, use the finger tips to check any visible change and to sense any bump just below the surface you may feel, but not see.

- Next, check the "clitoris" and surrounding area (directly above the vagina) by looking and by touch.
- Next, examine the "labia minora" (the smaller folds of skin just to the right and left of the vaginal opening). Look and touch by holding the skin between thumb and forefinger.
- Then look closely at the "labia majora" (the larger folds of skin just next to the labia minora). Examine both right and left just as you did the labia minora.

- Move down to the perineum (the area between the vagina and the anus) Check thoroughly.
- Finally, examine the area surrounding the anal opening as before by looking and touching.

Important note: Every woman should know the parts of the vulva (see illustration). You should also talk about the VSE with your physician or nurse practitioner, who can note what is "normal" for your individual anatomy. A well woman examination is a good time to ask questions.

Remember the basic rule: "Vulvar diseases are most easily safely and successfully treated when discovered early." Now you know ... and now you have yet another good way to help protect your own health ... the vulvar self-examination.

Source: Lawhead, R, and Allen Jr, M.D:. What Every Woman Should Know: Your Guide to the Benefits of Vulvar Self Examination." 1990.

SEXUALLY TRANSMITTED DISEASES

Anyone who is sexually active is at risk for acquiring a sexually transmitted disease (STD). The best approach to STDs is prevention. There is currently an epidemic of STDs in America, specifically in the 15- to 34-year-old age group. *Chlamydia,* gonorrhea, herpes, syphilis, genital warts, and HIV/AIDS are all STDs with related health risks. Safe sex protects against STDs, including AIDS.

What Is Safe Sex?

Safe sex means preventing the exchange of body fluids during sexual contact. It also means basic hygiene practices such as urinating and washing after sex. Safe sex means choosing your partners wisely and not being afraid to discuss the use of condoms before sexual contact. The following guidelines will help to reduce the risk of developing an STD:

- Limit the number of sexual partners ideally to one partner who is faithful to you.
- Be sure that a partner uses a condom, particularly one containing spermicide.
- Remember that the pill does not prevent STD.
- Do not engage in sexual activity with anyone who has symptoms of an STD.
- Talk to a partner about STD before sexual contact.
- Avoid high-risk activities that include exchanging body fluids with new partners. High-risk activities are unprotected vaginal intercourse, oral sex, and anal sex.
- Check your body frequently for signs of infection.
- Have regular Pap smears and checkups.

What Are the Symptoms of Sexually Transmitted Diseases?

The symptoms of STDs are:

- Abnormal vaginal discharge
- Pain with urination
- Burning or itching around the vagina
- Warts in the genital area
- Rashes, blisters, bumps, or sores in the pelvic area
- Pain in the pelvic area, fever, and chills
- Vaginal bleeding that is not your period
- Pain with intercourse

Sexual activity has *two* risks: pregnancy and STDs. If you believe that you have an STD, seek help; most county health departments have a special STD clinic.

If a Sexually Transmitted Disease Is Diagnosed ...

- Take all of the medication prescribed.
- Tell your sex partner(s).
- Return for follow-up care.

WOMEN AND HIV

What Is HIV?

HIV stands for human immunodeficiency virus. HIV is the virus that causes AIDS, or acquired immunodeficiency syndrome. Many people who acquire HIV develop AIDS. AIDS is considered to be a fatal disease. HIV alters the immune system, the system that fights off diseases, and the infected person dies of an AIDS-related disease such as cancer or serious infection.

Many people live for years after AIDS is diagnosed. The sooner a person gets treated after initial infection, the better the chances of postponing AIDS.

Women of reproductive age are the fastest-growing segment of the AIDS population. In the United States, AIDS is the sixth leading cause of death in women aged 25–44.

How Does a Person Get HIV?

In its early stages, infection with HIV causes no outward symptoms so that you cannot tell if a partner is infected. Having unprotected sex puts you at serious risk for the development of HIV infection that can lead to AIDS.

A person becomes infected by coming in contact with body fluids (blood, semen, vaginal fluids, breast milk) of an infected person. A woman can become infected by having unprotected vaginal, anal, or oral sex. Women can get HIV by sharing needles with an infected person. Pregnant women infected with HIV can pass the infection on to their babies.

Who Should Be Tested?

- Any woman who has injected drugs into herself with a needle
- Any woman who has had sex with an intravenous (IV) drug user
- Any woman diagnosed with a sexually transmitted disease
- Any woman who had a blood transfusion between 1970 and 1985
- Any woman who has been raped
- Any woman who has had unprotected sex
- Any woman who is pregnant or thinking about becoming pregnant

How Do I Protect Myself from HIV?

To protect yourself against HIV infection, never have unprotected sex with anyone. Use a latex condom every time you have sex.

How Do I Get Tested for HIV?

A simple blood test will tell you if you have been exposed to HIV. Look for an anonymous testing site. Anonymous testing means that your name is not used. There is no way to trace your name, address, or social security number. Many anonymous testing sites provide the testing service free of charge. The law requires that test results be kept confidential. Confidential means that your test results are told only to you.

What if the Test is Positive?

- Take steps to make sure that you do not pass on the virus.
- Get medical care so that you can stay healthy longer.
- Get treatment early for any illness that may occur.

What if the Test is Negative?

- Your HIV counselor will discuss when to be retested
- Your HIV counselor will discuss ways to decrease the risk of contracting HIV.

ENDOMETRIOSIS

A woman has endometriosis when small pieces of displaced tissue act like the tissue from inside the uterus so that every month or so it thickens and bleeds just as it would during menstruation. The displaced pieces of tissue can be found on the ovaries and fallopian tubes, on the rectum, on the outside of the uterus, and on the bladder. The bleeding from the pieces of tissue cannot leave the body via the vagina as menstrual blood does; it remains in the body and forms cysts and scars.

Symptoms of Endometriosis

Pain is the most common symptom—painful periods, painful sex, backache. Belly pain and pains with bowel movements are also common. The pain is worst at the start of menses (periods). The amount of pain does not always indicate the seriousness of the problem. Some women have little pain and some have severe pain. The amount of pain is not reflective of the amount of displaced tissue. Periods may be heavy, frequent, or irregular. Difficulty conceiving may be the first sign of endometriosis.

Diagnosis of Endometriosis

The only way to be sure that you have endometriosis is to see a doctor. He or she may schedule a test performed in the operating room to confirm that you have the displaced tissue inside the pelvis.

Treatment

Treatment for endometriosis includes:
- Pain-killing drugs
- Hormone drugs, including birth control pills
- Surgery to remove scar tissue and displaced tissue

FIBROIDS

Uterine fibroids are benign (not malignant) tumors of the uterus. They can create pelvic pain, abnormal vaginal bleeding, urinary frequency, constipation, pelvic pressure, and pain with intercourse. They most commonly occur during a woman's fertile years. They usually shrink during menopause.

The diagnosis of uterine fibroids is made with a test called an ultrasound. An ultrasound is performed in the x-ray department or in the doctor's office and provides a picture of the uterus.

Treatment of fibroids includes medication or surgery. Medication can reduce the size of the fibroid. Surgery can remove the fibroid only or the entire uterus. Sometimes, treatment involves waiting and watching for growth or shrinkage of the fibroid. Fibroids may be watched without the fear of cancer developing. Treatment will depend upon the symptoms the fibroid(s) are producing. Uterine fibroids do not appear to interfere with the ability to conceive.

INFERTILITY

Infertility is the failure to conceive after adequate attempts to become pregnant for 1 year. Some 10%–15% of couples are infertile. Half of infertility is related to the female partner, 30% to the male partner, and the rest to factors in both.

The evaluation for infertility is complex and involves both partners. Evaluations are performed in the doctor's office; rarely is hospitalization required.

The major factors causing infertility are:

- Inadequate sperm
- Lack of ovulation (egg production)
- Altered cervical (opening to the uterus) mucus
- Closure of the tubes that deliver the egg from the ovary
- Presence of pelvic adhesions (scar tissue in the pelvis of the woman)

The "work-up" for infertility depends on these factors. Testing includes:

- Analysis of semen (fluid containing sperm)
- Ovulation prediction tests and recording of body temperature to indicate ovulation
- Testing to determine the patency (opening) of the tubes
- Testing to rule out endometriosis that causes scarring in the pelvis
- Testing to observe cervical mucus at the time of ovulation

Treatment for infertility depends on the cause.

VAGINAL INFECTIONS

Bacterial Vaginosis

The most common form of infection of the vagina is bacterial vaginosis (BV). This infection is caused by a bacterium. Recent research suggests a nonsexual mode of transmission. BV does occur in sexually active women, however, and is related to premature labor and pelvic infection. BV can be found in male partners, but males do not develop a disease per se.

Women with BV may be without symptoms, or they may have vaginal discharge that smells badly. Often women report a foul odor from the vagina, which is most noticeable after intercourse.

BV is treated with an antibiotic. There is no need for sexual partner(s) to be treated.

Yeast Infection

Candida albicans, or a "yeast" infection, is a common vaginal infection that is not related to sexual activity. An upset in the balance in the vagina leads to yeast infection. This upset can be related to use of antibiotics, pregnancy, or diabetes.

Yeast infection creates vaginal itching, burning, and irritation. Burning when urine hits the inflamed tissue is common. Vaginal discharge is white and thick. Symptoms frequently worsen prior to a period.

Yeast is treated with an antifungal medication. There is no need to treat sexual partner(s).

Trichomoniasis

Trichomoniasis is a vaginal infection caused by an organism. The organism can live in both women and men. It is transmitted during intercourse. Trichomoniasis creates a foul-smelling, yellow-green, sometimes frothy vaginal discharge. This infection is treated with an antibiotic. Sexual partner(s) should also be treated.

General rules for women with vaginal infection:

- Do not douche when you have a vaginal infection.
- Keep clean by showering or bathing.
- Do not use feminine hygiene deodorant sprays.
- Take the entire course of medication as prescribed.
- Do not use tampons if medication is applied into the vagina because they will absorb the medication.
- Soak your diaphragm or cervical cap in a 70% alcohol or a Betadine solution for 30 minutes.
- Avoid intercourse for a least 1 week after treatment.

INDEX

An *f* following a page number indicates a figure; a *t* indicates a table.